AF738317

BRAIN METASTASES FROM PRIMARY TUMORS

BRAIN METASTASES FROM PRIMARY TUMORS

EPIDEMIOLOGY, BIOLOGY, AND THERAPY

VOLUME 1

Edited by

M.A. Hayat
Distinguished Professor
Biology Department
Kean University
Union, NJ, USA

ELSEVIER

AMSTERDAM • BOSTON • HEIDELBERG • LONDON
NEW YORK • OXFORD • PARIS • SAN DIEGO
SAN FRANCISCO • SINGAPORE • SYDNEY • TOKYO
Academic Press is an imprint of Elsevier

Academic Press is an imprint of Elsevier
32 Jamestown Road, London NW1 7BY, UK
225 Wyman Street, Waltham, MA 02451, USA
525 B Street, Suite 1800, San Diego, CA 92101-4495, USA

Copyright © 2014 Elsevier Inc. All rights reserved.

Legend for cover figure: Response to treatment after WBRT in a patient with multiple brain metastases from lung cancer. Left image: A 3.6 by 3.1 cm left cerebellar tumor is present before treatment. Right image: Two months post WBRT of 30 Gy in 10 daily fractions, the tumor shrunk to 2.5 by 2.0 cm. The patient also had an improvement in gait.

No part of this publication may be reproduced, stored in a retrieval system or transmitted in any form or by any means electronic, mechanical, photocopying, recording or otherwise without the prior written permission of the publisher.

Permissions may be sought directly from Elsevier's Science & Technology Rights, Department in Oxford, UK: phone (+44) (0) 1865 843830; fax (+44) (0) 1865 853333; email: permissions@elsevier.com. Alternatively, visit the Science and Technology Books website at www.elsevierdirect.com/rights for further information.

Notice
No responsibility is assumed by the publisher for any injury and/or damage to persons or property as a matter of products liability, negligence or otherwise, or from any use or operation of any methods, products, instructions or ideas contained in the material herein. Because of rapid advances in the medical sciences, in particular, independent verification of diagnoses and drug dosages should be made.

British Library Cataloguing-in-Publication Data
A catalogue record for this book is available from the British Library

Library of Congress Cataloging-in-Publication Data
A catalog record for this book is available from the Library of Congress

ISBN: 978-0-12-800896-6

For information on all Academic Press publications
visit our website at elsevierdirect.com

Typeset by MPS Limited, Chennai, India
www.adi-mps.com

Printed and bound by CPI Group (UK) Ltd, Croydon, CR0 4YY

14 15 16 17 10 9 8 7 6 5 4 3 2 1

Working together to grow libraries in developing countries

www.elsevier.com • www.bookaid.org

Contents

Preface ix
Contributors xi

I
GENERAL APPLICATIONS

1. Brain Metastases
ALBERT S. BRAVERMAN

Introduction 3
Origin of Primary Tumors 3
Neoplastic Cell Meningitis 4
Diagnosis 5
Pathogenesis 6
Therapy 7
The Future 9
References 9

2. Epidemiology of Central Nervous System Metastases
XIAO-TANG KONG, DANIELA ALEXANDRU AND DANIELA A. BOTA

Introduction 11
Incidence 12
Incidence by Demographic Features 13
Incidence by Specific Cancer Types – Adults 15
Incidence by Specific Cancer Types – Children 20
Conclusions 21
References 22

3. Involvement of the CXCL12/CXCR4/CXCR7 Axis in Brain Metastases
CHIARA CALATOZZOLO, EMILIO CIUSANI, ELENA CORSINI, FRANCESCO DI MECO, BIANCA POLLO AND ANDREA SALMAGGI

Introduction 25
CXCL12 and Its Receptors 26
CXCL12 Axis in Brain 28
CXCL12/CXCR4/CXCR7 and Metastasis 28
Brain Metastasis and CXCL12/CXCR4/CXCR7 31
Conclusions 33
References 34

4. Non-Uniform Distribution of Metastatic Intracranial Tumors in Cancer Patients
CARLO C. QUATTROCCHI, YURI ERRANTE, CARLO AUGUSTO MALLIO AND BRUNO BEOMONTE ZOBEL

Introduction 37
Brain Spatial Distribution of Metastases 43
Discussion 48
References 50

5. Targeting Angiogenesis, Enhancing Radiosensitization and Crossing the Blood–Brain Barrier for Brain Metastases
EMMANOUIL FOKAS

Introduction 53
Targeting Angiogenesis for Brain Metastases 54
Sensitizing Brain Metastases to Radiation 55
Crossing the Blood–Brain Barrier 56
Conclusion 58
References 58

6. Second Malignancies in Children Following Treatment for Neuroblastoma
ALBERTO GARAVENTA AND BRUNO DE BERNARDI

Introduction 61
Risk of SMN in Children Treated for Neuroblastoma 62
Incidence of Selected SMNs 63
Factors Increasing the Risk of SMNs 66
Survival After SMNs 71
Clinical Implications and Discussion 71
Conclusions 72
References 72

7. The Role of Chemotherapy in Metastatic Brain Tumors

LYNN MUBITA AND STEVEN N. KALKANIS

Introduction 75
Standard of Care for Brain Metastases 76
Current Chemotherapy Options for Brain Metastases 77
Non-Small Cell Lung Cancer 78
Breast Cancer 78
Melanoma 78
Other Tumors 78
Conclusion 79
References 79

8. Multiple Metastases to the Brain from Primary Cancers: Whole Brain Radiotherapy

HANY SOLIMAN, ARJUN SAHGAL AND MAY TSAO

Introduction 81
Whole Brain Radiation Therapy 82
Whole Brain Radiation Therapy with Other Therapies 84
Whole Brain Radiation Therapy Re-Irradiation 88
Side Effects 88
The Future of Whole Brain Radiation Therapy 89
References 90

9. Synovial Sarcoma Metastasized to the Brain

NIKOLAOS SAKELLARIDIS AND LYGERI SAKELLARIDI

Introduction 93
Brain Synovial Sarcomas 93
Synovial Sarcoma 94
Head and Neck Synovial Sarcomas 98
Does a Primary Brain Synovial Sarcoma Exist? 98
Metastases in Continuity Through the Skull Base 98
Hematogenous Metastases to the Brain 99
Brain Synovial Sarcoma Classification 99
Treatment of Intracranial Synovial Sarcomas 99
References 100

II

BRAIN METASTASES FROM NON-SMALL CELL LUNG CARCINOMA

10. Multiple Small Brain Metastases with Limited Focal Brain Edema from Non-Small Cell Lung Cancer with Epidermal Growth Factor Receptor Mutations

AKIMASA SEKINE

Introduction 106
Epidermal Growth Factor Receptor Mutations 106
Multiple Brain Metastases and EGFR Mutations: Influence of the Exon 19 Deletion on Radiographical Features 107
Miliary Brain Metastases and EGFR Mutations 108
Management of Brain Metastases from NSCLC with EGFR Mutations 108
Treatment of Multiple Brain Metastases from NSCLC with EGFR Mutations 109
References 110

11. Brain Metastasis of Patients with Lung Adenocarcinoma: Epidermal Growth Factor Receptor Mutations and Response to Whole-Brain Radiation Therapy

SHANG-GIN WU AND JIN-YUAN SHIH

Introduction 114
Brain Metastasis and EGFR Mutation 114
Preclinical Study and Mechanism 115
Clinical Study 116
Conclusion 119
References 119

12. Metastatic Spread of Lung Cancer to Brain and Liver: Role of CX3CR1

DAVID J. PINATO AND FRANCESCO A. MAURI

Introduction 123
Organotropic Spread of Lung Carcinoma: Role of Chemokine Signaling Pathways 124

CX3CR1 as a Molecular Determinant of Organotropic Diffusion of Lung Cancer 126
References 128

13. Solitary Brain Metastasis from Non-Small Cell Lung Cancer: Treatment with Linac-Based Stereotactic Radiosurgery

FILIPPO ALONGI, UMBERTO RICARDI AND MARTA SCORSETTI

Introduction 131
Technical and Technological Aspects 132
Radiobiological Issues and Clinical Data 134
Whole-Brain Radiation Therapy 135
Surgery 135
Patient Selection 136
Conclusion 137
References 137

14. Brain Metastases from Non-Small Cell Lung Cancer: Clinical Benefits of Erlotinib and Gefitinib

M. HOUMAN FEKRAZAD, OMID SANAEI, JULIE E. BAUMAN AND DENNIE V. JONES, Jr.

Introduction 142
Treatment Options for Brain Metastases 145
Targeted Therapy 146
Obstacles to Drug Activity within the CNS and Ways to Overcome 148
Clinical Implications of EGFR Mutations 150
Prophylactic Role of the Drugs 151
Adverse Reactions of Gefitinib and Erlotinib, Pros and Cons 151
Future Directions/Additional Agents 152
References 153

15. Bispecific Targeted Toxin DTATEGF Against Metastatic NSCLC Brain Tumors

WALTER A. HALL, JUN HUANG, YAN MICHAEL LI AND DANIEL A. VALLERA

Introduction 157
Diphtheria Toxin (DT) 159
DTATEGF 160
DTATEGF *in vitro* and *in vivo* Results 163
Discussion 164
References 166

16. Intracranial Disease in Patients with Non-Small Cell Lung Cancer: Treatment with Erlotinib

MAZHAR AJAZ, FIONA MCDONALD, JAISHREE BHOSLE, PAOLA BORDI AND MARY O'BRIEN

Introduction 170
First-Line Treatment for Advanced NSCLC 170
Development and Management of NSCLC Brain Metastases 171
Do EGFR Mutated NSCLC Patients Have a Higher Risk of Developing Brain Metastases? 172
Are Brain Metastases in EGFR-Mutated Patients Radiosensitive? 172
Erlotinib 172
Do EGFR TKIs Have Efficacy in Treatment and Prevention of Intracranial Disease from NSCLC? 174
What Is the Efficacy and Safety of Combining Erlotinib with Radiotherapy for Brain Metastases? 175
Is There a Role for Rechallenge and Pulsed Dose Escalation of Erlotinib? 176
Summary 176
References 177

17. Radiation Management of Synchronous Brain Metastases from Non-Small Cell Lung Cancer

ALLISON ASHWORTH, DAVID PALMA AND GEORGE RODRIGUES

Introduction 182
Management of Brain Metastases in Patients with NSCLC 182
Management of NSCLC Patients with Synchronous Brain Metastases 187
Conclusion 194
References 195

III

BRAIN METASTASES FROM SMALL CELL LUNG CARCINOMA

18. Brain Metastasis after Prophylactic Cranial Irradiation in Patients with Small Cell Lung Cancer

PATRICIA TAI, AVI ASSOULINE, KURIAN JOSEPH, JOSEPH SIU-KIE AU AND EDWARD YU

Introduction 200
Brain Metastasis after Prophylactic Cranial Irradiation 201
Treatment Options 206
Outcome and Conclusion 209
References 209

19. Brain Metastasis from Small-Cell Lung Cancer with High Levels of Placental Growth Factor

YU-HUA CHEN AND BO LI

Introduction 213
Placental Growth Factor 215
Roles of PLGF in SCLC Metastasis to the Brain 216
Discussion 221
Acknowledgments 224
References 224

20. Brain Metastases from Lung Cancer

AMOL J. GHIA AND RITSUKO KOMAKI

Introduction 227
Treatment Options 228
Toxicity of Radiation to the Brain 237
Conclusion 238
References 238

21. Lambert–Eaton Myesthenic Syndrome and Brain Metastasis from Occult Small Cell Lung Carcinoma: A Clinician's Perspective

ARUNANSU TALUKDAR, NIKHIL SONTHALIA, SAYANTAN RAY AND SUPRATIP KUNDU

Introduction 244
Lambert–Eaton Myesthenic Syndrome 244
Brain Metastasis 249
Our Experience 252
References 253

Index 255

Preface

Brain metastases outnumber all other primary intracranial tumors. Brain intracranial neoplasm occurs 5–10 times more frequently than primary tumors of the brain. Brain metastases are among the most devastating and debilitating complications of lung cancer, breast cancer, and melanoma. Lung cancer is the most common primary site, with 30–50% of patients developing brain metastases during the course of their disease, and often leads to serious deterioration in neurologic and neurocognitive functions. Brain metastases from non-small cell lung cancer (NSCLC) and small cell lung cancer are explained in this volume. Many patients with NSCLC metastatic to the brain either harbor or develop multiple lesions.

Overexpression of the epidermal growth factor receptor (EGFR), a transmembrane tyrosine kinase protein, is common in NSCLC. The presence of this receptor is associated with a poor prognosis. The use of EGFR-tyrosine kinase inhibitors (gefitinib, erlotinib) results in tumor response in patients even with advanced NSCLC. When erlotinib treatment follows previous chemotherapy, some increase in patient survival is achieved. Deletion of EGFR exon 19 using erlotinib tends to regress multiple intracranial brain metastases from NSCLC. In other words, this drug is site specific for intracranial metastases harboring EGFR exon 19. EGFR mutations and response to whole brain radiotherapy (WBRT) are discussed in this volume, so are the clinical benefits of these two drugs. A number of treatments, including WBRT, stereotactic radiosurgery, and chemotherapy are discussed. The advantages and limitations of these therapeutic methods are included.

WBRT is the standard care for patients with multiple brain lesions. The prevention and palliation of neurologic problems due to metastatic progression are important goals of treatment. There is controversy regarding the ideal management of this disease. An improvement in survival, however, might not be an ideal measure of the benefit of a local therapy because overall survival is commonly determined by extracranial disease. Tumor stage, size, number, and location, commodities, sterol use, previous therapies, age, ethnicity, and gender of the patient complicate the evaluation of clinical benefits. The contents of this volume are divided into General Applications, Brain Metastases from Non-Small Cell Lung Cancer, and Brain Metastases from Small Cell Lung Cancer for the convenience of the readers.

By bringing together a large number of experts (oncologists, neurosurgeons, physicians, medical research scientists, and pathologists) in the field of brain metastases from primary cancer, it is my hope that substantial progress will be made against this devastating disease inflicting humans. It is difficult for a single author to discuss effectively and comprehensively various aspects of an exceedingly complex process such as brain metastases. Another advantage of involving more than one author is to present different points of view on specific controversial aspects of the advantages and limitations of various treatments. I hope the information presented in this and other volumes will result in a better understanding of the molecular mechanisms underlying brain metastases and their cure and hopefully their prevention.

This volume was written by 61 contributors representing nine countries. I am grateful to them for their promptness in accepting my suggestions. Their thoughtful, practical experience highlights the very high quality of their writings, which should build and further the endeavors of the readers in this important medical field. I respect and appreciate the time-consuming hard work invested by the contributors. There exists a tremendous urgent demand by the public and the medical community to address the treatment of this complex disease. In the light of existing disease calamities, government funding must give priority to eradicating deadly malignancies over global military superiority.

I am grateful to Dr. Dawood Farahi and Mr. Phil Connelly for recognizing the importance of medical research and publishing through an institution of higher education. I am thankful to my students for their contribution to the final preparation of this volume.

M. A. Hayat
November 2013

Contributors

Mazhar Ajaz University of Surrey, Guildford UK

Daniela Alexandru Department of Neurosurgery, UC Irvine Medical Center, Orange, CA, USA

Filippo Alongi Radiation Oncology Department, Sacro Cuore-Don Calabria Hospital Negrar (Verona), Italy

Allison Ashworth Division of Radiation Oncology, Cancer Centre of Southeastern Ontario, Queen's University, Kingston, Ontario, Canada

Avi Assouline Radiation Oncology / Medical Oncology, Centre Clinique de la Porte de Saint Cloud, Boulogne-Billancourt, France

Joseph Siu-kie Au Radiation Oncology / Medical Oncology, Department of Clinical Oncology, Queen Elizabeth Hospital, Hong Kong, SAR China

Julie E. Bauman University of Pittsburgh Cancer Institute, Pittsburgh, PA, USA

Bruno Beomonte Zobel Unit of Diagnostic Imaging, Departmental Faculty of Medicine and Surgery, Center for Integrated Research, University Campus Bio-Medico of Rome, Rome, Italy

Jaishree Bhosle The Royal Marsden NHS Foundation Trust, Sutton, UK

Paola Bordi Medical Oncology Unit, University Hospital, Parma, Italy

Daniela A. Bota Department of Neurology, Department of Neurological Surgery and Chao Family Comprehensive Cancer Center, University of California-Irvine, Irvine, CA, USA

Albert S. Braverman Division of Hematology/ Oncology, Department of Medicine, Downstate Medical College of State University of New York, Brooklyn, NY, USA

Chiara Calatozzolo Fondazione IRCCS Istituto Neurologico C. Besta, Milano, Italy

Yu-Hua Chen Department of Developmental Cell Biology, Key Lab of Cell Biology, Ministry of Public Health of China, China Medical University, Shenyang, P. R. China

Emilio Ciusani Laboratory of Clinical Pathology and Medical Genetics, Fondazione Istituto Neurologico C. Besta, Milan, Italy

Elena Corsini Fondazione IRCCS Istituto Neurologico C. Besta, Milano, Italy

Bruno De Bernardi Department of Pediatric Hematology/Oncology, Istituto Giannina Gaslini, Genova, Italy

Francesco Di Meco Fondazione IRCCS Istituto Neurologico C. Besta, Milano, Italy

Yuri Errante Unit of Diagnostic Imaging, Departmental Faculty of Medicine and Surgery, Center for Integrated Research, University Campus Bio-Medico of Rome, Rome, Italy

M. Houman Fekrazad University of New Mexico, Cancer Research and Treatment Center, Albuquerque, NM, USA

Emmanouil Fokas Gray Institute for Radiation Oncology & Biology, Department of Oncology, University of Oxford, Oxford, UK

Alberto Garaventa Pediatric Oncology Unit, Istituto Giannina Gaslini, Genova, Italy

Amol J. Ghia Department of Radiation Oncology, The University of Texas, MD Anderson Cancer Center, Houston, TX, USA

Walter A. Hall SUNY Upstate Medical University, Syracuse, NY, USA

Jun Huang Xiangya Hospital of Central South University, P.R.China

Dennie V. Jones Division of Medical Oncology, University of Kentucky Markey Cancer Center, Lexington, KY, USA

Kurian Joseph Cross Cancer Institute, University of Alberta, Edmonton, AB, Canada

Steven N. Kalkanis Department of Neurosurgery, Henry Ford Health System, Detroit, MI, USA

Ritsuko Komaki The University of Texas, MD Anderson Cancer Center, Houston, TX, USA

Xiao-Tang Kong Neuro-Oncology Program, Department of Neurology, David Geffen School of Medicine at University of California, Los Angeles, Los Angeles, CA, USA

Supratip Kundu Department of Cardiology, Medical College and Hospital, Kolkata, West Bengal, India

Bo Li Department of Developmental Cell Biology, Key Lab of Cell Biology, Ministry of Public Health of China, China Medical University, Shenyang, P. R. China

Yan Michael Li The University of Texas, MD Anderson Cancer Center, Department of Neurosurgery, Houston, TX, USA

Carlo Augusto Mallio Unit of Diagnostic Imaging, Departmental Faculty of Medicine and Surgery, Center for Integrated Research, University Campus Bio-Medico of Rome, Rome, Italy

Francesco A. Mauri Department of Histopathology, Imperial College London, Hammersmith Campus, London, UK

Fiona McDonald The Royal Marsden Hospital, Sutton, Surrey, UK

Lynn Mubita Department of Neurosurgery, Henry Ford Health System, Detroit, MI, USA

Mary O'Brien Department of Medicine, Royal Marsden Hospital, Sutton, Surrey, UK

David Palma OICR London Regional Cancer Program, London, ONT, Canada

David J. Pinato Imperial Centre for Translational and Experimental Medicine (ICTEM), Imperial College London – Hammersmith Hospital, London, UK

Bianca Pollo Fondazione IRCCS Istituto Neurologico C. Besta, Milano, Italy

Carlo C. Quattrocchi Unit of Diagnostic Imaging, Departmental Faculty of Medicine and Surgery, Center for Integrated Research, University Campus Bio-Medico of Rome, Rome, Italy

Sayantan Ray Department of General Medicine, Calcutta National Medical College, Kolkata, West Bengal, India

Umberto Ricardi Radiation Oncology Department, University of Torino, Italy

George Rodrigues Departments of Oncology/ Epidemiology and Biostatistics, Radiation Oncology, Lawson Health Research Institute, London, ON, Canada

Arjun Sahgal Department of Radiation Oncology, Odette Cancer Centre, Toronto, ON, Canada

Lygeri Sakellaridi Department of Biology, University of Athens, Greece

Nikolaos Sakellaridis Department of Neurosurgery, Zaneio General Hospital, Piraeus, Greece

Andrea Salmaggi Department of Neurosciences, Alessandro Manzoni Hospital, Lecco, Italy

Omid Sanaei Golestan Research Center of Gastroenterology And Hepatology Golestan University of Medical Sciences Gorgan, Iran

Marta Scorsetti Radiation Oncology Department, Humanitas Cancer Center, Rozzano, Italy

Akimasa Sekine Department of Respiratory Medicine, Kanagawa Prefectural Cardiovascular and Respiratory Center, Yokohama, Japan

Hany Soliman Department of Radiation Oncology, Sunnybrook, Odette Cancer Centre, University of Toronto, ON, Canada

Nikhil Sonthalia Department of General Medicine, Medical College and Hospital, Kolkata, West Bengal, India

Patricia Tai University of Saskatchewan, Saskatoon, SK, Canada

Arunansu Talukdar Department of General Medicine, Medical College and Hospital Kolkata, West Bengal, India

May Tsao Odette Cancer Centre, Sunnybrook Health Sciences Centre, University of Toronto, ON, Canada

Daniel A. Vallera Section on Molecular Cancer Therapeutics, Professor of Radiation Oncology, University of Minnesota Masonic Cancer Center, Minneapolis, MN, USA

Shang-Gin Wu Department of Internal Medicine, National Taiwan University Hospital Yun-Lin Branch, Yun-Lin, Taiwan

Edward Yu Lawson Health Research Institute; Western University, London Health Science Center, London, ONT, Canada

Jin-Yuan Shih Division of Pulmonary and Critical Care Medicine, Department of Internal Medicine, National Taiwan University Hospital, Professor, Department of Internal Medicine, College of Medicine, National Taiwan University, Taipei, Taiwan

PART I

GENERAL APPLICATIONS

1. *Brain Metastases* 3

2. *Epidemiology of Central Nervous System Metastases* 11

3. *Involvement of the Cxcl12/Cxcr4/Cxcr7 Axis in Brain Metastases* 25

4. *Non-Uniform Distribution of Metastatic Intracranial Tumors in Cancer Patients* 37

5. *Targeting Angiogenesis, Enhancing Radiosensitization and Crossing the Blood–Brain Barrier for Brain Metastases* 53

6. *Second Malignancies in Children following Treatment for Neuroblastoma* 61

7. *The Role of Chemotherapy in Metastatic Brain Tumors* 75

8. *Multiple Metastases to the Brain from Primary Cancers: Whole Brain Radiotherapy* 81

9. *Synovial Sarcoma Metastasized to the Brain* 93

CHAPTER

1

Brain Metastases

Albert S. Braverman

OUTLINE

Introduction	3
Origin of Primary Tumors	3
Neoplastic Cell Meningitis	4
Diagnosis	5
Pathogenesis	6
Therapy	7
Surgery	7
Radiation	7
Systemic Therapy	8
Intrathecal Therapy	8
The Future	9
References	9

INTRODUCTION

Metastases to the brain are among the most clinically significant, because even a single one is likely to cause serious disability. Because most may be at least partially protected from otherwise effective systemic therapies by the blood–brain barrier, they present special management problems. But whether their pathogenesis differs from that of metastases at other sites is not known.

ORIGIN OF PRIMARY TUMORS

Since the first successful systemic treatment of a disseminated neoplasm – acute lymphoblastic leukemia (ALL) in children – the CNS has been recognized as a refuge for neoplastic cells. Permeation of the meninges at the base of the skull and spinal canal is mainly seen in certain types of lymphomas, though these occasionally produce nodular brain lesions. Such lesions are usually derived from epithelial neoplasms. Most are the result of hematogenous dissemination. The exceptions are those from prostatic carcinoma, and some breast cancers,

M.A. Hayat (ed): *Brain Metastases from Primary Tumors, Volume 1*
DOI: http://dx.doi.org/10.1016/B978-0-12-800896-6.00001-2

© 2014 Elsevier Inc. All rights reserved.

where tumor reaches the brain from skull lesions, or the dura attached to involved bone. This occurs only rarely in myeloma and lymphomas.

Of all epithelial tumors, both small and non-small cell lung cancer are associated with the highest incidence of brain metastases (BM), which occur in 30–60% of cases, and become manifest early in the course of the disease, often even before the primary tumor is diagnosed (Barnholtz-Sloan et al., 2004). Lung metastases may be especially likely to elicit edema, with ring enhancement and disruption of the blood–brain barrier, so that they produce focal deficits and other symptoms early (Hengel et al., 2013). Melanomas and renal cell carcinomas are also associated with a high incidence of BM (Schouten et al., 2002), but they are less common than breast or lung cancer.

Breast cancer is the second most common source of brain metastases, being a very common tumor in America; they ultimately develop in 35% of patients with metastatic disease (DiStefano et al., 1997). They mainly occur in HER2+ and triple negative breast cancer, arising less frequently from hormone receptor positive tumors (Lin and Winer, 2007; Foulkes et al., 2010). Their natural history differs from those due to lung cancer. They are not usually symptomatic until late in the course of the disease, after metastases to bone and lung become detectable. The number of metastases per brain in breast cancer patients appears, in some, but not all studies (Delattre et al., 1988; Hengel et al., 2013), significantly greater than those in the brains of lung cancer patients. But this may be, in part, due to gender; female lung cancer patients have been reported to have more metastases per brain than males (Yawn et al., 2003). The incidence of cerebellar metastases is highest in breast cancer patients (Yoshida and Takahashi, 2009), but this does not necessarily indicate a predilection for cerebellar involvement. The incidence of breast metastases in the cerebellum correlates strongly with the total number of brain metastases present (Hengel et al., 2013). Thus, the occurrence of metastases in a given brain region may be a function of the total number of BM which have occurred.

Most lung cancer patients present with incurable disease, and systemic therapies are only effective in a minority. But the majority of breast cancer patients are potentially curable at presentation, especially with adjuvant therapies. Breast cancer metastases at any site are far more sensitive to systemic chemotherapy than those from lung cancer, and also respond to endocrine therapy in tumors expressing hormone receptors. Such treatments may delay overt progression of micrometastases for years, and 50% of patients with bone and lung metastases may be controlled by systemic therapy for many months. But the drugs used in systemic therapies may not reach the brain, so that metastases there may accumulate while other metastases are suppressed by therapy (Hengel et al., 2012). Thus, in breast cancer, the brain may be a refuge for metastatic disease.

NEOPLASTIC CELL MENINGITIS

The leptomeninges are most often involved in ALL and certain lymphomas. This is assumed to be present in all ALL cases. It is rare in acute myeloblastic leukemia, though it occasionally occurs in the monoblastic subsets (M4 and M5). The lymphomas include Burkitt's, T-cell, and a subset of especially aggressive and high stage diffuse large B-cell lymphomas.

In the latter group, the presence of the typical 8;14 (myc) chromosome translocation should be ruled out, regardless of whether typical Burkitt's histology is observed, because a positive result implies an increased risk of meningeal involvement. Carcinomatous meningitis involvement is far less common. It is most frequently observed in small cell and breast carcinomas.

In fact, few such patients have a typical meningeal syndrome. They are usually alert, and without neck stiffness. The meninges at the bases of skull and cord are the most frequent sites of involvement. The usual clinical syndrome is that of mononeuritis multiplex, due to entrapment of nerve roots by meningeal growth. Ophthalmoplegias due to cranial nerve involvement are common, as are symptoms of lumbar root involvement.

DIAGNOSIS

Early BM are often clinically silent but, ultimately, cause focal neurologic deficits of gradual onset; they are sometimes associated with more diffuse problems, such as amnesia or dementia. Only occasionally do they present with seizures, and most never cause them. Nevertheless, anti-epileptic therapies are frequently prescribed. This may be based on experience with primary intracerebral brain tumors, surgical resection of which can result in epileptogenic foci. Although brain imaging is usually performed for brain-related symptoms, it is also indicated in all lung cancer patients regardless of whether symptoms are present (Gore et al., 2010). Asymptomatic metastases are often discovered in this way (Yokoi et al., 1999).

BM which have caused neurologic deficits are almost always detectable by imaging, which can usually readily distinguish them from primary brain tumors. The former are typically sharply circumscribed, though they often display ring enhancement (Barajas and Cha, 2012). Primary intracerebral brain tumors are diffusely permeative at their margins. In fact, when adequate imaging fails to demonstrate BM, a different cause for focal deficits is likely.

Pre-contrast computed tomography (CT) scanning cannot rule out BM, but occasionally rules them in. Post-contrast CT scanning usually detects BM which have reached the point of causing neurologic deficits. Magnetic resonance imaging (MRI) is the most sensitive and specific method of demonstrating brain metastases. It can often detect small asymptomatic lesions which are not apparent on post-contrast CT scanning, and is more effective in detecting posterior fossa metastases (Fink and Fink, 2013). If possible, it should be the primary diagnostic procedure of choice.

Biopsy of brain metastases is not usually necessary. In patients without a known neoplastic diagnosis, careful physical examination and imaging – especially of the chest – will disclose a source in many cases, and the diagnosis can be made by biopsy of a probable primary tumor. It is especially important to rule out apparently localized melanomas, which may metastasize early. Localized primary small cell tumors, whether bronchogenic or arising at other sites, are often found to have metastasized to the brain.

In patients at risk for primary brain lymphomas, such as those immunosuppressed post-transplant, or with AIDS, evaluation of cerebrospinal fluid Epstein–Barr DNA can help rule them in or out (Arribas et al., 2012). Clinical findings are of paramount importance in the diagnosis of neoplastic cell meningitis. It is not usually detected by CT scanning; MRI is positive in carcinomatous meningitis and about 50% of lymphomatous meningitis. Lumbar puncture to reveal neoplastic cells in the cerebrospinal fluid may be specific, but is quite insensitive. Examination of spinal fluid cells is diagnostic in less than 50% of cases, though flow cytometry may increase sensitivity. The presence of, for example, an abducens palsy is sufficient to establish the diagnosis.

PATHOGENESIS

BM are initially small, bland lesions which have not permeated adjacent parenchyma. Many are asymptomatic when imaging for staging detects them. But their growth is often associated with a local inflammatory, hypervascular reaction around them, denoted as *ring enhancing* by their appearance on imaging. The resulting edema is usually associated with neurologic deficits, and may lead to midline shift, herniation and sudden death. There is some evidence that BM from lung cancer acquire these changes more rapidly than those from other tumors (Hengel et al., 2013).

There is a possible anatomic explanation for the high incidence of BM in lung cancer. Cells from most tumors must pass through the pulmonary capillary circulation to reach organs other than the lung itself, which is the commonest site of metastases. Cells from primary lung cancers presumably enter the systemic circulation directly from draining veins. They thus reach the cerebral circulation without the interposition of other small vessels. Yet, specific cellular mechanisms which may facilitate the adhesion and growth of lung cancer cells in the brain still seem probable.

Studies in animal melanoma models revealed specific cell lineages from primary melanomas with a strong predilection for spread to the brain. Such cells were shown *in vitro* to bind to the surface of brain cells and to proliferate in this environment. A small population of primary tumor cells was shown to have a predilection for forming BM, and this population was enhanced by multiple *in vitro* passages (Brunson et al., 1978). The assumption was that such tumor cells had gained mutations enabling brain metastases. But the discovery of the epithelial–mesenchymal transition (Chafer et al., 2013) suggests that metastatic cells may not have gained mutations, but have acquired stem cell attributes. There is increasing evidence that metastatic cells do not necessarily acquire mutations additional to those in the primary tumors (Jones et al., 2008).

That human BM arise from tumor stem cells expressing specific brain markers is reasonable to assume but difficult to demonstrate (Nolte et al., 2013). Tissue from such lesions is usually obtained at post-mortem examinations, in which the metastases are devitalized, so that markers cease to be detectable. Perhaps the best evidence for the existence of such markers is the predilection of specific breast cancer subsets for the brain. Were it possible to characterize brain specific markers in subsets of the cells from any tumors, a pharmacologic approach to inhibiting brain metastases might be possible. Animal models of BM have provided information concerning marker expression (Mendes et al., 2005), and have also provided data on the relative roles of cooptation of pre-existing vessels and *de novo* angiogenesis in the development of BM vasculature (Bugyik et al., 2011). The lack of *de novo* angiogenesis in BM contrasts to its presence in primary brain tumors.

THERAPY

Surgery

Surgical resection has a limited role in the treatment of BM. Some indications for surgery are:

1. Occasional patients, usually with lung cancer, with potentially curable primary tumors and solitary brain metastases. MRI is essential to rule out additional small BM.
2. Incurable patients with good performance status, whose symptoms from a single brain metastasis cannot be controlled by radiation.
3. Occasionally, brain metastases may block ventricular outflow and lead to cerebral edema and death. This is a surgical emergency and usually requires the insertion of drains to prevent herniation, but not necessarily resection. In all cases, resection should only be considered if it is not likely to exacerbate or cause neurologic deficits. The size and position of the brain metastasis is important.

Radiation

Brain metastases are presumed to be resistant to systemic therapies because of the blood–brain barrier, and therefore require radiation. There are certain exceptions to this rule which will be discussed below. But, because of the disastrous consequences of delay in treatment, immediate radiation is usually indicated.

Glucocorticoid therapy averts metastasis edema due to radiation-induced tumor cell necrosis; it must be initiated immediately before radiation, and continued for 2–3 weeks. Without it, herniation may occur, but there are few controlled studies of this treatment (Ryken et al., 2010). A common error is to continue glucocorticoids for weeks or months after the completion of radiation. This is unnecessary and toxic. Tapering after radiation is appropriate and safe, unless manifestations of cerebral edema persist.

The brain is generally radio-resistant and acute changes during treatment are uncommon. There is a significant incidence of dementia within 3–4 years of treatment (Lisa et al., 1989), which most patients with brain metastases do not survive to experience. This is, however, a relative contraindication to prophylactic whole brain radiation, which is most often employed in patients with limited small cell carcinoma.

The following are the contexts in which radiation for BM is administered:

1. Whole brain prophylactic treatment in lung cancer patients, especially for those with small cell tumors.
2. Stereotactic radiation for single, large or a small number of BM. It may also be useful for individual BM which prove refractory to whole brain radiation (Sheehan et al., 2003).
3. Whole brain radiation for multiple BM (Tsao et al., 2005).
4. Adjuvant radiation after treatment of solitary BM. The ability of this treatment to improve prognosis is uncertain (Fuller et al., 1992; McPherson et al., 2010):
   a. after surgical resection
   b. after stereotactic radiotherapy.

These radiation treatments may result in symptomatic radionecrosis (Minniti et al., 2011) when the doses are high. The neurologic deficits of two-thirds of patients respond to radiation. Though most relapse in 3–6 months, a significant minority, if they do not succumb to their neoplastic disease at other sites, may remain relapse-free for a year or more. The interpretation of studies concerning the efficacy of brain radiation is complex. The endpoint of many is overall survival, a parameter which is strongly influenced by primary lung cancers and metastases likely to be present at other sites, and associated performance status. Only a few are based on the incidence of neurologic progression after treatment. Radiation is virtually never curative, except perhaps as prophylactic treatment. But because small cell lung patients are at very high risk for brain metastases, early imaging may detect small metastases, and radiation may provide longer control.

Systemic Therapy

BM from germ cell tumors respond to standard chemotherapy better than to radiation, which may not be indicated chemotherapy-naïve patients (Fossa et al., 1999). This may be because germ cell metastases at any site are among the most sensitive to chemotherapy. Because of local disruption of the blood–brain barrier, some amounts of drugs do probably enter most BM (Gerstner and Fine, 2007). The amount entering BM may be insufficient to control most BM but, because of their greater sensitivity, the small amount that enters germ cell BM may suffice. The blood–brain barrier in ring enhancing metastases has been shown to be disrupted, and such lesions may respond to systemic therapies, including endocrine drugs, appropriate for their primary tumors. But radiation is usually the primary treatment.

Those breast and prostate brain metastases which appear to arise from adjacent skull or dural lesions may respond to systemic therapies, as they are essentially systemic rather central nervous system lesions. This is especially important for patients who have not yet received potentially effective systemic therapies. Lapatinib is a specific tyrosine kinase inhibitor for breast cancer patients overexpressing epidermoid growth factor receptor 2 (HER2). Unlike the monoclonal trastuzumab, it crosses the blood–brain barrier, but its effect on established BM is modest (Lin et al., 2009).

Intrathecal Therapy

This is the treatment of choice for neoplastic cell meningitis. It is indicated prophylactically in all ALL, Burkitt's and T-cell lymphoma patients, but may be delayed until initial remission induction. It must be initiated immediately if there is clinical evidence of neoplastic cell meningitis. The two effective and well-tolerated drugs are methotrexate and cytarabine. These can be successfully administered by successive lumbar punctures; an Ommaya resevoir is more convenient and reliable, but its placement and presence are associated with complications, such as infection. In refractory cases – especially due to carcinomas – radiation may be necessary. It can often be limited to the base of the skull and cord. For nodular lymphomatous brain lesions radiation may be essential. If possible it should be avoided in patients with potentially curable neoplasms, such as ALL and lymphomas, because of the potential for long-term complications. High dose methotrexate with citrovorum rescue may ameliorate neoplastic cell meningitis, but intrathecal therapy is essential.

THE FUTURE

The key to prevention of BM is effective systemic therapies. More targeted therapies are now becoming available, as in breast cancer and previously refractory tumors, such as melanomas and lung cancer. There is now evidence that early detection of lung cancer in high-risk patients can increase cure rate, and this may significantly reduce the number of BM encountered in practice. In breast cancer, lapatinib can cross the blood–brain barrier, and may reduce the frequency of brain metastases when used prophylactically in HER2 overexpressing tumors. But, because of BM late development in breast cancer, studies will require prolonged treatment and follow up. Other drugs which can cross the barrier, such as nitrosoureas, are not generally effective. We cannot assume that subsets of tumor cells express markers which facilitate BM. If and when they are discovered, they may offer the possibility of pharamacologic prevention of tumor spread to the brain after primary tumor diagnosis.

In treating BM, attempts have been made to increase the permeability of the blood–brain barrier with polyethylene glycol, but their success has been modest. But, when systemic therapy is highly effective, as in germ cell tumors, it can play a major role in BM control. As systemic therapies improve they may improve BM treatment. As many BM are multiple, the role of surgical resection is likely to remain limited.

Stereotactic radiotherapy has been an important advance in treatment, and may be applied to multiple lesions. It may reduce the late development of dementia if it obviates the need for whole brain radiation. Prophylactic radiation therapy may prove to be useful in patients with HER2+ or triple negative breast tumors, especially when they are locally advanced. There may thus be an indication for periodic follow-up MRI brain scanning in such breast patients to detect sufficiently small BM to prevent neurologic deficits with radiation.

As our treatment of systemic disease improves, the concept of the central nervous system as a refuge for tumor cells, as is known to be the case in ALL, may become significant in other tumors. That is, treatment may not only avert or alleviate central nervous system symptoms, but may increase the chances of cure.

References

Arribas, J.R., Clifford, D.B., Fichtenbaum, C.J., Roberts`, R.L., Powderly, W.G., Storch, G.A., 2012. Detection of epstein-barr virus DNA in cerebrospinal fluid for diagnosis of AIDS-related central nervous system lymphoma. J. Clin. Microbiol. 33, 1580–1583.

Barajas Jr., R.F., Cha, S., 2012. Imaging diagnosis of brain metastasis. Prog. Neurol. Surg. 25, 55–73.

Barnholtz-Sloan, J.S., Sloan, A.E., Davis, F.G., Vigneau, F.D., Lai, P., Sawaya, R.E., 2004. Incidence proportions of brain metastases in patients diagnosed in the Metropolitan Detroit Cancer Surveillance System. J. Clin. Oncol. 22, 2865–2872.

Brunson, K.W., Beattie, G., Nicolson, G.L., 1978. Selection and altered properties of brain colonizing melanoma. Nature 272, 543–545.

Bugyik, E., Dezso, K., Reiniger, L., et al., 2011. Lack of angiogenesis in experimental brain metastases. Neuropathol. Exp. Neurol. 70, 979–991.

Chafer, C.L., Marjanovic, N.D., Lee, T., et al., 2013. Poised chromatin at the ZEB1 promoter enables breast cancer cell plasticity and enhances tumorgenicity. Cell 154, 61–74.

Delattre, J.Y., Krol, G., Thaler, H.T., 1988. Distribution of brain metastases. Arch. Neurol. 145, 741–744.

DiStefano, A., Yap, H.Y., Hortobabyi, G.N., 1997. The natural history of breast cancer patients with brain metastases. Cancer 44, 1913–1918.

Fink, K.R., Fink, J.R., 2013. Imaging of brain metastases. Surg. Neurol. Int. 4 (Suppl. 4), S209–219.
Fossa, S.D., Bokemyer, C., Gerl, A., 1999. Treatment outcome of patients with brain metastases from malignant germ cell tumors. Cancer 85, 988–997.
Foulkes, W.D., Smith, I.E., Reis-Filho, J.S., 2010. Triple negative breast cancer. N. Engl. J. Med. 363, 1938–1944.
Fuller, B.G., Kaplan, I.D., Adler, J., Cox, R.S., Bagshaw, M.A., 1992. Stereotaxic radiosurgery for brain metastases: The importance of adjuvant whole brain irradiation. Oncol. Biol. Phys. 23, 413–418.
Gerstner, E.R., Fine, R.L., 2007. Increased permeability of the blood-brain barrier to chemotherapy in metastatic brain tumors. J. Clin. Oncol. 25, 2306–2312.
Gore, E.M., Bae, K., Wong, S.J., et al., 2010. Phase III comparison of prophylactic cranial radiation in patients with locally advanced non-small cell lung cancer. J. Clin. Oncol. 29, 272–278.
Hengel, K., Sidhu, G., Choi, J., et al., 2013. Attributes of brain metastases from breast and lung cancer. Int. J. Clin. Oncol. 3, 396–401.
Jones, S., Chen, W.D., Parmigiani, G., et al., 2008. Comparative lesion sequencing provides insights into tumor evolution. Proc. Natl. Acad. Sci. USA 105, 4283–4288.
Lin, N.U., Diéras, V., Paul, D., et al., 2009. Multicenter phase II study of lapatinib in patients with brain metastases from HER2-positive breast cancer. Clin. Cancer Res. 15, 1452.
Lin, N.U., Winer, D.P., 2007. Brain metastases: the HER2 paradigm. Clin. Cancer Res. 13, 1648–1654.
Lisa, M., DeAngelis, M.D., Delattre, J.-Y., Posner, J.B., 1989. Radiation-induced dementia in patients cured of brain metastases. Neurology 39, 789.
McPherson, C.M., Suki, D., Feiz-Erfan, I., et al., 2010. Adjuvant whole-brain radiation therapy after surgical resection of single brain metastases. Neurol. Oncol. 12, 711–719.
Mendes, O., Kim, H.-T., Stoica, G., 2005. Expression of MMP2, 9 and 3 in breast cancer brain metastases in a rat model. Clin. Exp. Metastases 22, 237–246.
Minniti, G., Clarke, E., Lanzetta, G., Falchetto-Osti, M., et al., 2011. Stereotactic radiosurgery for brain metastases: analysis of outcome and risk of brain radionecrosis. Radiat. Oncol. 6, 48.
Nolte, S.M., Venugopal, C., McFarlane, N., et al., 2013. A cancer stem cell model for studying brain metastases from primary lung cancer. J. Natl. Cancer Inst. 105, 551–562.
Ryken, T.C., McDermott, M., Robinson, P.D., et al., 2010. The role of steroids in the management of brain metastases: a systematic review and evidence-based clinical practice guideline. J. Neurooncol. 96, 103–114.
Schouten, L.J., Rutten, J., Huveneers, H.A., 2002. Incidence of brain metastases in a cohort of patients with carcinoma of the breast, colon, kidney, and lung and melanoma. Cancer 94, 2698–2705.
Sheehan, J.P., Sun, M.H., Kondziolka, D., Flickinger, J., Lunsford, L.D., 2003. Radiosurgery in patients with renal cell carcinoma metastasis to the brain: long-term outcomes and prognostic factors influencing survival and local tumor control. Neurosurgery 98, 342–349.
Tsao, M.N., Lloyd, N.S., Wong, R.K., Rakovitch, E., Chow, E., Laperriere, N., 2005. Radiotherapeutic management of brain metastases: a systematic review and meta-analysis. Cancer Treat. Rev. 31, 256–273.
Yawn, B.P., Wollin, P.C., Schroeder, C., 2003. Temporal and gender-related trends in brain metastases from breast and lung cancer. Minn. Med. 86, 32–37.
Yokoi, K., Kamiya, N., Matsuguma, B., et al., 1999. Detection of brain metastases in potentially operable non-small cell lung cancer. Chest 115, 714–719.
Yoshida, S., Takahashi, H., 2009. Cerebellar metastases in patients with cancer. Surg. Neurol. 71, 184–187.

CHAPTER

2

Epidemiology of Central Nervous System Metastases

Xiao-Tang Kong, Daniela Alexandru and Daniela A. Bota

OUTLINE

Introduction 11

Incidence 12

Incidence by Demographic Features 13
Incidence by Race 13
Incidence by Gender 14
Incidence by Age 14
SEER Stage of the Cancer 14
Onset of Brain Metastases from Initial Diagnosis 14

Incidence by Specific Cancer Types – Adults 15
Lung Cancer 16
Breast Cancer 17
Melanoma 17
Renal Cancer 18
Colorectal Cancer 18
Prostate Cancer 18
Esophageal Cancer 19
Ovarian Cancer 19
Choriocarcinoma 19
Testicular Cancer 19

Incidence by Specific Cancer Types – Children 20

Conclusions 21

References 22

INTRODUCTION

Brain metastases are the most common type of brain tumors (Alexandru et al., 2012) and are associated with significant mortality and morbidity (Alexandru et al., 2012). The incidence of brain metastases varies by reporting institution, and different studies have reported different results. For example, the reported incidence varies from 2.8 to 14.3 individuals per 100000 population (Guomundsson, 1970; Percy et al., 1972; Walker et al., 1985;

M.A. Hayat (ed): *Brain Metastases from Primary Tumors, Volume 1*
DOI: http://dx.doi.org/10.1016/B978-0-12-800896-6.00002-4

© 2014 Elsevier Inc. All rights reserved.

Barnholtz-Sloan et al., 2004). At the same time, study-specific data indicate a rate of 9–17% of systemic cancers being complicated by brain metastases (Nayak et al., 2012). Autopsy studies also found that 8.7–24% of patients with systemic cancers had brain metastases (Posner and Chernik, 1978; Pickren et al., 1983).

With the advent of new imaging modalities, the incidence of brain metastases increased over time due to earlier detection of the lesions (Nayak et al., 2012). In addition, improved treatment for the systemic cancers increased survival and therefore the likelihood of the patient developing brain metastases over time (Barnholtz-Sloan et al., 2004; Nayak et al., 2012). The cohort study in Sweden found that the incidence of brain metastases doubled from 1987 to 2006 (Smedby et al., 2009).

The most common sources of brain metastases are lung cancer, breast cancer, melanoma, renal cancer, and colorectal cancer (Percy et al., 1972; Posner and Chernik, 1978; Pickren et al., 1983; Sawaya et al., 2001). However, virtually any cancer, including prostate cancer, ovarian cancer, and liver cancer can metastasize to the brain (Sawaya et al., 2001). Sometimes, patients can present with brain metastases without evidence of primary cancer (Alexandru et al., 2012). The primary tumor site, if eventually detected, is often the lung (Guomundsson, 1970; Sawaya et al., 2001; Nayak et al., 2012).

The incidence of brain metastases from various cancers changed over time. For example, during the 1980s, men had a higher incidence of brain metastases than women. This was likely due to a higher incidence of lung cancer in men at the time due to smoking (Walker et al., 1985). A more recent cohort study in Sweden reported that women had a higher incidence of brain metastases than men (Smedby et al., 2009). This study only investigated patients who were hospitalized and included all brain metastases. The reason for this change could be due to a decreased incidence of lung cancer in men due to smoking cessation and relative increase in incidence of lung cancer in women. In addition, a relative increase in the incidence of breast cancer in women over the study period from 1987 to 2006 also contributed to increased incidence of brain metastases. The incidence of breast cancer has increased slowly over the past 20 years. At the same time, it appeared that the incidence of brain metastases from breast cancer also increased (Smedby et al., 2009).

Smedby et al. (2009) reported that the median age at first admission due to brain metastases from systemic cancer was 67 years old among men and 64 years old among women. Half of the patients were admitted because of brain metastases as the primary diagnosis, 43% were admitted as other systemic cancers with secondary brain metastases while 7% were admitted due to other non-cancer disorders and found to have brain metastases incidentally (Smedby et al., 2009). Brain metastases are rare in children. The most common brain metastases in children are secondary to germ cell tumors, sarcoma, and neuroblastoma (Nayak et al., 2012).

INCIDENCE

Though the overall incidence of cancer as well as death due to cancer decreased recently between 2004 and 2012, there are still a total of 1638910 new cancer cases, and 577190 deaths from cancer projected to occur in the USA in 2012 (American Cancer Society, 2012). Brain metastases continue to remain the major type of brain tumor, about 3–5 times higher than the number of newly diagnosed primary malignant brain tumors each year (Sawaya et al., 2001). It was estimated that almost 70000 new brain metastases would occur over the remaining lifetime of individuals who received a diagnosis of primary invasive cancer in the USA in 2007 (Davis et al., 2012). Although the exact incidence of brain metastases is unknown, it is estimated that the incidence ranges from 2.8–11.1 per 100000 population in studies concluded before 1990 (Guomundsson, 1970; Percy et al., 1972; Fogelholm et al., 1984; Walker et al., 1985) to 7–14.3 per 100000 population in more recent studies (Counsell et al., 1996; Barnholtz-Sloan et al., 2004; Materljan et al., 2004; Smedby et al., 2009). The incidence of lifetime brain metastases from systemic cancers was estimated to increase yearly between 2003 and 2007 (Davis et al., 2012).

In 1970, Guomundsson performed a population based epidemiologic study in Iceland that covered brain metastasis between 1954 and 1963. The annual incidence was 2.8 per 100000 population (Guomundsson, 1970). A more extended study conducted from 1935 to 1968 by Percy et al. (1972) found the incidence in Minnesota in the USA was 11.1 per 100000 population. Studies in the 1970s and 1980s showed the incidence of 3.4 per 100000 population in Finland with 66 study subjects (1975–1983) (Fogelholm et al., 1984). More recent studies extended to the 1990s and 2000s showed a higher incidence than the studies conducted in the 1970s and 1980s. Materljan reported 9.9 per 100000 population with 80 study subjects in Croatia (Materljan et al., 2004). Counsell reported 14.3 per 100000 population with 214 study subjects in Scotland (Counsell et al., 1996). Smedby et al. (2009) studied a large population with 15517 subjects and clearly demonstrated that the incidence of brain metastases doubled from 7 per 100000 in 1987 to 14 per 100000 in 2006. Two other studies reported that the incidence proportion (also known as cumulative incidence) percentage (IP%) were 8.5% (1986–1995) in the Netherlands (Schouten et al., 2002) and 9.6% (1973–2001) in Michigan (Barnholtz-Sloan et al., 2004).

INCIDENCE BY DEMOGRAPHIC FEATURES

As the incidence of the primary tumors varies with different demographic characteristics, so does the incidence of brain metastases. Barnholtz-Sloan et al. (2004) described that race, gender and age influence the incidence of brain metastases. The study was conducted on a population-based MDCSS (Cancer Surveillance System for the Metropolitan Detroit Area) on 16210 patients who developed brain metastases after diagnosis with a single primary tumor between 1973 and 2001 (Barnholtz-Sloan et al., 2004). It compared the IP% among different race, sex, age at the diagnosis and Surveillance Epidemiology and End Results Program (SEER) stage of the primary cancer.

Incidence by Race

Barnholtz-Sloan et al. (2004) found that the IP% of brain metastases for African Americans was significantly higher compared with that for Caucasian patients for lung, melanoma, and breast cancers. However, IP% of brain metastases for renal cancers was lower in African American patients while the IP% of brain metastases for colorectal cancers was similar between African Americans and Caucasian patients (Barnholtz-Sloan et al., 2004).

Incidence by Gender

Investigation by Barnholtz-Sloan et al. (2004) found that men had higher IP% of brain metastases for each type of systemic cancer except breast cancer and lung cancer compared with women. In patients with lung cancer, the IP% for brain metastases for women was 21.8%, while IP% for men was 18.9% (Barnholtz-Sloan et al., 2004). The exception of the higher IP% of brain metastases in women can be attributed to the fact that during that same period the incidence of lung cancer was rising in women (Barnholtz-Sloan et al., 2004).

Incidence by Age

The IP% of brain metastases was the highest for the patients with lung cancer diagnosed at age 40–49 years; with primary melanoma, renal or colorectal cancer at age 50–59 years; and with primary breast cancer at age 20–39 years (Barnholtz-Sloan et al., 2004). The IP% was lowest for all primary cancers at the age group above 70 years, with the exception of melanoma. Melanoma had a similar percentage in patients over 70 years old as it did in patients who were 20–39 years old (Barnholtz-Sloan et al., 2004).

SEER Stage of the Cancer

SEER stage of the primary cancer is classified as localized, regional, distant and upstaged (Gavrilovic and Abrey, 2005). Barnholtz-Sloan et al. found that IP% increased as SEER stage of primary cancer increased (Barnholtz-Sloan et al., 2004). Compared to individuals with localized and regional stages, patients with the distant-stage of primary lung, melanoma, breast, colorectal and kidney cancers had the highest IP% of brain metastases (Gavrilovic and Abrey, 2005). Among the five kinds of primary cancers, melanoma had the highest IP% for brain metastases, consistent with the high propensity of the melanoma to metastasize to the brain (Gavrilovic and Abrey, 2005).

Onset of Brain Metastases from Initial Diagnosis

A large population study based on hospital admission found that the median time between diagnosis of the primary cancer and first admission with brain metastases varied among different cancers (Gavrilovic and Abrey, 2005). In patients with lung cancer, the median time was 2.6 months, in breast cancer 41.7 months, in melanoma 38.6 months, in colorectal cancer 25.2 months and in kidney cancer 17.0 months (Gavrilovic and Abrey, 2005; Davis et al., 2012). The time to admission was almost twice as long among women (16.3 months) as it was among men (8.8 months) (Gavrilovic and Abrey, 2005; Davis et al., 2012). With the exception of gender-specific malignancies, the time to admission was still longer in women when compared to men with lung cancer or malignant melanoma (Smedby et al., 2009; Davis et al., 2012). The time to admission was found to increase with age, more so in women than in men (Smedby et al., 2009; Davis et al., 2012). In a separate study, Schouten et al. (2002) found that 36% of patients with brain metastases were diagnosed within one month after their primary cancer diagnosis, 35% within 1 year of their primary cancer diagnosis, and 28% >1 year after their primary cancer diagnosis. Lung cancer was found to have the shortest interval between diagnosis and onset of brain metastases with 91% of brain metastases diagnosed within 1 year (Schouten et al., 2002).

INCIDENCE BY SPECIFIC CANCER TYPES – ADULTS

Primary lung cancer, breast cancer, melanoma, renal cancer, and colorectal cancer are the most common primary cancers responsible for brain metastasis (Table 2.1) (Posner and Chernik, 1978). Of all the primary tumors, lung cancer has the highest incidence of brain metastases. Melanoma, testicular and renal carcinomas have the greatest propensity to metastasize to the brain, but their relative rarity explains the low incidence of these neoplasms in large series of patients with brain metastases (Posner and Chernik, 1978). In 1994 and 1995, Posner reviewed 284 brain metastases from systemic carcinomas as defined by computed tomography (CT) or magnetic resonance imaging (MRI) scans. The investigators found that 38% of the metastases were from lung cancer, 19% from breast cancer, 13% from melanoma, 4% from renal cancer, and 1% were unknown (Posner and Chernik, 1978). Between 1986 and 1995 in the Netherlands, the IP% or percentage cumulative incidence of brain metastasis after 5 years from the first diagnosis was estimated to be 16.3% in patients with lung carcinoma, 9.8% in patients with renal carcinoma, 7.4% in patients with melanoma, 5.0% in patients with breast carcinoma, and 1.2% in patients with colorectal carcinoma (Fogelholm et al., 1984). The incidence was lower in patients with lung and breast carcinoma diagnosed before 1991 when compared with patients diagnosed after 1991 (Fogelholm et al., 1984). Another study, which analyzed patients over a period of 28 years from 1973 to 2001, found that the total IP% of brain metastases was the highest for lung cancer (19.9%) (Barnholtz-Sloan et al., 2004). This was followed by melanoma (6.9%), renal cancer (6.5%),

TABLE 2.1 Percentage of Brain Metastases from Different Primary Cancers in Adults

Authors	Posner et al.	Schouten et al.	Barnholtz-Sloan et al.	Smedby et al.	
Publication year	1996	2002	2004	2009	
Study years	1994–1995	1986–1995	1973–2001	1987–2006	
Sex	M and F	M and F	M and F	F	M
Lung cancer	38%	16.3	19.9	33	44
Breast cancer	19	5	5.1	33	
Melanoma	13	7.4	6.9	5.8	12.3
Renal cancer	4	9.8	6.5	4.7	7.8
Colorectal cancer	n/a	1.2	1.8	7.4	9
Other cancer	–	–	–	5.6*	8.6**
Unknown	1	–	–	10.5	18.2

*M: male; F: Female; *incidence rate of female genital cancer; **incidence rate of prostate cancer.*

breast cancer (5.1%), and colorectal cancer (1.8%) (Barnholtz-Sloan et al., 2004). Smedby et al. then reported the different incidence of brain metastases among men and women in Sweden (Smedby et al., 2009). Among patients with one primary solid tumor, the most common cancers causing brain metastases in men were lung cancer (44%), malignant melanoma (12%), colorectal cancer (9%) and prostate cancer (9%). Among women, the most common cancers causing brain metastases were lung (33%), breast (33%) and colorectal cancer (7%), and malignant melanoma (6%) (Smedby et al., 2009).

Lung Cancer

Lung cancer is the leading cause of cancer death in both men and women in the USA, accounting for 28% of all cancer deaths (Davis et al., 2012). Non-small cell lung cancer (NSCLC) comprises approximately 85% of lung cancer cases (Davis et al., 2012). In 2012, 226160 new cases of lung cancer and 160340 deaths from lung cancer were expected (Davis et al., 2012). The brain is one of the most common sites for cancer recurrence after definitive treatment for lung cancer. The risk of developing brain metastases for locally advanced (stage III) NSCLC is 24–55% (Schouten et al., 2002; Chen et al., 2007). An earlier study found that the incidence of brain metastases was 24% in a consecutive group of 259 patients with inoperable adenocarcinoma of the lung (Sorensen et al., 1988). More cases of brain metastases were identified at autopsy with 38 (44%) patients out of 87 autopsies presenting with brain metastases. Eleven of these patients (29%) were not diagnosed clinically before death. Patients younger than 60 years old and with initial performance status above 60% and patients responding to chemotherapy had higher risk for developing brain metastasis during treatment than other patients. This higher risk was very likely due to the fact that increased survival increases the risk of developing brain metastases, as seen in brain metastases from adenocarcinoma of the lung (Sorensen et al., 1988).

Chen et al. (2007) analyzed outcomes in 211 patients who were treated with neoadjuvant therapy for stage III NSCLC before surgical resection between 1990 and 2004 and found that the most common site of initial recurrence was the brain, with 22 (43%) patients developing brain metastasis as the site of first failure, which represented 71% of all isolated recurrences. Ultimately, 28 patients (55%) developed brain metastases at some point during their clinical course.

In early stages (Stage I and Stage II) of NSCLC, Hubbs et al. found that the 5-year actuarial risk of developing brain metastases was 10%, much lower compared with higher stages. Of patients developing brain metastases, the brain was the sole site of failure in 43%. On multivariate analysis, younger age, larger tumor size, lymphovascular space invasion, and hilar lymph node involvement were associated with an increased risk of developing brain metastases (Hubbs et al., 2010).

The propensity of brain metastasis varies among the pathological subtypes of lung cancer. Most studies concluded that NSCLC is the most common primary lung cancer to develop brain metastases (Barnholtz-Sloan et al., 2004). However, one autopsy study revealed that 40% of the patients with SCLC developed brain metastases while less than 20% of the patients in NSCLC have CNS involvement (Cairncross et al., 1980). Of NSCLC, non-squamous cell lung cancers were observed to have higher risk of developing brain metastasis. Shi et al. (2006) reviewed 181 lung cancer individuals with brain metastasis at initial staging. They found that patients with adenocarcinoma and large-cell carcinoma had greater risk of brain metastases than patients with squamous cell carcinoma. There was no correlation between the number/distribution of brain metastases and tumor histology (Shi et al., 2006). They reviewed 211 patients with stage III NSCLC and found that 63% (19/30) of patients with non-squamous lung cancer and 43% (9/21) with squamous lung cancer developed brain metastasis over a 5-year period.

As new treatments for NSCLC led to increased survival, it was noticed that the incidence of brain metastases was decreasing. Heon et al. (2010) found that the patients with somatic epidermal growth factor receptor (EGFR) mutations who received treatment with targeted tyrosine kinase inhibitors (gefitinib or erlotinib) had a lower incidence of brain metastases than the previously published rates. The EGFR somatic mutation was found to be associated both with increased response rates in patients treated with gefitinib or erlotinib and with longer median survival (Heon et al., 2010). Lung cancer is also the tumor most likely to spread to the brain with unknown primary tumor on presentation. More than two-thirds of the brain metastases with unknown primary tumor at initial work up were eventually found to originate from lung (Alexandru et al., 2012).

Breast Cancer

Breast cancer currently has the second highest incidence of brain metastases after lung cancer. New cases of breast cancer are estimated at 340650 in 2012 with 226870 in women and 2190 in men (American Cancer Society, 2012). Total incidence of brain metastases from breast cancer varies from 1.4% to 30% – depending on the data source (Frisk et al., 2012). Researchers noted that the incidence of breast cancer metastases was on the rise. This was very likely due to improved control of the systemic disease and to the consequent prolonged life span (Frisk et al., 2012). The interval between the diagnosis of primary breast cancer and the identification of brain metastases was an average of 2–3 years (Chen et al., 2007).

A large patient population study, with 50528 breast cancer patients followed over a median of 3.5 years, completed in Sweden, found that 1.4% of patients were admitted to hospital with brain metastases (Frisk et al., 2012). Compared with the period 1998–2000, patients diagnosed with breast cancer in 2004–2006 had a 44% increased risk of being admitted to hospital with brain metastases (Frisk et al., 2012). Pestalozzi et al. studied 9524 women with early breast cancer over a 13-year follow-up period between 1978 and 1999 without trastuzumab treatment. This study showed an incidence of 5.2% of brain metastases (Pestalozzi et al., 2006). The established risk factors for development of brain metastases from primary breast cancer were HER2-positive status, estrogen receptor negativity, high Ki-67 index/high grade, tumor size larger than 2cm, node positive disease, <35–50 years old, expression of EGFR and cytokeratin 5/6 (Pestalozzi et al., 2006). It was unclear whether trastuzumab treatment altered the risk for developing brain metastasis from primary breast cancer.

Melanoma

The total estimated new cases of melanoma in 2012 were 76250 with 44250 cases in men and 34350 in women (American Cancer Society, 2012). Melanoma is the second to third most common primary tumor that develops brain metastases, accounting for 5–21% of all metastatic brain tumors (Posner and Chernik, 1978; Schouten et al., 2002; Barnholtz-Sloan et al., 2004). The incidence of CNS metastases in advanced malignant melanoma was 46% when diagnosed clinically, and 75% when diagnosed through autopsy, as evaluated by a retrospective study of 122 patients seen at Wayne State University over a 12-year period (Schouten et al., 2002; Barnholtz-Sloan et al., 2004). Meningeal involvement was suspected clinically in 10.6% of the patients and it was found during autopsy in 52% of patients. The incidence was 6.7–8% when all stages of melanoma were included (Cohn-Cedermark et al., 1998; Barnholtz-Sloan et al., 2004). The study of 2516 patients with malignant melanoma showed that 201 (8%) developed CNS metastasis during a follow-up period of an average of 11 years (total follow up was between 7 and 18 years) (Cohn-Cedermark et al., 1998). The overall cumulative incidence at 5, 10 and 15 years was 7, 9, 9.5 % respectively. The median interval between initial diagnoses of malignant melanoma to the CNS metastasis was 2.6 years (0 day–20 years) (Cohn-Cedermark et al., 1998). At autopsy, 6.3% of the cases with metastatic melanoma were diagnosed.

Renal Cancer

Renal cancer accounts for approximately 3% of all cases of adult malignancies worldwide (Graus et al., 1983). In 2012, the estimated number of new renal cancer cases was 64 700 in both men and women. More cases were seen in men than women (40 250 vs. 24 520) (Paulino et al., 2003). Renal cell carcinoma (RCC) is the most common type of renal cancer (92%) and very frequently metastasizes to the brain with an incidence varying from 5.5% to 13.2%, (Schouten et al., 2002; Barnholtz-Sloan et al., 2004,). RCC is one of the cancers with high incidence of hemorrhagic brain metastases and large peritumoral vasogenic edema (Graus et al., 1983). Median interval between the initial treatment of the primary lesion and the diagnosis of brain metastasis was 1.6 years. The mean interval between the RCC diagnosis and identification of brain metastasis is approximately 1–2 years. However, RCC can have brain metastases occurring as late as 10–20 years after initial nephrectomy.

Colorectal Cancer

Colorectal cancer (CRC) is the third to fifth most common cancer in both men and women (Barnholtz-Sloan et al., 2004; Smedby et al., 2009). An estimated 103 170 cases of colon cancer and 40 290 cases of rectal cancer were expected to occur in 2012 (American Cancer Society, 2012). However, the incidence of brain metastases is low, being reported recently from 0.62% to 4% (Mongan et al., 2009). Mongan et al. (2009) reviewed colorectal carcinoma cases with brain metastases at Dartmouth-Hitchcock Medical Center between 1984 and 2006. They found that the incidence of brain metastases from CRC was 2.3%. The cerebellum was the most common area of brain involvement. Primary tumor in the left colon, long-standing pulmonary metastases, especially those with recent progression and CXCR4 expression by tumor cells were all associated with increased risk of brain metastases.

Prostate Cancer

Prostate cancer is the most common cancer in men in the USA. An estimated 241 740 new cases of prostate cancer occurred in the USA during 2012 (American Cancer Society, 2012).

The reported incidence of brain metastases from prostate cancer was 0.47% to 8.6%. According to this reported incidence, an estimate of 1136 to 20790 new cases of brain metastases from prostate cancer could be expected to occur in 2013.

Esophageal Cancer

The incidence rate for esophageal adenocarcinoma increased significantly among white men (1.8% per year), white women (2.1% per year) and Hispanic men (2.8% per year) during 1999–2008 (American Cancer Society, 2012). Although esophageal cancer is not one of the leading cancer etiologies and the estimated new cases in 2012 were only 17460 (American Cancer Society, 2012), the incidence of brain metastases from esophageal carcinoma (especially the adenocarcinoma subtype) is relatively high. Up to 16% of the patients with esophageal adenocarcinoma develop brain metastasis.

Ovarian Cancer

Ovarian cancer represents 3% of all cancers in women (American Cancer Society, 2012). The incidence of reported CNS metastases from ovarian cancers was low in the past. Among a large population study with 1316 ovarian cancer patients, only 14 patients had CNS metastasis (LeRoux et al., 1991). The incidence was 1.1%. Median interval from the diagnosis of ovarian carcinoma to the diagnosis of CNS metastases was 1.2–2.8 years.

Choriocarcinoma

Choriocarcinoma is an uncommon tumor but has a very high propensity to metastasize to the brain. This malignancy is seen in both men and women. In women, choriocarcinoma manifests as the gestational type or malignant gestational trophoblastic tumor related to a mole pregnancy. The overall reported incidence of choriocarcinoma was one per 24096 pregnancies between 1973 and 1982 (Alexandru et al., 2012). However, the numbers declined by 2.8% per year demonstrated by population-based data between 1973 and 1999. The incidence of CNS metastases from gestational choriocarcinoma varies from 8.8% to 9.3% (Athanassiou et al., 1983). They found that approximately half of the patients with choriocarcinoma had CNS metastases on presentation and the other half developed the metastases during therapy (Athanassiou et al., 1983). Patients with CNS metastases on presentation had a better prognosis than patients with late development of CNS metastases during therapy (Athanassiou et al., 1983). In men, choriocarcinoma manifests as a particular type of testicular germ cell carcinoma. The incidence of CNS metastases was reported as 30.8% (4/13) in a small patient population study (Alexandru et al., 2012; Frisk et al., 2012).

Testicular Cancer

Testicular cancer is not very common, but can metastasize to the brain. The incidence of CNS metastases was mainly obtained from studies in the 1970s and no recent large patient population study was conducted except for case reports. The incidence of brain metastases was 29.5% (23/78) from a study of 78 autopsied cases (Johnson et al., 1976). This study found that the patients had seminoma (6/19, 31.6%), embryonal carcinoma (6/21, 28.6%), teratocarcinoma (5/18, 27.8%), choriocarcinoma (1/4) and other mixed germinal carcinoma (5/16, 31.3%) (Johnson et al., 1976). The metastases included yolk sac carcinoma in addition to the testicular cancer subtypes reported in the above (Alexandru et al., 2012).

INCIDENCE BY SPECIFIC CANCER TYPES – CHILDREN

CNS metastases are an uncommon complication of systemic disease in children except in leukemia (Huang et al., 1996). Pediatric primary brain tumors are more common than metastatic tumors and, due to the rarity of metastatic brain tumors in children, the incidence of pediatric brain metastases is more difficult to estimate than the incidence in adults (Huang et al., 1996).

Prior autopsy studies established the incidence of brain metastasis in children to be between 6% and 13% (Vannucci and Baten, 1974). The Memorial Sloan Kettering Cancer Center autopsy data from 1951 to 1972 showed an incidence of brain metastases in children with malignant tumors of 6% (Vannucci and Baten, 1974). Another study performed between 1973 and 1982 in the same institute on post-mortem patients with solid tumors found that the incidence of brain metastases increased over time to 12.9% (18/139) (Graus et al., 1983). The same autopsy study demonstrated that osteogenic sarcoma and rhabdomyosarcoma (RMS) were the most frequent primary tumors causing brain metastases in patients younger than 15 years, and testicular germ cell tumor in patients between 15 and 21 years of age (Graus et al., 1983).

During clinical investigations, the incidence of brain metastases varied from 1.45% to 5.5% (see Table 2.2). Clinical studies showed a lower incidence of brain metastases from systemic cancer or solid tumors compared to autopsy studies. Huang et al. (1996) reviewed 200 pediatric patients with systemic malignancies including leukemia and found 11 patients (5.5%) had CNS including leptomeningeal and spinal metastases.

The incidence of CNS metastases from solid tumors was even less common. Bouffet et al. (1997) reported a 2.5% incidence of CNS metastases from solid tumors by reviewing brain metastases in 486 children during a 9-year period. Kebudi et al. (2005) reported that the incidence of brain metastases due to extracranial solid tumors including lymphomas was only 1.45%. Curless et al. (2002) reviewed 2035 children with solid tumors over 36 years in the literature and concluded the incidence of brain metastases was approximately 4%.

Paulino et al. (2003) studied 611 children with solid tumors including sarcoma, neuroblastoma and Wilm's tumor from 1965 to 2000. Among them, 4.9% were found to have brain metastasis. Twenty-six cases were diagnosed clinically and four cases were diagnosed by autopsy. Major clinical studies on incidence by specific cancer types found that the most common brain metastases in children were from neuroblastoma, sarcomas, including osteosarcoma, Ewing sarcoma (ES), rhabdomyosarcoma (RMS), and germ cell tumors (see Table 2.2) (Graus et al., 1983; Bouffet et al., 1997; Curless et al., 2002; Paulino et al., 2003; Kebudi et al., 2005).

Individual cancer type studies demonstrated that the incidence of brain metastases was 2.4% in RMS, 3.3% in ES and 4.3–5.5% in NB (Parasuraman et al., 1999; Matthay et al., 2003).

TABLE 2.2 Percentage of Brain Metastases from Different Primary Cancers in Children

Authors	Study Years	Number of Patients (n)	Primary Tumors	Percentage
Huang et al.	1991–1995	200 (<= 14 yo)	All pediatric tumors	0.5%
Kebudi et al.	1989–2002	1100 <= 16 yo	Solid tumors	1.45%
Parasuraman et al.	36 years	419 <= 18 yo	ES and RMS	3.3% and 2.4%
Bouffet et al.	1987–1995	486 <= 17 yo	Solid tumors	2.4%
Curless et al.	36 years	2040		
		429	Neuroblastoma	4.4%
		386	Osteosarcoma	6.5%
		487	ES	3.3%
		574	RMS	1.9%
		44	Melanoma	3.6%
		37	Germ cell tumors	13.5%
		78	Wilms tumor	1.3%
Paulino et al.	1965–2000	611 <= 20 yo	Solid tumor	4.9%
		113	NB	8%
		104	RMS	6.7%
		105	Ewing Sarcoma	5.7%
		106	Osteosarcoma	4.7%
		83	Non RMS soft tissue	2.4%
		100	Wilms tumor	1%
Kramer et al.	1980–1999	251	NB	4.3%
Matthay et al.	1985–2000	434 <= 21	NB	5.3%

ES: Ewing Sarcoma; RMS: Rhabdomyosarcoma; NB: Neuroblastoma.

Significant risk factors for CNS metastases from NB included lumbar puncture at diagnosis, age 2–3 years, and *MYCN* gene amplification (Parasuraman et al., 1999).

CONCLUSIONS

Brain metastases greatly outnumber primary brain tumors. They are also known to be the most common type of brain tumor and have a major impact on both quality of life and survival. Careful evaluation and early diagnosis of metastatic brain tumors are critically important for early intervention and optimal treatment choices. Today, with improved chemotherapeutic regimens, patients live longer and have improved control of their systemic cancer. Therefore, it is very likely that the cancer can evolve into metastatic brain tumors, as it can spread to areas where chemotherapeutics have poor penetration, like the central nervous system. As such, with new, more active treatments for various types of cancers, the incidence of brain metastases will also increase over time.

The incidence of brain metastases also increases due to new and improved imaging modalities for screening patients with systemic cancers. New evidence suggests that obtaining local control of CNS disease, either by surgical resection or stereotactic radiosurgery, improves both the quality of life and patient survival (Alexandru et al., 2012). Given the important role that the brain plays in all aspects of a patient's life, including personality and identity as well as independence, it is important to identify and treat brain metastases early to prevent decline in the patient's functional status and decrease in the patient's quality of life.

References

Alexandru, D., Bota, D.A., Linskey, M.E., 2012. Epidemiology of central nervous system metastases. Prog. Neurol. Surg. 25, 13–29.

American Cancer Society, 2012. American Cancer Society. Cancer Facts & Figures. Atlanta.

Athanassiou, A., Begent, R.H., Newlands, E.S., Parker, D., Rustin, G.J., Bagshawe, K.D., 1983. Central nervous system metastases of choriocarcinoma. 23 years' experience at Charing Cross Hospital. Cancer 52, 1728–1735.

Barnholtz-Sloan, J.S., Sloan, A.E., Davis, F.G., Vigneau, F.D., Lai, P., Sawaya, R.E., 2004. Incidence proportions of brain metastases in patients diagnosed (1973 to 2001) in the Metropolitan Detroit Cancer Surveillance System. J. Clin. Oncol. 22, 2865–2872.

Bouffet, E., Doumi, N., Thiesse, P., et al., 1997. Brain metastases in children with solid tumors. Cancer 79, 403–410.

Cairncross, J.G., Kim, J.H., Posner, J.B., 1980. Radiation therapy for brain metastases. Ann. Neurol. 7, 529–541.

Chen, A.M., Jahan, T.M., Jablons, D.M., Garcia, J., Larson, D.A., 2007. Risk of cerebral metastases and neurological death after pathological complete response to neoadjuvant therapy for locally advanced nonsmall-cell lung cancer: clinical implications for the subsequent management of the brain. Cancer 109, 1668–1675.

Cohn-Cedermark, G., Mansson-Brahme, E., Rutqvist, L.E., Larsson, O., Johansson, H., Ringborg, U., 1998. Central nervous system metastases of cutaneous malignant melanoma – a population-based study. Acta Oncol. 37, 463–470.

Counsell, C.E., Collie, D.A., Grant, R., 1996. Incidence of intracranial tumours in the Lothian region of Scotland, 1989–90. J. Neurol. Neurosurg. Psychiatr. 61, 143–150.

Curless, R.G., Toledano, S.R., Ragheb, J., Cleveland, W.W., Falcone, S., 2002. Hematogenous brain metastasis in children. Pediatr. Neurol. 26, 219–221.

Davis, F.G., Dolecek, T.A., Mccarthy, B.J., Villano, J.L., 2012. Toward determining the lifetime occurrence of metastatic brain tumors estimated from 2007 United States cancer incidence data. Neurol. Oncol. 14, 1171–1177.

Fogelholm, R., Uutela, T., Murros, K., 1984. Epidemiology of central nervous system neoplasms. A regional survey in Central Finland. Acta Neurol. Scand. 69, 129–136.

Frisk, G., Svensson, T., Backlund, L.M., Lidbrink, E., Blomqvist, P., Smedby, K.E., 2012. Incidence and time trends of brain metastases admissions among breast cancer patients in Sweden. Br. J. Cancer 106, 1850–1853.

Gavrilovic, I.T., Abrey, L.E., 2005. Diagnosis and treatment of primary central nervous system lymphoma. Curr. Oncol. Rep. 7, 47–54.

Graus, F., Walker, R.W., Allen, J.C., 1983. Brain metastases in children. J. Pediatr. 103, 558–561.

Guomundsson, K.R., 1970. A survey of tumors of the central nervous system in Iceland during the 10-year period 1954–1963. Acta Neurol. Scand. 46, 538–552.

Heon, S., Yeap, B.Y., Britt, G.J., et al., 2010. Development of central nervous system metastases in patients with advanced non-small cell lung cancer and somatic EGFR mutations treated with gefitinib or erlotinib. Clin. Cancer Res. 16, 5873–5882.

Huang, L.T., Hsiao, C.C., Weng, H.H., Lui, C.C., 1996. Neurologic complications of pediatric systemic malignancies. J. Formos. Med. Assoc. 95, 209–212.

Hubbs, J.L., Boyd, J.A., Hollis, D., Chino, J.P., Saynak, M., Kelsey, C.R., 2010. Factors associated with the development of brain metastases: analysis of 975 patients with early stage nonsmall cell lung cancer. Cancer 116, 5038–5046.

Johnson, D.E., Appelt, G., Samuels, M.L., Luna, M., 1976. Metastases from testicular carcinoma. Study of 78 autopsied cases. Urology 8, 234–239.

Kebudi, R., Ayan, I., Gorgun, O., Agaoglu, F.Y., Vural, S., Darendeliler, E., 2005. Brain metastasis in pediatric extracranial solid tumors: survey and literature review. J. Neurooncol. 71, 43–48.

Leroux, P.D., Berger, M.S., Elliott, J.P., Tamimi, H.K., 1991. Cerebral metastases from ovarian carcinoma. Cancer 67, 2194–2199.

Materljan, E., Materljan, B., Sepcic, J., Tuskan-Mohar, L., Zamolo, G., Erman-Baldini, I., 2004. Epidemiology of central nervous system tumors in Labin area, Croatia, 1974–2001. Croat. Med. J. 45, 206–212.

Matthay, K.K., Brisse, H., Couanet, D., et al., 2003. Central nervous system metastases in neuroblastoma: radiologic, clinical, and biologic features in 23 patients. Cancer 98, 155–165.

Mongan, J.P., Fadul, C.E., Cole, B.F., et al., 2009. Brain metastases from colorectal cancer: risk factors, incidence, and the possible role of chemokines. Clin. Colorectal Cancer 8, 100–105.

Nayak, L., Lee, E.Q., Wen, P.Y., 2012. Epidemiology of brain metastases. Curr. Oncol. Rep. 14, 48–54.

Parasuraman, S., Langston, J., Rao, B.N., et al., 1999. Brain metastases in pediatric Ewing sarcoma and rhabdomyosarcoma: the St Jude Children's Research Hospital experience. J. Pediatr. Hematol. Oncol. 21, 370–377.

Paulino, A.C., Nguyen, T.X., Barker Jr., J.L., 2003. Brain metastasis in children with sarcoma, neuroblastoma, and Wilms' tumor. Int. J. Radiat. Oncol. Biol. Phys. 57, 177–183.

Percy, A.K., Elveback, L.R., Okazaki, H., Kurland, L.T., 1972. Neoplasms of the central nervous system. Epidemiologic considerations. Neurology 22, 40–48.

Pestalozzi, B.C., Zahrieh, D., Price, K.N., International Breast Cancer Study Group, 2006. Identifying breast cancer patients at risk for Central Nervous System (CNS) metastases in trials of the International Breast Cancer Study Group (IBCSG). Ann. Oncol. 17, 935–944.

Pickren, J.W., Lopez, G., Tsukada, Y., et al., 1983. Brain metastases: An autopsy study. Cancer Treat. Symp. 2, 295–313.

Posner, J.B., Chernik, N.L., 1978. Intracranial metastases from systemic cancer. Adv. Neurol. 19, 579–592.

Sawaya, R., Bindal, R.K., Lang, F.F., Abi-Said, D., 2001. Metastatic brain tumors. In: El, K. (Ed.), Brain Tumors: An Encyclopedic Approach, 2nd edn. Churchill Livingstone, London.

Schouten, L.J., Rutten, J., Huveneers, H.A., Twijnstra, A., 2002. Incidence of brain metastases in a cohort of patients with carcinoma of the breast, colon, kidney, and lung and melanoma. Cancer 94, 2698–2705.

Shi, A.A., Digumarthy, S.R., Temel, J.S., Halpern, E.F., Kuester, L.B., Aquino, S.L., 2006. Does initial staging or tumor histology better identify asymptomatic brain metastases in patients with non-small cell lung cancer? J. Thorac. Oncol. 1, 205–210.

Smedby, K.E., Brandt, L., Backlund, M.L., Blomqvist, P., 2009. Brain metastases admissions in Sweden between 1987 and 2006. Br. J. Cancer 101, 1919–1924.

Sorensen, J.B., Hansen, H.H., Hansen, M., Dombernowsky, P., 1988. Brain metastases in adenocarcinoma of the lung: frequency, risk groups, and prognosis. J. Clin. Oncol. 6, 1474–1480.

Vannucci, R.C., Baten, M., 1974. Cerebral metastatic disease in childhood. Neurology 24, 981–985.

Walker, A.E., Robins, M., Weinfeld, F.D., 1985. Epidemiology of brain tumors: the national survey of intracranial neoplasms. Neurology 35, 219–226.

CHAPTER

3

Involvement of the CXCL12/CXCR4/CXCR7 Axis in Brain Metastases

Chiara Calatozzolo, Emilio Ciusani, Elena Corsini, Francesco Di Meco, Bianca Pollo and Andrea Salmaggi

OUTLINE

Introduction 25

CXCL12 and its Receptors 26

CXCL12 Axis in Brain 28

CXCL12/CXCR4/CXCR7 and Metastasis 28

Brain Metastasis and CXCL12/CXCR4/CXCR7 31

Conclusions 33

References 34

INTRODUCTION

Chemokines are a superfamily of small cytokines (8–12 kDa) with chemotactic properties. They bind to specific receptors and are involved in cell trafficking, activation and differentiation.

More than 50 different chemokines have been identified and are classified into four families based on the position of four conserved cysteine residues. The first group, so-called CC chemokines because of two adjacent cysteines near the amino terminus, has 28 members; the second group, CXC chemokines, include proteins characterized by the presence of a

M.A. Hayat (ed): Brain Metastases from Primary Tumors, Volume 1
DOI: http://dx.doi.org/10.1016/B978-0-12-800896-6.00003-6

© 2014 Elsevier Inc. All rights reserved.

single variable amino acidic residue between the two cysteines and consists of 17 members. The other two chemokine families each have a single member: CX3C, that has three variable amino acidic residues between the cysteines and XC, in which the first and third cysteines are lacking.

Based on the presence or absence of a specific amino acidic motif "glu-leu-arg" (ELR, using the single letter code), CXC chemokines can be subgrouped into ELR^+ and ERL^-. CXC–ERL^+ chemokines preferentially attract neutrophils and are pro-angiogenic factors (CXCL1, 2, 3, 5, 6, 7, 8,) while ERL^- act on lymphocytes and, with the exception of CXCL12, inhibit the formation of vasculature (Bonecchi et al., 2009).

Physiologically, chemokines bind to specific G protein-coupled receptors (GPCRs). Chemokine receptors have a conserved structure with seven transmembrane domains, three extracellular and three intracellular loops with the C-terminus in the cytoplasm. Several chemokines may bind to various receptors and the same receptor may bind different chemokines. At present, we know seven CXC receptors (CXCR1–7), 10 CC receptors (CCR1–10), XCR1 and CX3CR1. In addition, there are decoy receptors that bind multiple chemokines without triggering signal transduction (D6, DARC, CCX–CKR) (Mantovani et al., 2006). Chemokine receptors act through heterotrimeric G-proteins which activate various signal transduction pathways, such as phosphoinositide 3-kinase (PI3K), phospholipase-C (PLC), mitogen-activated protein kinases (MAPK), protein kinase C (PKC) and RAS or Rho GTPases (Thelen and Stein, 2008).

Chemokines also interact with glycosaminoglycans (GAGs) that are required for presentation of chemokines by endothelial cells and extracellular matrix, making the formation of a chemotactic gradient that directs leukocyte and tumor cell migration *in vivo* possible.

Chemokines were initially identified as potent chemotactic agents for inflammatory cells, as leukocytes, monocytes and neutrophils. Their regulatory role in development, homeostasis and various pathological processes was discovered subsequently. Recently, a role in cancer progression and metastasization was proposed for chemokines: tumor cells expressing chemokine receptors could be attracted by chemokines produced by target organs and chemokines produced by tumor cells could recruit endothelial cells and tumor-associated stromal and inflammatory cells (Lazennec and Richmond, 2010).

CXCL12 AND ITS RECEPTORS

Stromal cell-derived factor (SDF-1, CXCL12) is a CXC chemokine widely expressed in many tissue types where it regulates hematopoietic cell trafficking. This role of CXCL12 is crucial not only in adult life, but also in embryo development. Due to the impairment in migration of hematopoietic stem cells from the fetal liver and major defects in brain and heart development, CXCL12 gene knockout in mice is lethal.

CXCL12, produced by osteoblasts, plays an important role in CD34+ cell migration to bone marrow and its function has been attributed to the receptor CXCR4.

Due to alternative splicing, CXCL12 has two major isoforms, α and β: CXCL12α is the most diffused and it is secreted by marrow stromal cells and endothelial cells; CXCL12β is expressed by highly vascularized organs such as liver, spleen, and kidneys, it is pro-angiogenic and more resistant than the α isoform to blood proteolysis. Additional splicing variants are CXCL12γ, CXCL12δ, CXCL12ε and CXCL12φ, all with chemotactic actvities.

CXCL12 expression is enhanced in hypoxic or damaged tissues because of elevated levels of HIF-1α that acts on its binding sites on the CXCL12 promoter, leading to chemoattraction of CXCR4-positive cells involved in tissue regeneration (Ceradini et al., 2004).

After binding with its receptor CXCR4, CXCL12 forms a complex with the Gαi-subunit resulting in Gβγ-subunit dissociation. The Gαi-subunit acts by inhibiting cAMP production by adenylyl cyclase and stimulating intracellular calcium mobilization. The Gβγ-subunit in turn activates PI3K and PLC leading to activation of downstream pathways such as MAPK, ERK1/2, JNK and AKT (Roland et al., 2003). These effectors induce actin polymerization and cytoskeletal rearrangements responsible for chemotaxis and expression and activation of integrins involved in adhesion to endothelial cells. These processes are essential for leukocyte activities in the immune response, but they are also implicated in the metastatic process and in local invasion of tumor cells.

CXCR4 was extensively studied as co-receptor for HIV infecting CD4+ T cells.

As CXCL12, CXCR4 plays an essential role in hematopoiesis, and in brain and heart development. The role in hematopoiesis is maintained in adult life: the CXCR4 inhibitor AMD3100 was recently approved as an immunostimulant to induce hematopoietic stem cell mobilization in hematological diseases (Keating, 2011).

While CXCR4 expression is low or absent in many healthy tissues, it was demonstrated to be upregulated in over 23 types of cancer, including melanoma, breast, ovarian and prostate cancer, and gliomas. CXCR4 expression is induced by vascular endothelial growth factor (VEGF) and hypoxia-inducible factor 1α (HIF1α), thus, in hypoxic regions of tumor, the CXCL12/CXCR4 axis may promote survival and metastasization.

Until recently, CXCR4 was believed to be the unique CXCL12 receptor. However, a second receptor was identified recently: the orphan receptor RDC1, now called CXCR7. CXCR7 binds CXCL12 with higher affinity than CXCR4, and it also binds another chemokine, CXCL11/I-TAC, previously known as a CXCR3 ligand, even if with lower affinity than CXCL12 (Balabanian et al., 2005, Burns et al., 2006).

CXCR7 gene maps on chromosome 2 in humans, as CXCR4. It is expressed and plays an important role in the hematopoietic system, heart, bone, kidney and brain (Sierro et al., 2007). Like CXCR4, CXCR7 was found expressed in a variety of tumors, such as lymphoma, breast, lung and prostate cancer. It is involved in the inhibition of apoptosis and in the adhesion to endothelial cells and metastasis. CXCR7 is also expressed in activated endothelial cells and in tumor vasculature stimulated by hypoxia (Burns et al., 2006, Miao et al., 2007).

Initially, CXCR7 was considered a decoy receptor because it does not elicit typical signaling pathways of G-protein-coupled receptors such as CXCR4. It was shown that it causes CXCL12 sequestration generating the chemokine gradient essential for proper migration of CXCR4-positive primordial germ cells in embryos (Boldajipour et al., 2008). Another mechanism of action proposed for CXCR7 is regulation of CXCR4 activity through the formation of functional CXCR4/CXCR7 heterodimers. Recently, it has been demonstrated that CXCR4/CXCR7 heterodimers can recruit β-arrestin activating ERK1/2, p38 MAPK, and SAPK and enhancing cell migration in response to CXCL12 stimulation (Décaillot et al., 2011).

CXCL12 AXIS IN BRAIN

CXCL12 and its receptor CXCR4 are expressed in embryonic life and play a major role in development of the cerebellum, neocortex and hippocampal dentate gyrus: CXCL12 acts as a chemoattractive cue for CXCR4 positive precursor cells regulating neuronal migration (Lazarini et al., 2003). CXCR4 is also expressed in neural stem cells in adult life: its mRNA is abundant in the subventricular zone neural stem cells in adult mice. More recently, CXCR7 has also been investigated for its role in neurogenesis: both CXCR4 and CXCR7 are involved in protecting neural progenitor cells from apoptosis in response to CXCL12 (Zhu et al., 2012).

In the central nervous system (CNS), CXCR4 is expressed in astrocytes, endothelial cells, neurons and microglia. CXCL12 is known to promote astrocyte proliferation via CXCR4 activation and MAPK and Erk1/2 signaling. More recently, Ödemis and colleagues showed that CXCR7 also activates traditional G-protein transduction pathways, such as Erk and Akt, involved in cell proliferation and migration, in astrocytes (Ödemis et al., 2012). This observation is in contrast with previous works that excluded CXCR7-mediated G-protein activation, suggesting different mechanisms of action of this receptor depending on cell type.

CXCL12 is also involved in repair processes after CNS trauma (Jaerve and Müller, 2012).

CXCR4 and CXCL12 are overexpressed in brain tumors, such as gliomas (Bajetto et al., 2006a), medulloblastomas (Yang et al., 2007) and meningiomas (Bajetto et al., 2006b). In glioblastoma, CXCL12 and CXCR4 are associated to areas of necrosis and angiogenesis (Rempel et al., 2000), promote tumor proliferation and chemotaxis (Bajetto et al., 2006a), and angiogenesis (Li and Ransohoff, 2009). CXCL12 was found to be associated with poor prognosis in glioblastomas and in low-grade gliomas (Salmaggi et al., 2004, 2005). Recent studies have shown that CXCR7 is also expressed in gliomas and a role in promoting survival of tumor cells has been proposed (Calatozzolo et al., 2011).

Overall, the complex interactions between CXCL12 and its two receptors may be implicated in tumor cell survival and in the mechanisms of tumor invasion. Their role in brain tumor metastasis remains so far less clearly defined.

CXCL12/CXCR4/CXCR7 AND METASTASIS

The chemokine CXCL12 and its receptors CXCR4 and CXCR7 have been described to play a pivotal role in tumor growth, in metastatic dissemination and in the cross-talk between neoplastic and support cells in the tumor microenvironment (reviewed in Sun et al., 2010). It has been suggested by recent works that the two receptors could make different contributions to tumor progression (Hernandez et al., 2011).

It is well known that expression of specific adhesion molecules, chemokines and receptors on tumor cells as well as on target organs are essential for organotropism in metastasis.

In physiological conditions, CXCL12 is constitutively expressed in a variety of tissue types and organs, including bone marrow, liver, lung and lymph nodes that represent common organs for metastasis homing. Moreover, both tumor cells and tumor-associated stromal cells contribute to create a microenvironment able to promote the metastatic process. Orimo and co-workers showed that, in breast cancer, high levels of CXCL12, released by tumor cells and tumor-associated stromal cells, directly stimulated the proliferation and invasiveness of cancer cells by autocrine and paracrine mechanisms (Orimo et al., 2005). In *in vitro* experiments, high amounts of CXCL12 released by CAFs (cancer associated fibroblasts lines, isolated from non-small cell lung cancer) induced an increased colony-forming capacity and extracellular signal-regulated kinase phosphorylation in cancer cells (Wald et al., 2011). The CXCR4/CXCL12 axis has been also reported to regulate immune cell infiltrates into tumors which, in turn, may promote neoangiogenesis and tumor progression.

Interestingly, antineoplastic agents commonly used in tumor treatment, such as irradiation, cyclophospamide and 5-fluorouracil, may increase CXCL12 expression in stem cells. However, CXCL12 production in the tumor context may exert an antimetastatic effect. As a matter of fact, experiments performed in mammary cancer cells leading to an epigenetic silencing of CXCL12, showed an increase of metastatic potential of colorectal and melanoma tumor cells and exogenous administration of CXCL12 increased survival of tumor-bearing mice because of a reduced metastatic ability of tumor cells (Wendt et al., 2008). The authors speculated that CXCL12 production by tumor cells could have an antimetastatic effect shielding the primary tumor by distant chemokine gradient.

Enhanced CXCR4 expression is reported in many different types of cancers (Sun et al., 2010), including breast, ovarian and prostate cancer, pancreatic adenocarcinoma, small cell lung cancer (SCLC), melanoma, neuroblastoma and glioma (Calatozzolo et al., 2011), while CXCR4 expression is low or absent in most normal tissues. CXCR4 expression on tumor cells is correlated with a poor prognosis in cancer patients.

Hypoxia-induced HIF-1α activation and VEGF release have been described among the mechanisms inducing the increase in CXCR4 expression in glioma cells, while stimulation with interleukin-5 (IL5) and interferon-γ (IFN-γ), produced by stromal cells, increases CXCR4 expression in neuroblastoma cells. In addition, radiotherapy has also been reported to produce the undesirable side effect of increasing CXCR4 expression (Kuonen et al., 2012).

After CXCL12 binding, CXCR4 signaling promotes actin polymerization, pseudopodia formation and chemotactic response in breast cancer cells. In SCLC cells, CXCL12 elicited an activation of phospho-p44/42 mitogen-activated protein kinase and induced tumor cell invasion into extracellular matrix and firm adhesion to marrow stromal cells, suggesting that CXCR4 can induce integrin activation on SCLC cells (Burger and Kipps, 2006).

The central role of the CXCR4/CXCL12 pathway in metastasis was also demonstrated in preclinical studies in melanoma, pancreatic, thyroid, prostate, and colon cancer models, showing that directed metastasis of cancer cells is mediated by CXCR4 activation and migration of tumor cells towards CXCL12 expressing organs.

The importance of CXCR4/CXCL12 axis in tumor growth and metastatic process was confirmed by data showing that CXCR4 antagonists or neutralizing antibodies affect tumor growth and invasiveness both in *in vitro* and in experimental models.

Small interfering RNA (siRNA)-mediated inhibition of CXCR4 expression in breast cancer cells decreased both their invasion capacity in *in vitro* invasion assay and metastasis development in a murine model (Liang et al., 2005). In an animal model of prostatic cancer, neutralizing antibody against CXCR4 has been reported to reduce the extent of bone metastasis (Sun et al., 2005).

In a murine model, D'Alterio et al. studied the effect of genetic CXCR4 reduction on the development of lung metastasis of melanoma cells (D'Alterio et al., 2012). After injection of murine melanoma B16 cells in $CXCR4^{+/+}$ and $CXCR4^{+/-}$ C57Bl/6 mice, they observed smaller metastasis in the latter. The authors suggested that the reduction may be partially due to a significant decrease in LY6G myeloid cells in the tumor context in $CXCR4^{+/-}$ mice when compared to $CXCR4^{+/+}$ mice, leading to a reduction of p38 MAPK activation. The administration of AMD3100 (plerixafor), a CXCR4 antagonist, further reduced the size and the number of lung metastases, but it was more effective in $CXCR4^{+/-}$ mice.

CXCR7 has been described to be expressed on fetal liver cells, activated endothelial cells and a variety of tumor cells (Burns et al., 2006; Miao et al., 2007; Wang et al., 2008), while its expression on T lymphocytes is controversial (Balabanian et al., 2005; Burns et al., 2006). CXCR7 is highly expressed on tumor-associated vasculature and it may be upregulated on endothelial cells by tumor necrosis factor α (TNFα), IL1β (Burns et al., 2006) and by hypoxia.

Transfection-induced CXCR7 expression has been described to increase cell proliferation in the human breast cancer cell line MDA-MB-435. Moreover, the anti-apoptotic effect exerted by CXCR7 was abrogated in a dose-dependent manner by the CXCR7 antagonist CCX754.

In vitro adhesion experiments on cytokine-stimulated human umbilical vein endothelial cells demonstrated an increased adherence of CXCR7-transfected tumor cells (Burns et al., 2006). Similar results on cell survival, as well as on adhesion ability, were obtained on CXCR7-expressing prostate cancer cell lines. Moreover, CXCR7 overexpression has been reported to increase the invasive abilities of cancer cells in *in vitro* invasion assays (Wang et al., 2008). Strong CXCR7 expression, observed both on cancer and endothelial cells in brain metastasis of different solid tumors, suggests an important role of this receptor in promoting migration of tumor cells through the blood–brain barrier (Salmaggi et al., 2009). In addition, CXCR7 was described to increase the expression of VEGF and IL-8, supporting its relevant contribution to the growth of tumor vasculature (Wang et al., 2008). In experimental models, CXCR7 expression enhanced the ability of breast cancer cells to produce lung metastasis (Miao et al., 2007).

These findings on CXCR4 and CXCR7, in some cases apparently contradictory, need further studies, aimed to clarify the individual contribution of the two receptors and especially their reciprocal interactions.

In an interesting study, Hernandez et al. (2011) investigated the roles of the two receptors in the different steps of metastasis. The authors evaluated the effect of overexpression of CXCR4, CXCR7 and both receptors (double transductant) in the rat mammary adenocarcinoma cell line MTLn3, analyzing invasiveness, entry into the bloodstream and lung metastasis development. While CXCR4 overexpression enhanced the chemotactic and invasive ability of the tumor cells in response to CXCL12, as well as intravasation (associated also to an increase in MMP12 production), CXCR7 overexpression further increased chemotactic response only if associated with high CXCR4 expression. The authors suggested that CXCR7 binds monomeric CXCL12, leaving dimeric CXCL12 to bind CXCR4 and mediate signalling through β-arrestin, as reported by other studies (Rajagopal et al., 2010).

On the other hand, CXCR7 overexpression has been reported to inhibit invasion and intravasation of tumor cells, probably following a decreased expression of the metalloprotease MMP12, leading to an inhibition of the ability to degrade extracellular matrix (Hernandez et al., 2011). However, unexpectedly, in this mouse model both CXCR4 and CXCR7 overexpression was not reported to increase the number of lung metastases.

BRAIN METASTASIS AND CXCL12/CXCR4/CXCR7

There is clinical evidence that the incidence of brain metastases has doubled in the last decade compared to the 1990s.

Although the exact incidence is unknown and varies depending on the primary site of cancer, on the design of studies (autopsy data versus clinical studies and trials versus population studies), metastasization to the brain by systemic tumors is not so uncommon, (Kamar and Posner, 2010). The most common sources of brain metastases are lung and breast cancer, but also renal carcinoma and melanoma are rather frequent.

A role for chemokines in homing organ-specific metastasization has been theorized. As chemokines attract hematopoietic cells in the site of inflammation, they work in a similar manner in the metastatic context. Therefore, chemokines expressed in the brain act on circulating tumor cells expressing the corresponding receptor promoting their adhesion, migration, and proliferation.

A recent review by Preusser and colleagues (Preusser et al., 2012) has reported the few papers dealing with the role of CXCR4 and CXCL12 in metastasization to the brain of breast and small cell lung cancer.

According to the "seed and soil" hypothesis at the basis of metastasization, the brain – as an organ rich in CXCL12 – might well attract tumor cells positive for one of the two receptors of this chemokine. Although this mechanism is by no means likely to be the most relevant in all tumors metastasizing to the brain, it may indeed give a relevant contribution in at least a subset of tumors/patients with brain metastatic disease.

In our experience, we performed an immunohistochemical analysis of CXCL12, CXCR4 and CXCR7 expression on a group of 56 brain metastases (Salmaggi et al., 2009). Of the 56 patients included in the study, 18 had a primary breast cancer, 17 a primary lung cancer, eight a kidney cancer, five each a colorectal and an ovarian cancer, two a prostate cancer and one a thyroid cancer.

CXCL12 was expressed in tumor and endothelial cells, with different distributions according to primary tumor (Figure 3.1). The chemokine was also expressed in the brain parenchyma surrounding the tumor in only a few endothelial cells. CXCR7 was diffusely expressed in metastatic cells and tumor-associated vessels, with some differences related to primary tumor (Figures 3.1 and 3.2). In the periphery of the tumor, astrocytes showed focal positivity for CXCR7, while it was intensely expressed in endothelial cells. CXCR4 was expressed in tumor and endothelial cells in all samples (Figure 3.2).

We evaluated the impact of clinical data on survival and we observed, as expected, that RPA class, single versus multiple metastasis, early versus delayed or no post-surgery radiotherapy and treatment versus no treatment at recurrence were significantly predictive of a longer survival.

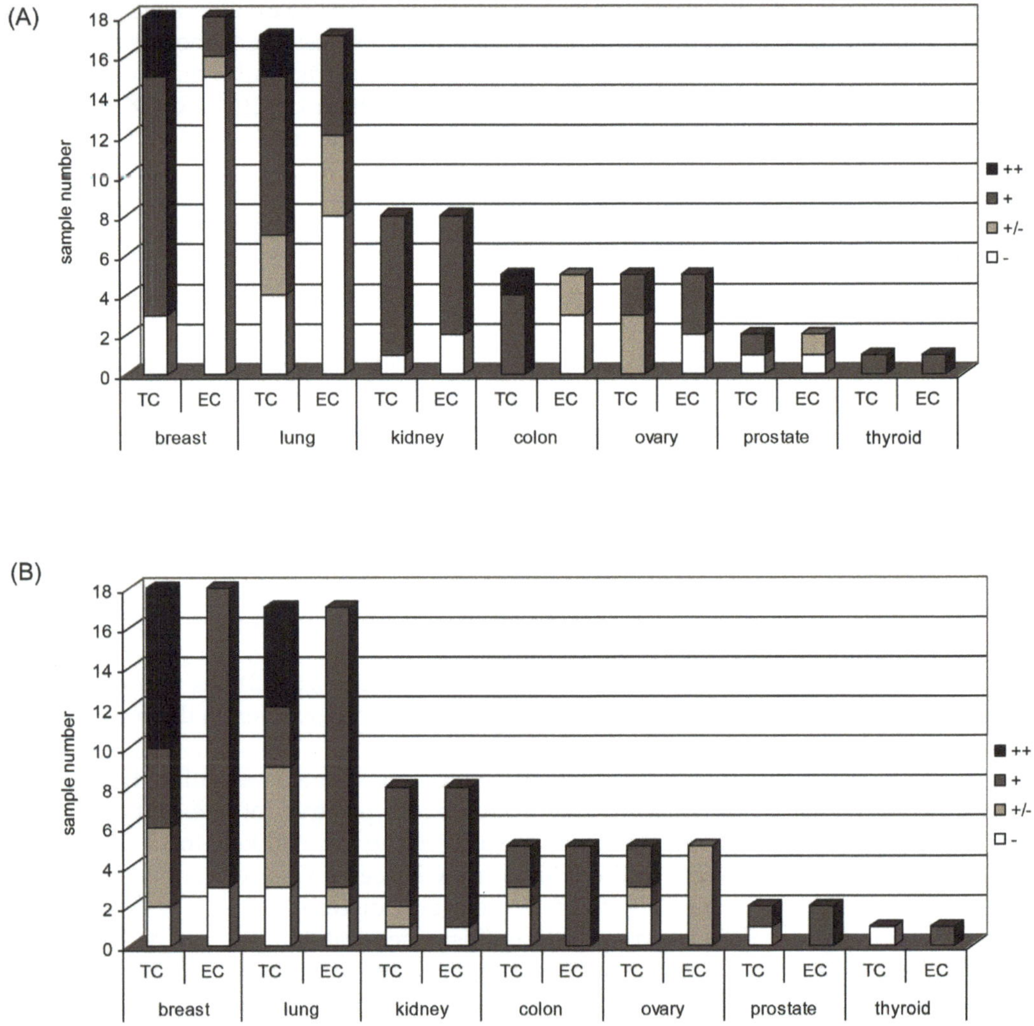

FIGURE 3.1 Intensity of CXCL12 (A) and CXCR7 (B) immunoreactivity in tumor and endothelial cells in brain metastases classified by primary tumor. TCs: tumor cells; Ecs: endothelial cells. *(Salmaggi A. et al. Cancer Biol Ther. 2009; 8(17):1608–14.)*

Among immunohistochemical parameters, CXCL12 expression in endothelial cells was found associated with a worse outcome (Figure 3.3).

CXCR7 expression in tumor and endothelial cells observed in our samples could facilitate the passage across the blood–brain barrier of CXCR7 positive metastatic cells. As observed by Burns and colleagues in *in vitro* models, CXCR7 expression in both tumor and endothelial cells improves adhesion of tumor cells to vessels supporting the metastasization process (Burns et al., 2006).

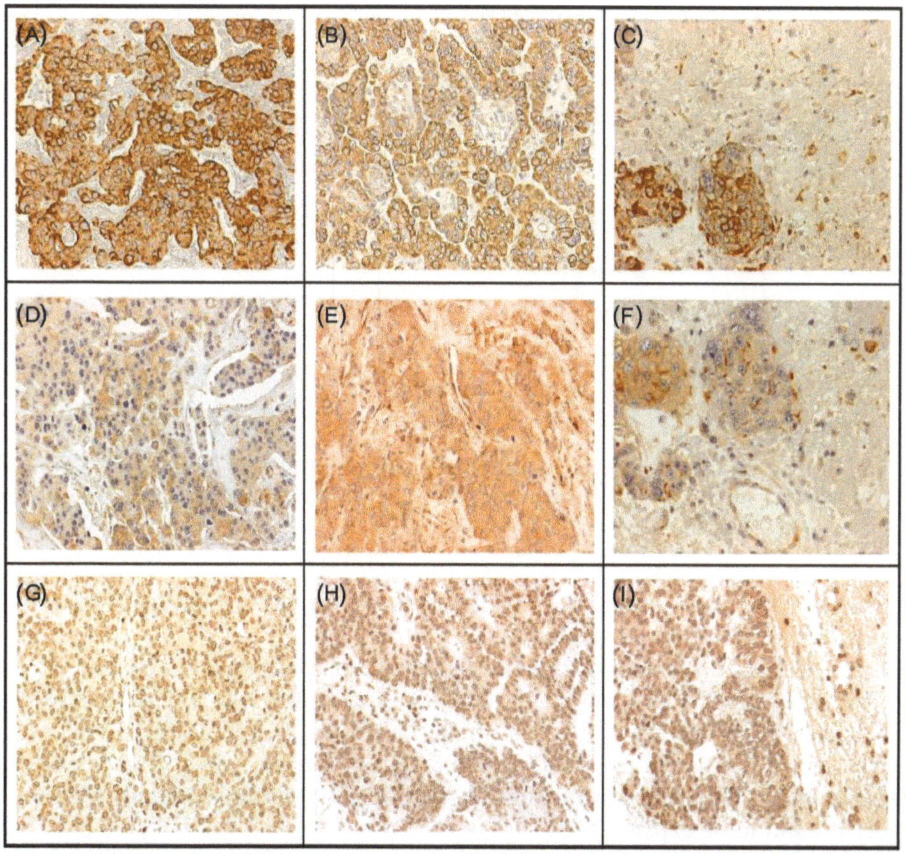

FIGURE 3.2 Expression of the chemokine CXCL12 (A–C) and its receptors CXCR7 (D–F) and CXCR4 (G–I) nuclear staining in all cases, respectively in metastases from breast (A, D and H) and lung carcinoma (B, E and H) and in brain parenchyma surrounding the metastatic lesions (C, F and I). Magnification is ×200. *(Salmaggi A. et al. Cancer Biol Ther. 2009; 8(17):1608–14.)*

Concerning the impact of the investigated molecules on clinical outcome, only CXCL12 expression in endothelial cells showed a statistically significant correlation with worse outcome, stressing the relevance of this chemokine in brain metastasis progression.

CONCLUSIONS

The CXCR4/CXCR7/CXCL12 pathway is involved in the complex scenario of tumor progression and the two receptors CXCR4 and CXCR7 play different and complementary functions in the metastatic process. While CXCR4 is mainly implicated in invasion and chemotaxis, CXCR7 promotes angiogenesis, regulates the interaction between endothelial cells and tumor cells in intra- and extravasation and exerts an anti-apoptotic action.

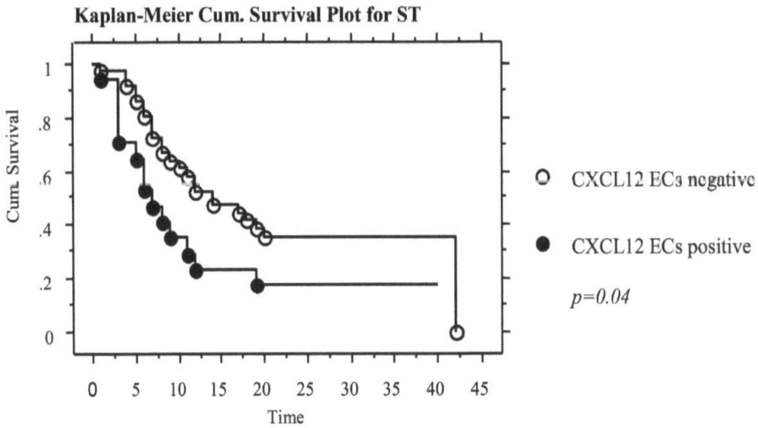

FIGURE 3.3 Kaplan–Meier curve shows correlation of patient survival with CXCL12 expression assessed by immunohistochemistry in endothelial cells (p=0.04 log-rank). CXCL12 ECs, CXCL12 expression in endothelial cells. *(Salmaggi A. et al. Cancer Biol Ther. 2009; 8(17):1608–14.)*

In vivo data are sometimes conflicting, but differences in experimental conditions and/or models may partially explain these results.

There are sufficient data supporting the fact that this pathway is also "at work" in the CNS. On the other hand, there are many data supporting the role of this axis in metastatic diffusion of tumors outside the CNS. The interaction of CXCL12 with its two receptors is certainly one of the pathways involved in migration of tumor cells within the CNS, even if the molecular mechanisms regulating the metastatic diffusion of systemic tumors into the CNS largely remain to be explored.

Both receptors are promising therapeutic targets and several agents inhibiting the CXCL12 pathway are currently available. Although further *in vivo* studies are needed better to explain the partially conflicting data, the clinical use of these agents could contribute to reduce the brain-specific metastatic potential of many solid tumors.

References

Bajetto, A., Barbieri, F., Dorcaratto, A., et al., 2006a. Expression of CXC chemokine receptors 1–5 and their ligands in human glioma tissues: role of CXCR4 and SDF1 in glioma cell proliferation and migration. Neurochem. Int. 49, 423–432.

Bajetto, A., Barbieri, F., Pattarozzi, A., et al., 2006b. CXCR4 and SDF1 expression in human meningiomas: a proliferative role in tumoral meningothelial cells in vitro. Neuro Oncol. 9, 3–11.

Balabanian, K., Lagane, B., Infantino, S., et al., 2005. The chemokine sdf-1/cxcl12 binds to and signals through the orphan receptor rdc1 in t lymphocytes. J. Biol. Chem. 280, 35760–35766.

Boldajipour, B., Mahabaleshwar, H., Kardash, E., et al., 2008. Control of chemokine-guided cell migration by ligand sequestration. Cell 132, 463–473.

Bonecchi, R., Galliera, E., Borroni, E.M., Corsi, M.M., Locati, M., Mantovani, A., 2009. Chemokines and chemokine receptors: an overview. Front. Biosci. 14, 540–551.

Burger, J.A., Kipps, T.J., 2006. CXCR4: a key receptor in the crosstalk between tumor cells and their microenvironment. Blood 107, 1761–1767.

Burns, J.M., Summers, B.C., Wang, Y., et al., 2006. A novel chemokine receptor for sdf-1 and i-tac involved in cell survival, cell adhesion, and tumor development. J. Exp. Med. 203, 2201–2213.

Calatozzolo, C., Canazza, A., Pollo, B., et al., 2011. Expression of the new CXCL12 receptor, CXCR7, in gliomas. Cancer Biol. Ther. 11, 242–253.

Ceradini, D.J., Kulkarni, A.R., Callaghan, M.J., et al., 2004. Progenitor cell trafficking is regulated by hypoxic gradients through hif-1 induction of sdf-1. Nat. Med. 10, 858–864.

D'Alterio, C., Barbieri, A., Portella, L., et al., 2012. Inhibition of stromal CXCR4 impairs development of lung metastases. Cancer Immunol. Immunother. 61, 1713–1720.

Décaillot, F.M., Kazmi, M.A., Lin, Y., Ray-Saha, S., Sakmar, T.P., Sachdev, P., 2011. CXCR7/CXCR4 heterodimer constitutively recruits beta-arrestin to enhance cell migration. J. Biol. Chem. 286, 32188–32197.

Hernandez, L., Magalhaes, M.A., Coniglio, S.J., Condeelis, J.S., Segall, J.E., 2011. Opposing roles of CXCR4 and CXCR7 in breast cancer metastasis. Breast Cancer Res. 13, R128.

Jaerve, A., Müller, H.W., 2012. Chemokines in CNS injury and repair. Cell Tissue Res. 349, 229–248.

Kamar, F.G., Posner, J.B., 2010. Brain metastases. Semin. Neurol. 30, 217–235.

Keating, G.M., 2011. Plerixafor: a review of its use in stem-cell mobilization in patients with lymphoma or multiple myeloma. Drugs 71, 1623–1647.

Kuonen, F., Secondini, C., Rüegg, C., 2012. Molecular pathways: emerging pathways mediating growth, invasion, and metastasis of tumors progressing in an irradiated microenvironment. Clin. Cancer Res. 18, 5196–5202.

Lazarini, F.O., Tham, O., Casanova, P., Arenzana-Seisedos, F., Dubois-Dalcq, M., 2003. Role of the chemokine stromal cell-derived factor (SDF-1) in the developing and mature central nervous system. Glia 42, 139–148.

Lazennec, G., Richmond, A., 2010. Chemokines and chemokine receptors: new insights into cancer-related inflammation. Trends Mol. Med. 16, 133–144.

Li, M., Ransohoff, R.M., 2009. The roles of chemokine CXCL12 in embryonic and brain tumor angiogenesis. Semin. Cancer Biol. 19, 111–115.

Liang, Z., Yoon, Y., Votaw, J., Goodman, M.M., Williams, L., Shim, H., 2005. Silencing of CXCR4 blocks breast cancer metastasis. Cancer Res. 65, 967–971.

Mantovani, A., Bonecchi, R., Locati, M., 2006. Tuning inflammation and immunity by chemokine sequestration: decoys and more. Nat. Rev. Immunol. 6, 907–918.

Miao, Z., Luker, K.E., Summers, B.C., et al., 2007. CXCR7 (RDC1) promotes breast and lung tumor growth in vivo and is expressed on tumor-associated vasculature. Proc. Natl. Acad. Sci. USA 104, 15735–15740.

Ödemis, V., Lipfert, J., Kraft, R., et al., 2012. The presumed atypical chemokine receptor CXCR7 signals through G(i/o) proteins in primary rodent astrocytes and human glioma cells. Glia 60, 372–381.

Orimo, A., Gupta, P.B., Sgroi, D.C., et al., 2005. Stromal fibroblasts present in invasive human breast carcinomas promote tumor growth and angiogenesis through elevated SDF-1/CXCL12 secretion. Cell 121, 335–348.

Preusser, M., Capper, D., Ilhan-Mutlu, A., et al., 2012. Brain metastases: pathobiology and emerging targeted therapies. Acta Neuropathol. 123, 205–222.

Rajagopal, S., Kim, J., Ahn, S., et al., 2010. Beta-arrestin- but not G protein-mediated signaling by the "decoy" receptor CXCR7. Proc. Natl. Acad. Sci. USA 107, 628–632.

Rempel, S.A., Dudas, S., Ge, S., Gutierrez, J.A., 2000. Identification and localization of the cytokine SDF1 and its receptor, CXC chemokine receptor 4, to regions of necrosis and angiogenesis in human glioblastoma. Clin. Cancer Res. 6, 102–111.

Roland, J., Murphy, B.J., Ahr, B., et al., 2003. Role of the intracellular domains of cxcr4 in sdf-1-mediated signaling. Blood 101, 399–406.

Salmaggi, A., Gelati, M., Pollo, B., et al., 2004. CXCL12 in malignant glial tumors: a possible role in angiogenesis and cross-talk between endothelial and tumoral cells. J. Neurooncol. 67, 305–317.

Salmaggi, A., Gelati, M., Pollo, B., et al., 2005. CXCL12 expression is predictive of a shorter time to tumor progression in low-grade glioma: a single-institution study in 50 patients. J. Neurooncol. 74, 287–293.

Salmaggi, A., Maderna, E., Calatozzolo, C., et al., 2009. CXCL12, CXCR4 and CXCR7 expression in brain metastases. Cancer Biol. Ther. 8, 1608–1614.

Sierro, F., Biben, C., Martínez-Muñoz, L., et al., 2007. Disrupted cardiac development but normal hematopoiesis in mice deficient in the second CXCL12/SDF-1 receptor, CXCR7. Proc. Natl. Acad. Sci. USA 104, 14759–14764.

Sun, X., Cheng, G., Hao, M., et al., 2010. CXCL12/CXCR4/CXCR7 chemokine axis and cancer progression. Cancer Metastasis Rev. 29, 709–722.

Sun, Y.X., Schneider, A., Jung, Y., et al., 2005. Skeletal localization and neutralization of the SDF-1(CXCL12)/CXCR4 axis blocks prostate cancer metastasis and growth in osseous sites in vivo. J. Bone Miner. Res. 20, 318–329.

Thelen, M., Stein, J.V., 2008. How chemokines invite leukocytes to dance. Nat. Immunol. 9, 953–959.

Wald, O., Izhar, U., Amir, G., et al., 2011. Interaction between neoplastic cells and cancer-associated fibroblasts through the CXCL12/CXCR4 axis: role in non-small cell lung cancer tumor proliferation. J. Thorac. Cardiovasc. Surg. 141, 1503–1512.

Wang, Z., Ma, Q., Liu, Q., et al., 2008. Blockade of SDF-1/CXCR4 signalling inhibits pancreatic cancer progression in vitro via inactivation of canonical Wnt pathway. Br. J. Cancer 99, 1695–1703.

Wendt, M.K., Cooper, A.N., Dwinell, M.B., 2008. Epigenetic silencing of CXCL12 increases the metastatic potential of mammary carcinoma cells. Oncogene 27, 1461–1471.

Yang, L., Jackson, E., Woerner, B.M., Perry, A., Piwnica-Worms, D., Rubin, J.B., 2007. Blocking CXCR4-mediated cyclic AMP suppression inhibits brain tumor growth in vivo. Cancer Res. 67, 651–658.

Zhu, B., Xu, D., Deng, X., et al., 2012. CXCL12 enhances human neural progenitor cell survival through a CXCR7- and CXCR4-mediated endocytotic signaling pathway. Stem Cells 30, 2571–2583.

CHAPTER

4

Non-Uniform Distribution of Metastatic Intracranial Tumors in Cancer Patients

Carlo C. Quattrocchi, Yuri Errante, Carlo Augusto Mallio and Bruno Beomonte Zobel

OUTLINE

Introduction 37
Epidemiology and Clinical Presentation of Brain Metastases 37
Intra-axial Metastases: Pathogenesis and Neuroimaging 38
Extra-axial Metastases: Pathogenesis and Neuroimaging 41
Pachymeningeal Metastases 41
Leptomeningeal Metastases 41

Brain Spatial Distribution of Metastases 43
Role of the Primary Tumor on the Distribution 45
Brain Local Vulnerability/Resistance to Metastases 46
Recurrent Metastases 46

Discussion 48

References 50

INTRODUCTION

Epidemiology and Clinical Presentation of Brain Metastases

Brain metastases (BMs) occur in 20–40% of adult cancer patients with an incidence of >170 000 new cases per year in the USA (Suh, 2010) and become symptomatic during life in 60–75% of the patients. Thus, they represent the most common tumors of the central nervous system (CNS).

Although the exact incidence is unknown because some brain metastatic patients are neurologically asymptomatic, the frequency of the diagnosis of BMs has increased in recent

M.A. Hayat (ed): *Brain Metastases from Primary Tumors, Volume 1*
DOI: http://dx.doi.org/10.1016/B978-0-12-800896-6.00004-8

© 2014 Elsevier Inc. All rights reserved.

years probably due to an increased sensitivity of imaging techniques (Qian et al., 2008), particularly when lesions are located in the posterior cranial fossa or they are very small. Other explanations may be the increase of the overall survival in oncologic patients due to the advent of more effective systemic treatments and an acquired resistance of metastatic tumor cells in the brain to escape the effects of those chemotherapeutic agents that, although partially, pass the blood–brain barrier.

The most common primary tumors responsible for BMs are lung cancer in men and breast cancer in women. Other primary tumors include melanoma, renal cell cancer, colon cancer, pelvic tumors and unknown primary tumors (Johnson and Young, 1996). In addition to the cerebral and cerebellar parenchyma, other sites of intracranial metastases include the meninges, the pituitary and pineal glands and the choroid plexus (Kishi et al., 1982).

Brain metastases are more often diagnosed in patients with known malignancy (metachronous presentation). Less frequently (up to 30%), brain metastases are diagnosed either at the time of the diagnosis of the primary tumor (synchronous presentation) or before the discovery of the primary tumor (precocious presentation). The primary site is unknown in up to 15% of patients. Neoplastic disease prognosis worsens tremendously when a patient receives the diagnosis of brain metastasis. Median survival of patients after the identification of symptomatic brain metastases is, in fact, generally short from about 4 months in breast cancer (Distefano et al., 1979) to 4–12 months in lung cancer (Lagerwaard et al., 1999) patients.

Intra-axial Metastases: Pathogenesis and Neuroimaging

Two main biological mechanisms have been considered to explain the occurrence of brain intra-axial metastases in the last 120 years: mechanical trapping of tumor emboli and the "seed and soil" hypothesis. The "seed and soil" hypothesis is the dominant current explanation of metastasis (Fidler et al., 2002). This hypothesis states that successful outgrowth of metastatic tumors depends on the cross-talk and permissible interactions between the tumor cells and the site-specific microenvironment in the host organs. Currently, this hypothesis is based on the principle that neoplasms are biologically heterogeneous and contain subpopulations of cells with different angiogenic, invasive, and metastatic properties. On this basis, the process of metastasis is selective for cells that succeed in promoting angiogenesis, invasion, embolization, survival in the circulation, arrest in distant capillary beds, extravasation and multiplication within the brain tissue. An emerging paradigm is that tumors are able to produce factors that induce the formation of pre-metastatic niches in organs where metastases will ultimately develop (Kaplan et al., 2005). The interaction with metastatic tumor cells in the brain is largely based on the neoplastic angiogenesis/vascular remodeling as in other organs and on three other unique properties that differentiate the brain from other organs.

1. Angiogenesis/vascular remodeling: the potent angiogenesis/permeability factor, vascular endothelial growth factor (VEGF) plays a crucial role in the development of pathological neovascularization and in the increase of microvessel density. Whether tumor-associated blood vessels are formed by new vessel formation or by co-option of existing highly dense vessels is not yet clear. In murine models, metastases did not show an increase of vessel density, but microvessel luminal dilation as a form of vascular remodeling in which the division of endothelial cells increases the surface and the size of the vessels (Fidler et al., 2002).

2. **2.** Blood–brain and blood–tumor barriers: the microvasculature of the brain parenchyma is lined with a continuous, non-fenestrated endothelium with tight junctions and little pinocytic vesicle activity. This structure, known as the blood–brain barrier (BBB), limits the entrance of circulating macromolecules into the brain parenchyma. Experiments on transgenic and knockout mice clearly demonstrated that the pericytes surrounding the brain blood vessels play an intimate role in the formation and maintenance of BBB integrity, challenging the conventional view that astroglial cells play the major role in regulating the BBB. Activation of adhesion molecules, such as tumor cell integrin aVb3, seems to control brain metastases through the regulation of VEGF expression (Lorger et al., 2009). Also, the role of the basement membrane proteins such as collagen, laminins and integrins have been demonstrated (Carbonell et al., 2009).
3. High energy consumption: the dense network of blood vessels in the brain provides it with an abundant supply of oxygen and nutrients. High-throughput proteomic analysis of experimental models of brain metastatic cells has shown profiles towards the elevated expression of proteins involved in promoting energy utilization. Moreover, microarray expression profiles on laser-captured tumor cells from surgically resected human breast cancer brain metastasis samples showed hexokinase 2 (HK2), (an enzyme that mediates the first step in glucose metabolism by phosphorylating glucose to produce glucose-6-phosphate), as a candidate gene upregulated in brain metastasis (Palmieri et al., 2009).
4. Immune-privileged site: despite the brain being considered an immune privileged sanctuary, glial cells play immune functions in the brain. Microglia are a specialized population of glial cells that are regarded as the resident macrophages in the brain. Like macrophages, under proper conditions, microglia are phagocytic, able to present antigens and seem constantly to remodel their processes in apparent attempts to survey the brain parenchymal environment (Davalos et al., 2005). Also astroglial cells may be involved in defense of the cellular infiltration. Immunohistochemistry studies have shown that both microglia and astrocytes are activated even at the early stages of the metastatic cascade in response to the arrival and migration of cancer cells in the brain, indicating that the surveillance system of glial cells is very sensitive in detecting metastatic tumor cells (Lorger and Felding-Habermann, 2010).

The most common primary sites of cancer for intra-axial metastases are lung cancer, breast cancer and melanoma. Other primary tumors include colon cancer, kidney cancer and pelvic malignancies.

In the current clinical setting, intra-axial metastases are identified by conventional magnetic resonance imaging (MRI) with a 3mm spatial resolution. Gadolinium-enhanced MRI is superior to contrast-enhanced computed tomography (CT) in the diagnosis of brain metastases, because of higher spatial resolution, higher contrast resolution, higher sensitivity with paramagnetic contrast agents, no bone artifacts in the images and less partial-volume artifacts for the detection of lesions adjacent to bones. In this context, contrast-enhanced MRI is known to be more sensitive than contrast-enhanced CT (including double-dose delayed contrast) or than unenhanced MRI in detecting brain metastases, particularly when located in the posterior fossa or very small (Schellinger et al., 1999). Double or triple doses of gadolinium-based contrast agents are, in this respect, better than single doses, but increasing the dose may lead to an increased number of false-positive findings (Sze et al., 1998).

On MRI T1-weighted images, lesions are isointense to mildly hypointense and are hyperintense on T2-weighted and fluid attenuation inversion recovery (FLAIR) images.

In cases of a mucinous content, the lesions may be hypointense on T2-weighted images. Hemorrhagic metastases are hyperintense on T1-weighted images and may also show hypointensity on turbo spin echo and gradient echo T2-weighted images, owing to the extravasation and/or deposition of blood products, respectively. Usually metastatic lesions show marked vasogenic edema and mass effect. Surrounding edema is hyperintense on FLAIR and relatively hypointense on T1-weighted images and is usually wide in comparison to the size of the lesion. Following administration of a gadolinium-based contrast agent, solid, nodular, or irregular ring patterns of enhancement are seen (Figure 4.1).

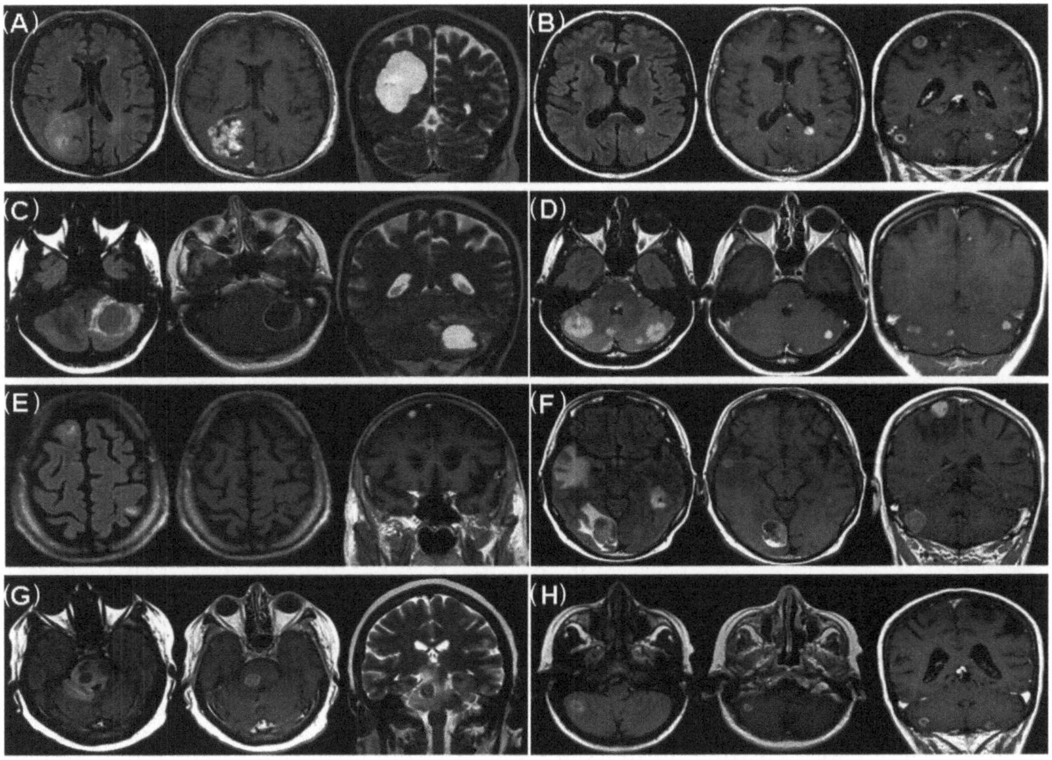

FIGURE 4.1 Intra-axial metastases. (A and B): Patients with lung cancer. (A) A 60-year-old woman with a right occipital solitary metastasis from a bronchiolo-alveolar lung carcinoma; (B) a 64-year-old man with multiple brain metastases from a lung adenocarcinoma. (C and D): Patients with breast cancer. (C) A 51-year-old woman with a left cerebellar metastasis from a ductal infiltrating carcinoma; (D) a 43-year-old woman with multiple metastases from an infiltrating ductal carcinoma. (E and F): Patients with melanoma. (E) A 77-year-old man with multiple low-melanin metastases; (F) a 58-year-old man with multiple high-melanin metastases (compare middle panels: hyperintense lesions with melanin expression are detected on unenhanced T1-weighted images in F as compared to E). (G and H): Patients with colon cancer. (G) A 52-year-old woman with a right pontine solitary metastasis; (H) a 58-year-old man with multiple cerebellar metastases. In A, C and G: left panel = axial FLAIR; middle panel = gadolinium-enhanced axial T1-weighted image; right panel = coronal T2-weighted image. In B, D and H: left panel = axial FLAIR; middle panel = gadolinium-enhanced axial T1-weighted image; right panel = gadolinium-enhanced coronal T1-weighted image. In E and F: left panel = axial FLAIR; middle panel = unenhanced axial T1-weighted image; right panel = gadolinium-enhanced coronal T1-weighted image.

Extra-axial Metastases: Pathogenesis and Neuroimaging

Extra-axial metastases include lesions that directly do not involve the brain parenchyma; thus, lesions may be located in the skull, in the pachymeningeal (dural) and in the leptomeningeal compartments. Here, we discuss the lesions that primarily develop in the meningeal compartments.

Pachymeningeal Metastases

Dural metastases may occupy the epidural space, usually by direct extension from skull metastases, or the subdural space either by direct extension from an epidural metastasis or by hematogenous spread. Dural metastases occur in up to 9–10% of all patients with cancer, as based on autopsy reports, and represent the only site of intracranial metastases in about 4% of cases (Nayak et al., 2009). The most common primary sites of cancer are the breast, prostate, lung (small cell and non-small cell), head and neck and hematologic malignancies such as lymphoma and leukemia. Other tumor types include renal cell cancer, neuroblastoma, thyroid cancer, thymic cancer, leiomyosarcoma, carcinoid, melanoma, squamous cell cancer of skin, and adenocarcinoma of unknown primary origin. The most common locations are parietal and frontal whereas the infratentorial location is most commonly affected through perineural dissemination from head and neck tumors with intracranial extension. When large in size, lesions may cause vasogenic intra-axial edema and, at times, may invade the intra-axial structures. If lesions are located proximal to dural venous sinuses, patients may experience symptoms from occlusion of the sinuses or from compression of cranial nerves, such as III, IV and VI in the cavernous sinus.

Patients usually complain of headache and/or cranial neuropathy at onset, followed by visual changes, alterations in mental status, and seizures. About one-tenth of patients are asymptomatic and are diagnosed incidentally by neuroimaging. At the first diagnosis, patients have progressive and systemic neoplastic disease with bone, lymph nodes, liver and lungs as the most commonly involved sites. The median survival of patients with dural metastases is about 10 months, which is favorable compared to the 4–6 months of patients with intra-axial metastases and to the 2 months of those with leptomeningeal metastases.

Gadolinium-enhanced brain MRI is the study of choice for the diagnosis of dural metastases, especially using 3D high resolution T1-weighted imaging with isotropic voxels. The lesions may appear as focal meningeal plaques with or without an enhancing dural tail or as lenticular nodules (Figure 4.2). The lesions may be single or multiple, sometimes appearing as diffuse dural thickening with nodular areas. Sometimes, in women with breast cancer, it is a true diagnostic challenge to establish the differential diagnosis between a dural metastasis and a meningioma (Wilms et al., 1991). Diffuse dural enhancement may also be challenging: differentials include a reactive response following a lumbar puncture, a reactive response to skull metastases, infectious or inflammatory etiologies and idiopathic pachymeningeal thickening.

Leptomeningeal Metastases

Leptomeningeal metastases are the result of the seeding of tumor cells to the leptomeninges (the pia and the arachnoid) via the cerebrospinal fluid, represent the third most common metastatic complication of the central nervous system and are increasingly common as

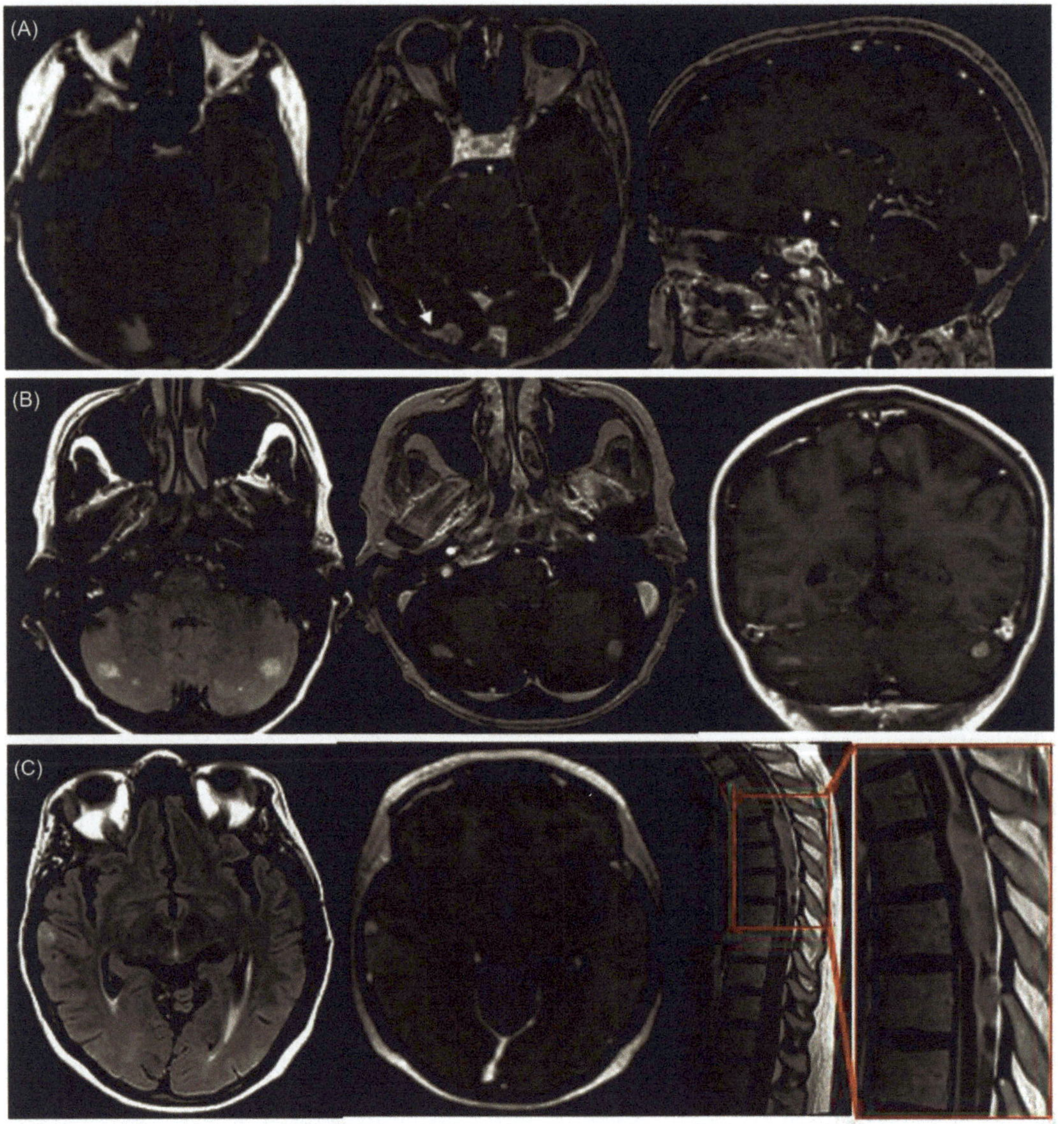

FIGURE 4.2 Extra-axial metastases. (A) A 62-year-old woman with lung cancer, extra-axial enhancing nodule with dural tail enhancement (arrow in the middle panel) is indicative of pachymeningeal infiltration. Left panel = axial FLAIR; middle panel = gadolinium-enhanced axial T1-weighted image; right panel = gadolinium-enhanced sagittal T1-weighted image. (B) Leptomeningeal metastases in a 65-year-old woman with lung cancer. Left panel = axial FLAIR; middle panel = gadolinium-enhanced axial T1-weighted image; right panel = gadolinium-enhanced coronal T1-weighted image. (C) Leptomeningeal metastases in a 53-year-old woman with melanoma. Left panel = axial FLAIR; middle panel = gadolinium-enhanced axial T1-weighted image; right panel = gadolinium-enhanced sagittal T1-weighted image of the spine, indicative of extra-axial seeding.

cancer patients live longer. Leptomeningeal metastases are found in 1–5% of patients with solid tumors (carcinomatous meningitis), 5–15% of patients with leukemia (leukemic meningitis) and lymphoma (lymphomatous meningitis), and 1–2% of patients with primary brain tumors (Chamberlain, 2010).

Autopsy studies revealed that 19% of patients with cancer and neurologic signs and symptoms have evidence of leptomeningeal involvement. Breast, lung, and melanoma are the most common primary tumors to metastasize to the leptomeninges. Similarly to dural metastases, leptomeningeal metastases most often present in patients with disseminated and progressive systemic neoplastic disease (>70%), but can present after a disease-free interval (20%) and even be the first manifestation of cancer (5–10%). Leptomeninges may be reached by cancer cells through: (1) hematogenous spread; (2) direct extension from contiguous tumor; or (3) centripetal migration along perineural or perivascular spaces (Gleissner and Chamberlain, 2006). Once cancer cells have entered the subarachnoid space, they are passively transported by the CSF bulk flow resulting in the often observed multifocal seeding (see Figure 4.2). The most common sites are the base of the brain, the dorsal surface of the spinal cord, and the cauda equina (Gleissner and Chamberlain, 2006). Hydrocephalus may occur at any level of the neuraxis and is due to obstruction of the CSF outflow, either dependent on compression or on traction of the ventricular foramina/sylvian aqueduct. Clinical manifestations depend on the involvement of the cerebral hemispheres, the cranial nerves, and the spinal cord and roots. Signs on examination generally exceed symptoms reported by the patient.

The most useful laboratory test in the diagnosis of leptomeningeal metastasis is the lumbar puncture. The presence of malignant cells in the CSF is diagnostic of leptomeningeal metastasis but the diagnosis of primary tumor, especially if it is occult, is often not possible.

Magnetic resonance imaging with gadolinium enhancement is the technique of choice to evaluate patients with suspected leptomeningeal metastasis. Because leptomeningeal metastasis involves the entire neuraxis, imaging of the entire CNS is required. FLAIR images may show inhomogeneous CSF signal saturation that leads to the suspicion of CSF bulk flow alterations in the subarachnoid spaces. Cranial nerve enhancement and subarachnoid enhancing nodules can be considered diagnostic of leptomeningeal metastasis in patients with cancer (Figure 4.3). Nonetheless, gadolinium-enhanced imaging has a more than 30% incidence of false-negative results so that a normal study does not exclude the diagnosis of leptomeningeal metastases. Due to the dural–arachnoid enhancement that may be observed after lumbar puncture, imaging should be obtained prior to the procedure.

BRAIN SPATIAL DISTRIBUTION OF METASTASES

A preferential distribution of extra-axial metastases has not been described, except the caudal location in the dural sac of the lesions that are defined as "drop" metastases, thus reflecting a gravity/CSF flow-dependent mechanism. The spatial distribution of intra-axial BMs has been studied in several series, leading to the concept of a non-random distribution in the brain. In a CT retrospective study, using standard sheets as anatomical reference, Delattre et al. found solitary metastases in the posterior fossa in 50% of patients with pelvic or gastrointestinal tumors and only in 10% of patients with other primary tumors

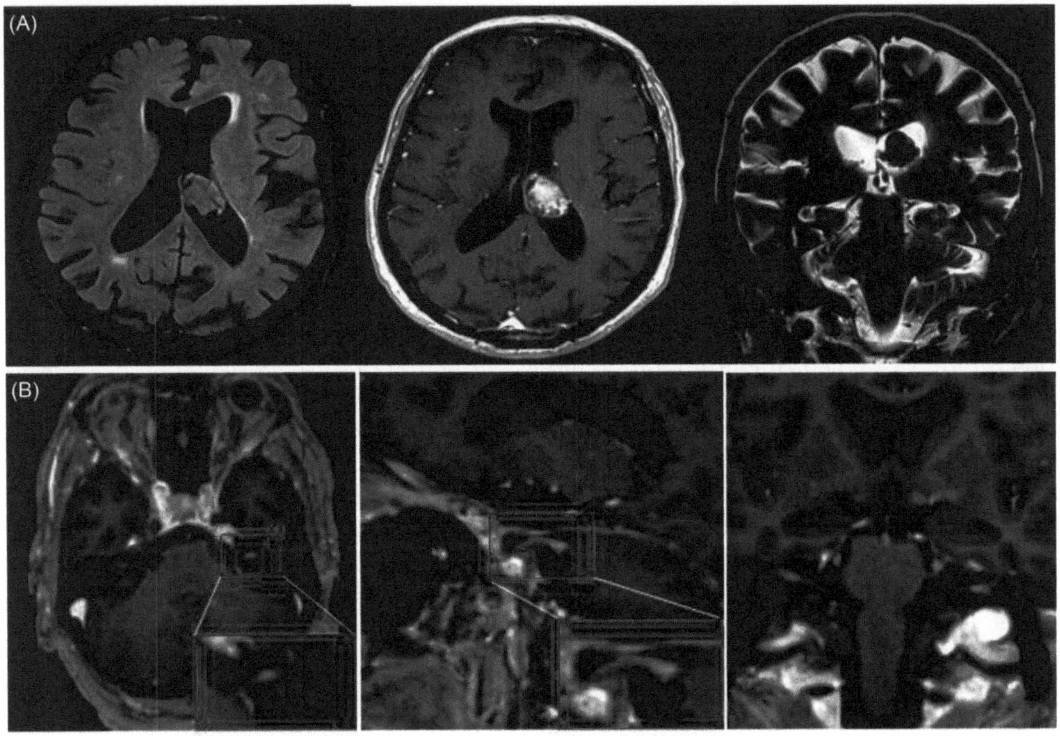

FIGURE 4.3 Other intracranial sites of metastasis. (A) An 81-year-old man with colon cancer and a left choroid plexus metastasis. Left panel = axial FLAIR; middle panel = gadolinium-enhanced axial T1-weighted image; right panel = coronal T2-weighted image. (B) A 62-year-old woman with breast cancer and multiple cranial nerve metastases. Left panel = gadolinium-enhanced axial T1-weighted image demonstrating enhancement of the VII–VIII cranial nerves (left bottom inlet); middle panel = gadolinium-enhanced sagittal T1-weighted image demonstrating enhancement of the right V cranial nerve (left bottom inlet); right panel = gadolinium-enhanced coronal T1-weighted image.

(Delattre et al., 1988). Hwang et al. (1996), using both CT and MRI scans and predetermined standard sheets as anatomical reference, highlighted the predominant involvement of the arterial border zones, demonstrating a preferential occurrence of lesions in anterior border zones, rather than posterior and cerebellar border zones.

Autopsy studies have shown that breast cancer metastases are more frequent in the cerebellum and in the basal ganglia and that non-small cell lung cancer metastases are preferentially distributed in the occipital lobe and in the cerebellum (Graf et al., 1988). Other more recent studies reported, for lung and breast cancer, that there is a higher probability of cerebellar metastases than what would be predicted based solely on brain volume (Bender and Tomé, 2011) and, for breast cancer, high frequency of lesions in the cerebellum (Hengel et al., 2012).

Using a voxel-based approach, we recently reported that the cerebellum is predominantly involved in breast cancer patients and that the occipital lobes and the cerebellum are the most frequent sites of BMs in lung cancer patients (Figure 4.4) (Quattrocchi et al., 2012).

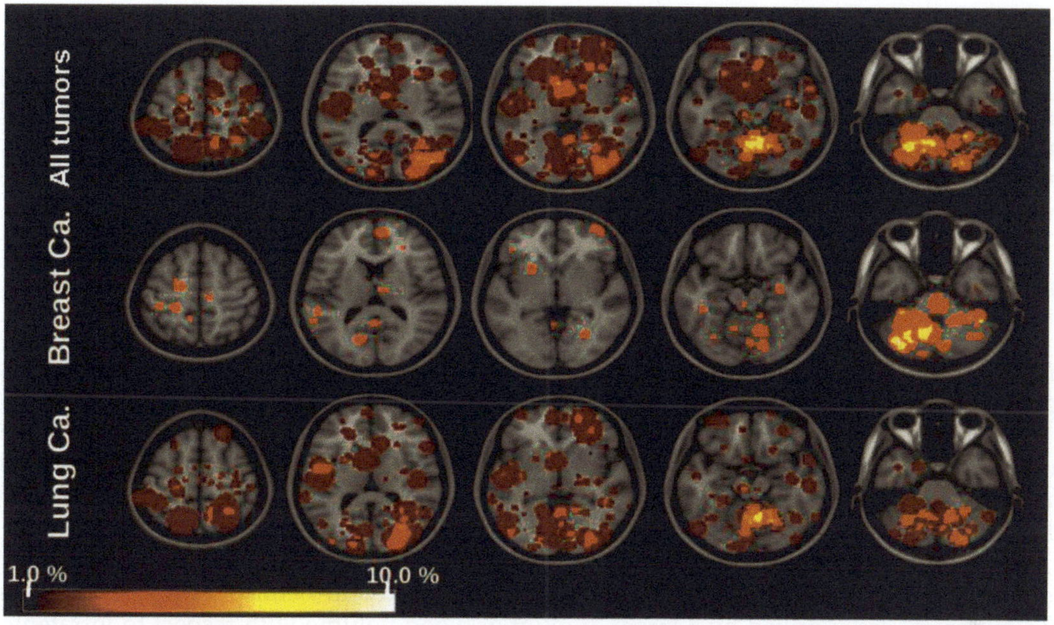

FIGURE 4.4 Brain spatial distribution of intra-axial metastases. Mean lesion frequency maps of intra-axial metastases in a group of 811 lesions from all primary tumors, of 136 lesions from breast cancer and of 611 lesions from non-small cell lung cancer patients. The color bar represents the lesion frequency; voxels with a lesion frequency <1% are not shown.

Role of the Primary Tumor on the Distribution

The risk of developing brain metastases has been extensively estimated on the basis of intrinsic clinicopathological properties of the primary tumor. However, brain vulnerability has not been deeply investigated, especially in the clinical context. Particularly, clinicopathological nomograms have been developed to predict the occurrence of brain metastases.

For breast cancer, younger age, stage at the initial diagnosis, higher grade, negative status of estrogen receptor, overexpression of human epidermal growth factor receptor 2, extracerebral metastatic sites and short disease-free survival (Graesslin et al., 2010) as well as BRCA1 mutations have been associated with a higher incidence of brain metastases, but not with a differential distribution in the brain. During treatment of systemic disease from breast cancer, protocols including trastuzumab in HER-2 expressing breast cancer have been associated with longer times to brain metastases than those not treated with trastuzumab and triple negative breast cancer (Ahn et al., 2013).

For lung cancer, primary tumor size, cell type (non-squamous cell) and lymph node staging and ratio (metastatic lymph nodes/examined lymph nodes) have been associated with a higher probability of incurring brain metastasis (Mujoomdar et al., 2007).

In colon cancer patients, although the prevalence is rare, primary tumor in the left colon, long-standing pulmonary metastases, especially those with recent progression, and CXCR4 expression by tumor cells have been associated with an increased risk of brain metastases (Mongan et al., 2009).

In patients with melanoma, elevated staging and lactic acid dehydrogenase at diagnosis of unresectable stage III/IV disease independently predict the risk of developing CNS metastasis from the time of diagnosis. The location, especially if unknown, and pathological Clark level of the primary melanoma can independently predict CNS metastasis-free interval from the time of diagnosis of the primary tumor (Bedikian et al., 2011).

Brain Local Vulnerability/Resistance to Metastases

Despite the risk of developing brain metastases being extensively estimated on the basis of intrinsic clinicopathological properties of the primary tumor, much less effort has been spent on the study of brain vulnerability, especially in the clinical context.

From the clinical point of view, a large portion of patients with breast cancer, lung cancer and melanoma do not develop brain metastases over the course of their disease, suggesting that the brain local microenvironment may play a crucial role and limit or stop the attempt of cancer cells to invade the brain and develop macroscopic metastases.

Among the factors that affect intracranial location of brain metastases, tissue and blood volume are crucial factors. The supratentorial areas (cerebral hemispheres, diencephalon and midbrain) are supplied by a larger amount of blood volume with respect to infratentorial structures (cerebellum, pons and medulla). Thus, in a randomly expected distribution, brain metastases should more often be located in the supratentorial areas. Most brain metastases are found at the gray–white junction of the brain parenchyma. This is the area where the caliber of blood vessels changes suddenly with consequent trapping of tumor emboli. Eighty percent of brain metastases occur in the arterial border zones of the cerebral hemispheres (Hwang et al., 1996) whereas only 1% of the metastases are reported to occur in the posterior circulation and in the cerebellum and only 3% of the metastases involve the brainstem. To date, only the grade of small vessel ischemic disease of the brain has been demonstrated to be a protective factor against the development of brain metastases (Mazzone et al., 2009), especially in lung cancer patients (Quattrocchi et al., 2013).

Recurrent Metastases

The current therapeutic strategy for brain metastases includes surgery and/or radiation therapy. Stereotactic radiosurgery is used for solitary intra-axial metastases and, in some centers, for oligometastatic patients (to a maximum of three to four lesions). Whole brain radiation therapy (WBRT) is used with a prophylactic purpose in small cell lung cancer patients, considered at high risk to develop brain metastases and has been also proposed in non-small cell lung cancer patients. In non-oligometastatic patients (i.e. more than three or four lesions, depending on the study group), WBRT is considered to be an effective technique also because systemic therapies partially or inadequately penetrate the blood–brain barrier.

Recurrence after surgical resection may be observed as a regrowth at the same site or as extra-axial lesions originating from seeding of cells in the meningeal compartments (Figure 4.5).

Following radiosurgery, the regrowth of the lesion is rare at the site of treatment, due to the clinical target volumes being larger than the contrast-enhancing lesions.

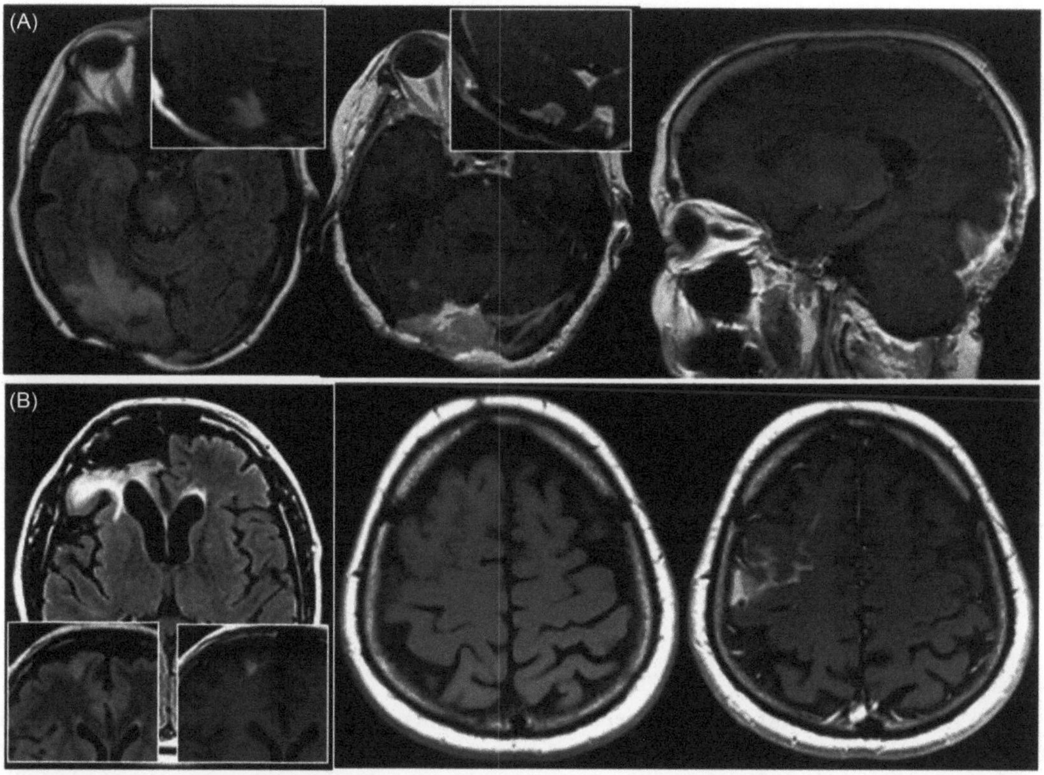

FIGURE 4.5 Post-surgery recurrent extra-axial metastases. (A) A 62-year-old woman with lung cancer; recurrent extra-axial enhancing solid tissue 3 months after surgery (same patient as in Figure 4.2A). Left panel = axial FLAIR (pre-surgery FLAIR in the right upper inlet); middle panel = gadolinium-enhanced axial T1-weighted image (pre-surgery enhanced T1-weighted image in the right upper inlet); right panel = gadolinium-enhanced sagittal T1-weighted image. (B) A 60-year-old man with lung cancer; recurrent extra-axial enhancement 6 months after surgery. Left panel = axial FLAIR (pre-surgery FLAIR and gadolinium-enhanced axial T1-weighted image in the left and right bottom inlets); middle panel = gadolinium-unenhanced axial T1-weighted image; right panel = gadolinium-enhanced axial T1-weighted image confirms extra-axial seeding.

As regards WBRT, radiation commonly decreases growth rates of the existing lesions in non-oligometastatic patients. In high-risk cancer patients, although prophylactic treatments are known to decrease the risk of brain metastases, the long-term effects on the distribution of new intra-axial lesions are not known.

One of the most common complications of WBRT is the neurocognitive toxicity. This phenomenon is usually classified as early-onset or late-onset toxicity. Early neurocognitive toxicity involves verbal and short-term memory disturbances and is reported to occur within the first 4 months. Late neurocognitive toxicity is typically characterized by the onset of severe dementia and cerebellar involvement even years after WBRT. Hippocampal radiation-induced damage has been associated with neurocognitive decline. In order to reduce the neurocognitive toxicity, a radiotherapy approach which spares the hippocampus and the peri-hippocampal region (hippocampus + 5 mm margin), has been proposed and discussed due to the potential risk of disease progression in these regions. Regarding this issue, several studies have been performed to quantify the exact incidence of metastases within the hippocampal tissues. Marsh et al. found that only 16/697 metastases (2.29%) involved the hippocampus; however, in this study the incidence of hippocampal metastases in oligometastatic patients (those with one to three metastases) was 0.97% (1/103) (Marsh et al., 2010). Gondi et al. identified metastases within 5 mm of the hippocampus in 8.6% of patients and in 3% of brain metastases; however, none of the metastases were located within the hippocampus (Gondi et al., 2010). Wan and colleagues (Wan et al., 2013) recently reported 7/2270 metastases (0.3%) to be located within the hippocampus albeit only 1/7 (14.3%) was found in oligometastatic patients (those with one to four lesions) while 6/7 (85.7%) were identified in non-oligometastatic patients.

Nevertheless, there are insufficient data to understand whether there is a specific tropism for certain tumor histotypes to metastasize within the hippocampus. Furthermore, the problem of cognitive decline has not been fully investigated and appears to be a multifactorial problem. In these patients, it is still not clear to what extent the cognitive decline is affected by comorbidities such as primary or secondary neurodegenerative diseases, the brain metastatic load, the radiation-induced damage and the neurotoxicity resulting from systemic therapies.

DISCUSSION

Brain metastases (BMs) are the most common tumors of the central nervous system. The multistep metastatic process includes primary tumor cell embolization, survival of cancer circulating cells, endothelial invasion, extravasation, angiogenesis, resistance to the glial immune surveillance and proliferation within the brain parenchyma.

The risk of developing BMs has been extensively estimated on the basis of clinicopathological properties of the primary tumor. An emerging paradigm is that tumors are able to produce factors that induce the formation of the so-called pre-metastatic niches in organs where metastases will ultimately develop. These pre-metastatic niches are thought to provide an appropriate environment for the development of secondary tumors. The notion that tumors can have remote effects on the microenvironment of organs in which metastases will form has the potential to revolutionize our understanding about how the microenvironment of a particular organ regulates metastasis formation, and why particular patterns of metastasis occur for certain tumors. Although the risk of developing BMs may be estimated on demographic and primary tumor features, the BMs-free survival time and the metastatic lesion load at first diagnosis are not confidently predictable.

There is evidence of a preferential distribution of BMs in patients with breast cancer and lung cancer, confirmed by means of both autopsy and MRI studies. In fact, autoptic studies have shown that breast cancer metastases are more frequent in the cerebellum and in the basal ganglia and that non-small cell lung cancer metastases are preferentially distributed in the occipital lobe and in the cerebellum (Graf et al., 1988; Hengel et al., 2012; Quattrocchi et al., 2012). Other more recent studies reported, for lung and breast cancer, that there is a higher probability of cerebellar metastases than what would be predicted based solely on brain volume (Bender and Tomé, 2011; Quattrocchi et al., 2012).

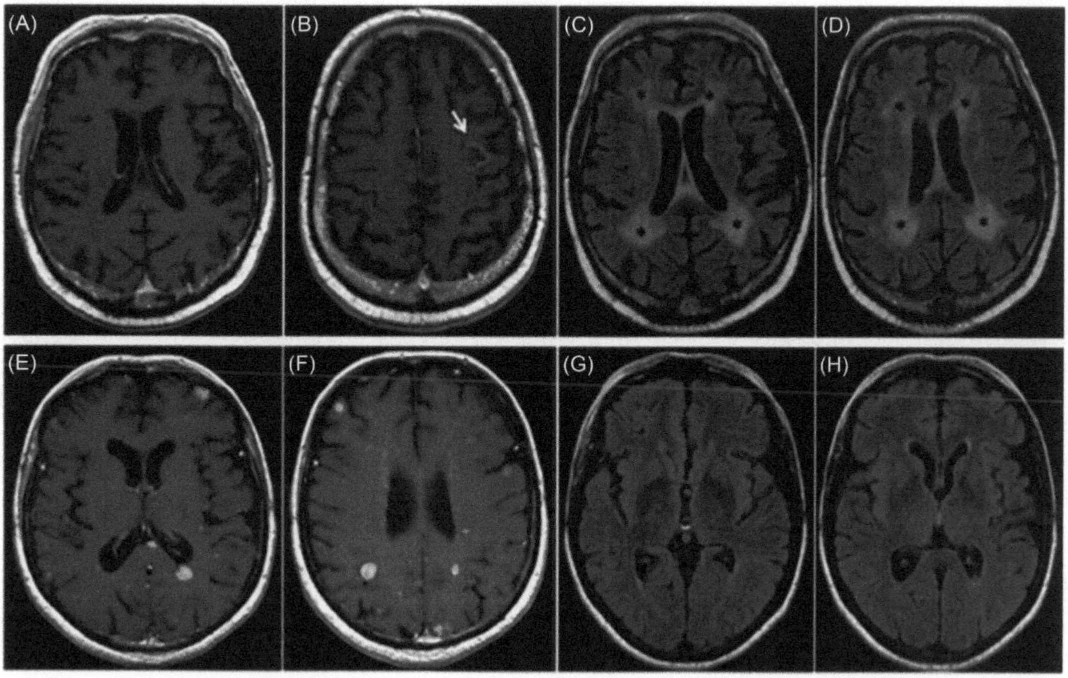

FIGURE 4.6 Inverse comorbidity between small vessel ischemic disease and brain metastatic load. (A–D) A 72-year-old man with lung adenocarcinoma shows a left frontal solitary metastasis (white arrow in B) on contrast-enhanced T1-weighted images (A and B) and a diffuse pattern of hyperintense bilateral lesions on FLAIR images (black asterisks in C and D). (E–H) Conversely, a 64-year-old woman with lung adenocarcinoma shows multiple metastases bilaterally on contrast-enhanced T1-weighted images (E and F) and absence of hyperintense lesions on FLAIR images (G and H).

The non-uniform distribution of brain metastases suggests the existence of mechanisms of brain-specific vulnerability to metastasis. One of the mechanisms could be related to different regional blood perfusion volumes and times between the posterior and the anterior circulation and/or to different regional vasomotor responses to tumor-induced vasoconstriction and vasodilation.

Brain vulnerability to BMs is a feature that is somehow linked with the concept of the pre-metastatic niches. As it is for vulnerability, brain-specific resistance to metastases should be considered. Small vessel ischemic disease (SVID) has been shown to be protective against the development of BMs in lung cancer patients (Mazzone et al., 2009; Quattrocchi et al., 2013) (Figure 4.6). Brain white matter lesions due to SVID are a frequent MRI finding in adults, both in asymptomatic and in cancer patients. These lesions are the common consequence of chronic ischemic events related to hypertension, arteriolosclerosis, small vessel spasms, cardioemboli, arterial wall thickening and may remain asymptomatic during the entire life span.

Several pathologic studies have shown that the histological correlate of SVID is a combination of reactive gliosis with a local increase of astrocytic and microglial cells, oligodendroglial loss and axonal loss, lipohyalinosis, arteriolosclerosis, vessel wall leakage and collagen deposition in venular walls.

As regards vascularization and perfusion, evidence exists on lower vessel density and on lower cerebral blood volume at the level of SVID compared to the healthy white matter.

The blood–brain barrier (BBB) is well established as the filter that limits the entrance of circulating macromolecules into the brain parenchyma. Its barrier role is not only passive due to the structural properties of the endothelial tight junctions but also active because of the presence of astroglial cells and pericytes that, surrounding the brain blood vessels, form and maintain the BBB integrity. Moreover, the role of the basement membrane composed of a balance of extracellular scaffold proteins such as collagen, laminins and integrins has been demonstrated. Changes of the basement membrane and of the interstitial extracellular space have a crucial protective role and make difficult for metastatic cell clones to invade and to proliferate within the brain parenchyma. Indeed, the known low vessel density in areas of SVID determines a local reduction of cerebral blood volume. These phenomena may generate a hostile microenvironment to BMs. Moreover, the tissue enrichment of glial cells at sites of SVID may determine a site-specific rise of immune surveillance, because of the local increase of antigen presenting cells such as astrocytes and microglial cells.

Finally, the mechanisms of brain vulnerability and resistance to metastases have been poorly explored; there is need for further studies on this subject as cancer patients live longer and challenge neuro-oncologists, neuroradiologists, radiation therapists and neurosurgeons for effective therapeutic approaches.

References

Ahn, H.K., Park, Y.H., Lee, S.J., et al., 2013. Clinical implication of Time To Brain Metastasis (TTBM) according to breast cancer subtypes. Springerplus 2, 136.

Bedikian, A.Y., Wei, C., Detry, M., et al., 2011. Predictive factors for the development of brain metastasis in advanced unresectable metastatic melanoma. Am. J. Clin. Oncol. 34, 603–610.

Bender, E.T., Tomé, W.A., 2011. Distribution of brain metastases: implications for non-uniform dose prescriptions. Br. J. Radiol. 84, 649–658.

Carbonell, W.S., Ansorge, O., Sibson, N., Muschel, R., 2009. The vascular basement membrane as "soil" in brain metastasis. PloSOne 4, e5857.

Chamberlain, M.C., 2010. Leptomeningeal metastasis. Curr. Opin. Oncol. 22, 627–635.

Davalos, D., Grutzendler, J., Yang, G., et al., 2005. ATP mediates rapid microglial response to local brain injury *in vivo*. Nat. Neurosci. 8, 752–758.

Delattre, J.Y., Krol, G., Thaler, H.T., et al., 1988. Distribution of brain metastases. Arch. Neurol. 45, 741–744.

Distefano, A., Yap, H.Y., Hortobagyi, G.N., Blumenschein, G.R., 1979. The natural history of breast cancer patients with brain metastases. Cancer 44, 1913–1918.

Fidler, I.J., Yano, S., Zhang, R.D., Fujimaki, T., Bucana, C.D., 2002. The seed and soil hypothesis: vascularisation and brain metastases. Lancet Oncol. 3, 53–57.

Gleissner, B., Chamberlain, M.C., 2006. Neoplastic meningitis. Lancet Neurol. 5, 443–452.

Gondi, V., Tome, W.A., Marsh, J., et al., 2010. Estimated risk of perihippocampal disease progression after hippocampal avoidance during whole-brain radiotherapy: safety profile for RTOG 0933. Radiother. Oncol. 95, 327–331.

Graesslin, O., Abdulkarim, B.S., Coutant, C., et al., 2010. Nomogram to predict subsequent brain metastasis in patients with metastatic breast cancer. J. Clin. Oncol. 28, 2032–2037.

Graf, A.H., Buchberger, W., Langmayr, H., et al., 1988. Site preference of metastatic tumors of the brain. Virchows Arch. A Pathol. Anat. Histopathol. 412, 493–498.

Hengel, K., Sidhu, G., Choi, J., et al., 2012. Attributes of brain metastases from breast and lung cancer. Int. J. Clin. Oncol. [Epub ahead of print].

Hwang, T.L., Close, T.P., Grego, J.M., et al., 1996. Predilection of brain metastases in grey and white matter junction and vascular border zones. Cancer 77, 1551–1555.

Johnson, J.D., Young, B., 1996. Demographic of brain metastasis. Neurosurg. Clin. N. Am. 7, 337–344.

Kaplan, R.N., Riba, R.D., Zacharoulis, S., et al., 2005. VEGFR1-positive haematopoietic bone marrow progenitors initiate the pre-metastatic niche. Nature 438, 820–827.

Kishi, K., Nomura, K., Mihi, Y., et al., 1982. Metastatic brain tumor: A clinical and pathological analysis of 101 cases with biopsy. Arch. Pathol. Lab. Med. 106, 133–135.

Lagerwaard, F.J., Levendaq, P.Q., Nowak, P.J., et al., 1999. Identification of prognostic factors in patients with brain metastases: a review of 1292 patients. Int. J. Radiat. Oncol. Biol. Phys. 43, 795–803.

Lorger, M., Felding-Habermann, B., 2010. Capturing changes in the brain microenvironment during initial steps of breast cancer brain metastasis. Am. J. Pathol. 176, 2958–2971.

Lorger, M., Krueger, J.S., O'Neal, M., Staflin, K., Felding-Habermann, B., 2009. Activation of tumor cell integrin alphavbeta3 controls angiogenesis and metastatic growth in the brain. Proc. Natl. Acad. Sci. USA 106, 10666–10671.

Marsh, J.C., Herskovic, A.M., Gielda, B.T., et al., 2010. Intracranial metastatic disease spares the limbic circuit: a review of 697 metastatic lesions in 107 patients. Int. J. Radiat. Oncol. Biol. Phys. 76, 504–512.

Mazzone, P.J., Marchi, N., Fazio, V., et al., 2009. Small vessel ischemic disease of the brain and brain metastases in lung cancer patients. PloSOne 4, e7242.

Mongan, J.P., Fadul, C.E., Cole, B.F., et al., 2009. Brain metastases from colorectal cancer: risk factors, incidence, and the possible role of chemokines. Clin. Colorectal Cancer 8, 100–105.

Mujoomdar, A., Austin, J.H., Malhotra, R., et al., 2007. Clinical predictors of metastatic disease to the brain from non-small cell lung carcinoma: primary tumor size, cell type, and lymph node metastases. Radiology 242, 882–888.

Nayak, L., Abrey, L.E., Iwamoto, F.M., 2009. Intracranial dural metastases. Cancer 115, 1947–1953.

Palmieri, D., Fitzgerald, D., Shreeve, S.M., et al., 2009. Analyses of resected human brain metastases of breast cancer reveal the association between up-regulation of hexokinase 2 and poor prognosis. Mol. Cancer Res. 7, 1438–1445.

Qian, Y.-F., Yu, C.-L., Zhang, C., et al., 2008. MR T1-weighted inversion recovery imaging in detecting brain metastases: could it replace T1-weighted spin-echo imaging? Am. J. Neuroradiol. 29, 701–704.

Quattrocchi, C.C., Errante, Y., Gaudino, C., et al., 2012. Spatial brain distribution of intra-axial metastatic lesions in breast and lung cancer patients. J. Neurooncol. 110, 79–87.

Quattrocchi, C.C., Errante, Y., Mallio, C.A., Santini, D., Tonini, G., Zobel, B.B., 2013. Brain metastatic volume and white matter lesions in advanced cancer patients. J. Neurooncol. [Epub ahead of print].

Schellinger, P.D., Meinck, H.M., Thron, A., 1999. Diagnostic accuracy of MRI compared to CCT in patients with brain metastases. J. Neurooncol. 44, 275–281.

Suh, J.H., 2010. Stereotactic radiosurgery for the management of brain metastases. N. Engl. J. Med. 362, 1119–1127.

Sze, G., Johnson, C., Kawamura, Y., et al., 1998. Comparison of single- and triple-dose contrast material in the MR screening of brain metastases. Am. J. Neuroradiol. 19, 821–828.

Wan, J.F., Zhang, S.J., Wang, L., Zhao, K.L., 2013. Implications for preserving neural stem cells in whole brain radiotherapy and prophylactic cranial irradiation: a review of 2270 metastases in 488 patients. J. Radiat. Res. 54, 285–291.

Wilms, G., Lammens, M., Marchal, G., et al., 1991. Prominent dural enhancement adjacent to nonmeningiomatous malignant lesions on contrast-enhanced MR images. Am. J. Neuroradiol. 12, 761–764.

CHAPTER

5

Targeting Angiogenesis, Enhancing Radiosensitization and Crossing the Blood–Brain Barrier for Brain Metastases

Emmanouil Fokas

OUTLINE

Introduction	53
Targeting Angiogenesis for Brain Metastases	54
Sensitizing Brain Metastases to Radiation	55
Crossing the Blood–Brain Barrier	56
Conclusion	58
References	58

INTRODUCTION

Brain metastases (BM) constitute a significant disease burden and have a major impact on patient morbidity and mortality (Walker et al., 1985). Recent progress in the preclinical and clinical development of molecular targeted drugs has revealed that some of them have potent therapeutic efficacy for BM. Here the preclinical and clinical knowledge on the role of targeting angiogenesis in BM is discussed. In addition, the potential of sensitizing BM to radiation and increasing blood–brain barrier penetrability to improve the outcome of this devastating disease is examined.

M.A. Hayat (ed): *Brain Metastases from Primary Tumors, Volume 1*
DOI: http://dx.doi.org/10.1016/B978-0-12-800896-6.00005-X

© 2014 Elsevier Inc. All rights reserved.

TARGETING ANGIOGENESIS FOR BRAIN METASTASES

Angiogenesis is essential for the development and survival of cancer. The formation of new blood vessels plays an important role in tumor progression, metastasis and resistance to chemoradiation (Kerbel, 2008). Since the pioneering work of Folkman (1971), there has been intense research into the development of anti-angiogenic cancer therapies in primary tumors and a large number of angiogenesis inhibitors are currently in clinical development.

The impact of targeting angiogenesis in BM is less well studied and conflicting findings have been reported. Kim et al. (2004) showed that vascular endothelial growth factor (VEGF) promoted the growth of breast cancer BM in nude mice. Targeting the VEGF receptor with the tyrosine kinase inhibitor PTK787/Z222584 led to a significant decrease in BM growth and vascular density (Kim et al., 2004). Transfection of colon and lung adenocarcinoma cells with the antisense-VEGF165 gene significantly reduced the incidence of BM after intracarotid injection (Yano et al., 2000). Overexpression of VEGF165 induced significant progression of melanoma BM that was associated with brain vessel co-option rather than sprouting angiogenesis, highlighting VEGF as an important therapeutic target for the treatment of BM (Yano et al., 2000). Carbonell et al. (2009) used different human and murine tumor cells lines to study BM in SCID, syngeneic BALB/c and syngeneic C3H/He mice. They showed that 95% of early micrometastases demonstrated vascular co-option with little evidence for isolated neurotropic growth. The vascular basement membrane promoted adhesion and invasion of malignant cells and was sufficient for tumor growth prior to any evidence of angiogenesis. Blockade of β1 integrin in tumor cells prevented adhesion to vascular basement membrane and decreased BM development and growth. Hence, β1 integrin could be a useful therapeutic strategy for BM (Carbonell et al., 2009). In an elegant study using a mouse model with a cranial window, Kienast et al. (2010) showed that tumor cells, upon extravasation, closely correlated with microvessels, either by direct angiogenesis (lung cancer) or vessel co-option (melanoma). Blockade of VEGF-A by bevacizumab inhibited angiogenesis and resulted in prolonged dormancy of lung cancer but not melanoma (Kienast et al., 2010). In contrast, targeting VEGFR-2 by ZD6474 inhibited angiogenesis but resulted in sustained BM progression via brain vessel co-option (Leenders et al., 2004). Magnetic resonance imaging (MRI) demonstrated substantially reduced central blood volumes in large BM, derived from a prostate cancer model, after treatment with the VEGFR inhibitor AZD2171 (Juan Yin et al., 2009). A rim of elevated blood volume was retained at the tumor–brain interface while small tumors displayed a static response (Juan Yin et al., 2009). These data underlie that the outcome of treatment with anti-angiogenic therapies might also depend on the histological type, which should be taken into consideration before deciding to initiate clinical trials with these agents.

Hemorrhagic episodes were recorded in the early clinical studies conducted in patients with metastatic disease, including BM, after treatment with bevacizumab (Carden et al., 2008). In consequence, the use of anti-angiogenic drugs such as bevacizumab had been contraindicated for a long time. Hence, patients with BM have been excluded from participating in clinical trials testing the efficacy of anti-angiogenics, even though the exact risk of intracranial bleeding remained largely uninvestigated (Carden et al., 2008). However, recent studies and meta-analyses in over 10000 patients indicated that VEGF targeting therapies are safe for use in patients with BM, as intracranial bleeding incidence is low (0.8–3.3%) and does not exceed baseline (De Braganca et al., 2010). These reports have prompted the

European Medicines Agency to reconsider the decision to contraindicate the administration of bevacizumab and allow its use in patients with non-small cell lung cancer (NSCLC), renal cell carcinoma (RCC), colorectal and breast cancer that develop BM (Besse et al., 2010). The new guidelines now indicate that treatment decisions should be made after carefully assessing the potential benefits and risks for individual patients (De Braganca et al., 2010). It is expected that the contraindication will also be removed in the USA in the near future.

As a result of the exclusion of patients with active BM from clinical studies, there are only scarce data regarding the efficacy of anti-angiogenic agents in this tumor entity. In a retrospective analysis, De Braganca et al. (2010) identified six patients with NSCLC and treatment naïve or progressive BM who had previously received bevacizumab. The best central nervous system (CNS) response was partial in two, stable disease in three, and progression in one. Bevacizumab treatment resulted in clinical improvement of patient symptomatology and reduced corticosteroid dependence (De Braganca et al., 2010). In an open-label, expanded access study conducted in 212 patients with BM from RCC, sunitinib treatment resulted in an objective response in 26 (12%) patients, without increased toxicity compared to that in the metastatic RCC population (Gore et al., 2011). Similar findings were also reported for sorafenib (Stadler et al., 2010). In a phase III study, the addition of the anti-angiogenic agent thalidomide to whole brain radiation therapy provided no survival benefit in patients with BM and was associated with high toxicity (Knisely et al., 2008). Notably, the alterations in blood flow during and after treatment were not monitored in that study.

Important lessons have been learned from the preclinical and clinical use of anti-VEGF strategies in the treatment of glioblastoma multiforme (GBM) which could possibly also have applications in BM. Administration of cediranib in mice can alleviate brain edema and prolong survival, despite continuous tumor growth (Carmeliet and Jain, 2011). In humans, it decreases corticosteroid dependence but whether this can improve patient outcome remains to be defined (Carmeliet and Jain, 2011). Additionally, special attention should be paid when assessing the response of BM using MRI as the reduction in contrast media uptake may overestimate regression of cerebral lesions (Quant and Wen, 2011). Several clinical trials testing the efficacy of anti-angiogenic agents, either as monotherapy or in combination with radiation and/or chemotherapy, have been initiated in patients with BM. The results of these studies are awaited with great interest and will provide important insight on the efficacy and safety of anti-angiogenic therapies.

SENSITIZING BRAIN METASTASES TO RADIATION

Radiotherapy, either in the form of whole brain radiotherapy (WBRT) and/or stereotactic radiosurgery (SRS), is the cornerstone of treatment. However, local or intracerebal recurrence after radiotherapy is not uncommon and has a negative impact on neurocognitive function. Hence, it is important to explore further the potential of new targeted therapies that enhance radiation efficacy to achieve long-term control of BM while minimizing side effects.

Over a decade ago, montexafin gadolinium (MGd), an MRI-detectable agent, drew significant interest as a potential radiosensitizing agent for patients with BM treated with radiotherapy as it is taken up in tumors at higher concentrations compared to normal tissues (Magda and Miller, 2006). Although its precise mechanism of action remains unclear, it plays a role in electron scavenging and disrupts cellular metabolism by inhibiting key proteins, such as thioredoxin reductase, leading to generation of reactive oxygen species (Magda and Miller, 2006). In a randomized controlled study, the addition of MGd to WBRT failed to improve survival in 401 patients with BM induced by various histological types (Mehta et al., 2003). The authors of the study reported a small delay in the time to neurologic progression in the combination group in patients with BM originating from lung cancer (Mehta et al., 2003). In a multicenter randomized phase III clinical trial, 554 patients with NSCLC received WBRT or WBRT plus MGd and the time to neurologic progression was examined (Mehta et al., 2009). Again, the incorporation of MGd to WBRT failed to meet its primary endpoint. Interestingly, an older preclinical study had failed to demonstrate a radiosensitizing effect for MGd in various tumor cells or xenograft models, raising questions about the efficacy of MGd as a radiosensitizing agent (Bernhard et al., 2000).

Efaproxiral has also been investigated as a radiosensitizer as it reduces hemoglobin's oxygen binding affinity, leading to increased oxygen release into tissues (Rosenberg and Knox, 2006). In a phase II clinical study that recruited 57 patients with BM, the combination of efaproxiral with WBRT ($10 \times 3\,Gy$) resulted in a median survival of 6.5 months (Shaw et al., 2003). Following this, a phase III study in 515 patients with BM was initiated. However, the addition of efaproxiral to WBRT failed to improve survival compared to WBRT alone (Suh et al., 2006). Similarly, a confirmatory phase III trial in breast cancer patients did not show any survival benefit for the combination arm (Scott et al., 2007). Hence, neither MGd nor efaproxiral improve neurologic outcome or survival in patients with BM treated with WBRT.

In a prospective randomized trial, lonidamine, an indazole carboxylic acid, was given with WBRT in patients with BM (DeAngelis et al., 1989). Survival and response rate were unaffected by the presence or absence of lonidamine. Similarly, the addition of the hypoxic cell radiosensitizers metronidazole and misonidazole or the proliferation marker bromodeoxyuridine failed to improve the outcome in patients with BM who received WBRT (Eyre et al., 1984; DeAngelis et al., 1989; Komarnicky et al., 1991; Phillips et al., 1995).

Despite the significant effort in evaluating chemotherapeutics, either alone or in combination with radiotherapy, for BM, level I evidence has shown no survival benefit of the alkylating agent temozolomide, nitrosoureas, carboplatin, or tegafur in this disease (Olson et al., 2010).

Vorinostat, a histone deacetylase inhibitor, sensitizes tumor cells to radiation. In a recent preclinical study, Baschnagel et al. (2009) showed that vorinostat enhanced the response of MDA-MB-231BR breast cancer BM to radiation and prolonged overall survival in mice. Currently, a phase I clinical trial is investigating the radiosensitizing potential of vorinostat in patients with BM, induced by various primary sites, in combination with WBRT. A further phase I study examines the combination of vorinostat with SRS for BM in patients with non-small cell lung cancer and the results are awaited with interest.

CROSSING THE BLOOD–BRAIN BARRIER

The blood–brain barrier (BBB) has a unique architecture that functions as a barrier between brain and systemic circulation, limiting access of many molecules to the cerebrospinal fluid. It consists of specialized endothelial cells that line cerebral blood vessels in conjuction with perivascular astrocytes and pericytes (Pardridge, 2005). The transportation of molecules across the BBB occurs directly through the endothelial cells and it is mediated by tight junctions and complex transport systems found on the luminal and abluminal membranes (Pardridge, 2005).

The BBB plays a major role in the treatment of BM. Several clinical studies and meta-analyses have shown that BM respond poorly to chemotherapy. Even though BM resistance to chemotherapy could account for this outcome, at least in part, it is now clear the BBB impairs adequate delivery of chemotherapy drugs to cerebral secondaries (Deeken and Loscher, 2007). Small lipophilic molecules readily pass through the BBB. In contrast, large hydrophilic molecules, such as many chemotherapeutic and some targeted agents, do not cross the BBB. Furthermore, a plethora of drug efflux pumps like P-glycoprotein (PgP) and other multidrug resistance proteins rapidly remove some of these molecules outside the CNS (Deeken and Loscher, 2007). Agarwal et al. (2010) elegantly demonstrated the role of efflux transporters in restricting the brain distribution of chemotherapeutic drugs. The uptake of gefitinib was profoundly increased in knockout mice for the efflux pumps Abcb1 and Abcg2 (Agarwal et al., 2010). Additionally, elacridar, an inhibitor of both pumps, increased uptake of sorafenib concentration in the brain, highlighting the importance of efflux pumps in mediating drug delivery to the BM (Lagas et al., 2010).

BM result in disruption of the BBB that occurs when BM grow larger than 1–2 mm in diameter. In a preclinical study, Zhang et al. (1992) investigated the selective BBB permeability induced by BM from eight different tumor cell lines. Lesions up to 0.2 mm diameter presented an intact BBB while larger secondaries were characterized by increased contrast agent leakage, indicating a functionally compromised BBB (Zhang et al., 1992). Similarly, in patients with BM, there is enhancement of the gadolinium contrast on MRI, indicating a disrupted BBB (Fortin, 2012). However, patients at the time of diagnosis likely have very small lesions with an intact BBB that fail to take up contrast agents and thus they cannot be diagnosed by MRI (Deeken and Loscher, 2007). These lesions likely contribute to intracerebral recurrence and provide an additional rationale for the development of strategies to overcome the BBB.

During the last decades, there has been progressively increasing interest in designing drugs that will improve BBB permeability. One approach is the exploitation of receptors that are normally expressed on the BBB endothelium (Deeken and Loscher, 2007; Fortin, 2012). Antibodies and peptides against transferin or insulin receptors and the receptor lipoprotein receptor-related protein (LRP-1) have been tested in preclinical studies. LRP-1 plays a role in the transport of various proteins along the BBB and it is upregulated in brain tumors (Deeken and Loscher, 2007). ANG1005 is a novel agent consisting of paclitaxel that is bound to a ligand of LRP-1, angiopep 2 and it is currently in phase I clinical studies for patients with BM or glioblastoma. A recent study showed that ANG1005 can prolong survival in mice with intracerebral tumors and leads to a 54-fold improved delivery of paclitaxel across the BBB, compared to unconjugated paclitaxel (Thomas et al., 2009). Furthermore, the phosphodiesterase 5 inhibitor, vardenafil, enhances uptake and efficacy of trastuzumab in mouse BM breast tumor model (Hu et al., 2010).

An alternative strategy is the direct disruption of the BBB. Brain irradiation has a high potential to increase BBB permeability but the precise mechanisms of action have not been well characterized (Fortin, 2012). This potential of radiation is probably the result of diverse effects such as loss of tight junctions and endothelial cell, astrocytic reaction and chemotactic attraction of leukocytes to the site of damaged endothelium in association with VEGF production and downregulation of P-glycoprotein (Deeken and Loscher, 2007; Fortin, 2012). However, how and when radiation should be applied to improve BBB penetrability remains unclear.

CONCLUSION

In conclusion, preclinical and clinical evidence suggests that targeting angiogenesis might be beneficial in the prevention and treatment of brain metastases, but this effect might depend on the histological type. Large meta-analyses indicate that the risk of intracerebal bleeding in patients with BM receiving bevacizumab is similar to the baseline. Similarly to GBM, the impact of these agents on BM microenvironment parameters, such as hypoxia and blood flow, should be investigated in large clinical studies to assess their efficacy and predictive value throughout the treatment of BM. The toxicity of anti-angiogenic agents should be monitored closely, especially when combined with other cytotoxic therapies. Although considerable effort has been put into the development of novel radiosensitizing agents in the treatment of BM, the results from testing these compounds in clinical studies have been disappointing. These data indicate that we need to focus towards new directions in BM management to improve the therapeutic ratio in these patients. The development of an agent that will sensitize BM to radiation without increasing toxicity to normal brain tissue remains imperative. Finally, the BBB continues to pose a challenge in the management of BM. The assessment of new ways to improve BBB penetrability of chemotherapeutics should be encouraged to enhance the survival of patients with this disease. Special attention should be paid in closely monitoring possible adverse reactions of combination treatments as the clinical experience with application of these agents in patients with BM remains limited.

References

Agarwal, S., Sane, R., Gallardo, J.L., Ohlfest, J.R., Elmquist, W.F., 2010. Distribution of gefitinib to the brain is limited by P-glycoprotein (ABCB1) and breast cancer resistance protein (ABCG2)-mediated active efflux. J. Pharmacol. Exp. Ther. 334, 147–155.

Baschnagel, A., Russo, A., Burgan, W.E., et al., 2009. Vorinostat enhances the radiosensitivity of a breast cancer brain metastatic cell line grown in vitro and as intracranial xenografts. Mol. Cancer Ther. 8, 1589–1595.

Bernhard, E.J., Mitchell, J.B., Deen, D., Cardell, M., Rosenthal, D.I., Brown, J.M., 2000. Re-evaluating gadolinium(III) texaphyrin as a radiosensitizing agent. Cancer Res. 60, 86–91.

Besse, B., Lasserre, S.F., Compton, P., Huang, J., Augustus, S., Rohr, U.P., 2010. Bevacizumab safety in patients with central nervous system metastases. Clin. Cancer Res. 16, 269–278.

Carbonell, W.S., Ansorge, O., Sibson, N., Muschel, R., 2009. The vascular basement membrane as "soil" in brain metastasis. PLoS One 4, e5857.

Carden, C.P., Larkin, J.M., Rosenthal, M.A., 2008. What is the risk of intracranial bleeding during anti-VEGF therapy? Neuro Oncol. 10, 624–630.

Carmeliet, P., Jain, R.K., 2011. Principles and mechanisms of vessel normalization for cancer and other angiogenic diseases. Nat. Rev. Drug Discov. 10, 417–427.

De Angelis, L.M., Currie, V.E., Kim, J.H., et al., 1989. The combined use of radiation therapy and lonidamine in the treatment of brain metastases. J. Neurooncol. 7, 241–247.

De Braganca, K.C., Janjigian, Y.Y., Azzoli, C.G., et al., 2010. Efficacy and safety of bevacizumab in active brain metastases from non-small cell lung cancer. J. Neurooncol. 100, 443–447.

Deeken, J.F., Loscher, W., 2007. The blood-brain barrier and cancer: transporters, treatment, and Trojan horses. Clin. Cancer Res. 13, 1663–1674.

Eyre, H.J., Ohlsen, J.D., Frank, J., et al., 1984. Randomized trial of radiotherapy versus radiotherapy plus metronidazole for the treatment metastatic cancer to brain. A Southwest Oncology Group study. J. Neurooncol. 2, 325–330.

Folkman, J., 1971. Tumor angiogenesis: therapeutic implications. N. Engl. J. Med. 285, 1182–1186.

Fortin, D., 2012. The blood-brain barrier: its influence in the treatment of brain tumors metastases. Curr. Cancer Drug Targets 12, 247–259.

Gore, M.E., Hariharan, S., Porta, C., et al., 2011. Sunitinib in metastatic renal cell carcinoma patients with brain metastases. Cancer 117, 501–509.

Hu, J., Ljubimova, J.Y., Inoue, S., et al., 2010. Phosphodiesterase type 5 inhibitors increase Herceptin transport and treatment efficacy in mouse metastatic brain tumor models. PLoS One 5, e10108.

Juan Yin, J., Tracy, K., Zhang, L., et al., 2009. Noninvasive imaging of the functional effects of anti-VEGF therapy on tumor cell extravasation and regional blood volume in an experimental brain metastasis model. Clin. Exp. Metastasis 26, 403–414.

Kerbel, R.S., 2008. Tumor angiogenesis. N. Engl. J. Med. 358, 2039–2049.

Kienast, Y., von Baumgarten, L., Fuhrmann, M., et al., 2010. Real-time imaging reveals the single steps of brain metastasis formation. Nat. Med. 16, 116–122.

Kim, L.S., Huang, S., Lu, W., Lev, D.C., Price, J.E., 2004. Vascular endothelial growth factor expression promotes the growth of breast cancer brain metastases in nude mice. Clin. Exp. Metastasis 21, 107–118.

Knisely, J.P., Berkey, B., Chakravarti, A., et al., 2008. A phase III study of conventional radiation therapy plus thalidomide versus conventional radiation therapy for multiple brain metastases (RTOG 0118). Int. J. Radiat. Oncol. Biol. Phys. 71, 79–86.

Komarnicky, L.T., Phillips, T.L., Martz, K., Asbell, S., Isaacson, S., Urtasun, R., 1991. A randomized phase III protocol for the evaluation of misonidazole combined with radiation in the treatment of patients with brain metastases (RTOG-7916). Int. J. Radiat. Oncol. Biol. Phys. 20, 53–58.

Lagas, J.S., van Waterschoot, R.A., Sparidans, R.W., Wagenaar, E., Beijnen, J.H., Schinkel, A.H., 2010. Breast cancer resistance protein and P-glycoprotein limit sorafenib brain accumulation. Mol. Cancer Ther. 9, 319–326.

Leenders, W.P., Kusters, B., Verrijp, K., et al., 2004. Antiangiogenic therapy of cerebral melanoma metastases results in sustained tumor progression via vessel co-option. Clin. Cancer Res. 10, 6222–6230.

Magda, D., Miller, R.A., 2006. Motexafin gadolinium: a novel redox active drug for cancer therapy. Semin. Cancer Biol. 16, 466–476.

Mehta, M.P., Rodrigus, P., Terhaard, C.H., et al., 2003. Survival and neurologic outcomes in a randomized trial of motexafin gadolinium and whole-brain radiation therapy in brain metastases. J. Clin. Oncol. 21, 2529–2536.

Mehta, M.P., Shapiro, W.R., Phan, S.C., et al., 2009. Motexafin gadolinium combined with prompt whole brain radiotherapy prolongs time to neurologic progression in non-small-cell lung cancer patients with brain metastases: results of a phase III trial. Int. J. Radiat. Oncol. Biol. Phys. 73, 1069–1076.

Olson, J.J., Paleologos, N.A., Gaspar, L.E., et al., 2010. The role of emerging and investigational therapies for metastatic brain tumors: a systematic review and evidence-based clinical practice guideline of selected topics. J. Neurooncol. 96, 115–142.

Pardridge, W.M., 2005. Molecular biology of the blood-brain barrier. Mol. Biotechnol. 30, 57–70.

Phillips, T.L., Scott, C.B., Leibel, S.A., Rotman, M., Weigensberg, I.J., 1995. Results of a randomized comparison of radiotherapy and bromodeoxyuridine with radiotherapy alone for brain metastases: report of RTOG trial 89-05. Int. J. Radiat. Oncol. Biol. Phys. 33, 339–348.

Quant, E.C., Wen, P.Y., 2011. Response assessment in neuro-oncology. Curr. Oncol. Rep. 13, 50–56.

Rosenberg, A., Knox, S., 2006. Radiation sensitization with redox modulators: a promising approach. Int. J. Radiat. Oncol. Biol. Phys. 64, 343–354.

Scott, C., Suh, J., Stea, B., Nabid, A., Hackman, J., 2007. Improved survival, quality of life, and quality-adjusted survival in breast cancer patients treated with efaproxiral (Efaproxyn) plus whole-brain radiation therapy for brain metastases. Am. J. Clin. Oncol. 30, 580–587.

Shaw, E., Scott, C., Suh, J., et al., 2003. RSR13 plus cranial radiation therapy in patients with brain metastases: comparison with the Radiation Therapy Oncology Group Recursive Partitioning Analysis Brain Metastases Database. J. Clin. Oncol. 21, 2364–2371.
Stadler, W.M., Figlin, R.A., McDermott, D.F., et al., 2010. Safety and efficacy results of the advanced renal cell carcinoma sorafenib expanded access program in North America. Cancer 116, 1272–1280.
Suh, J.H., Stea, B., Nabid, A., et al., 2006. Phase III study of efaproxiral as an adjunct to whole-brain radiation therapy for brain metastases. J. Clin. Oncol. 24, 106–114.
Thomas, F.C., Taskar, K., Rudraraju, V., et al., 2009. Uptake of ANG1005, a novel paclitaxel derivative, through the blood-brain barrier into brain and experimental brain metastases of breast cancer. Pharm. Res. 26, 2486–2494.
Walker, A.E., Robins, M., Weinfeld, F.D., 1985. Epidemiology of brain tumors: the national survey of intracranial neoplasms. Neurology 35, 219–226.
Yano, S., Shinohara, H., Herbst, R.S., et al., 2000. Expression of vascular endothelial growth factor is necessary but not sufficient for production and growth of brain metastasis. Cancer Res. 60, 4959–4967.
Zhang, R.D., Price, J.E., Fujimaki, T., Bucana, C.D., Fidler, I.J., 1992. Differential permeability of the blood-brain barrier in experimental brain metastases produced by human neoplasms implanted into nude mice. Am. J. Pathol. 141, 1115–1124.

CHAPTER

6

Second Malignancies in Children Following Treatment for Neuroblastoma

Alberto Garaventa and Bruno De Bernardi

OUTLINE

Introduction 61

Risk of SMN in Children Treated for Neuroblastoma 62

Incidence of Selected SMNs 63
- *Leukemias and Lymphomas* 63
- *Solid Tumors* 66

Factors Increasing the Risk of SMNs 66
- *Genomic Aberrations and Second Malignancies* 67
- *Chemotherapy* 68
- *High-Dose Chemotherapy* 68
- *Radiotherapy* 69
- *Metabolic MIBG Radiation Therapy* 70

Survival After SMNs 71

Clinical Implications and Discussion 71

Conclusions 72

References 72

INTRODUCTION

Treatment for childhood cancer has become progressively more effective in the last few decades leading to a remarkable increase in both 5- and 10-year overall survival for these patients, which now approaches 80% overall (Smith et al., 2010). However, the mortality due to recurrence or progression of the original tumor after these time periods remains a relevant problem (Reulen et al., 2010). In addition, long-term survivors of cancer diagnosed in childhood do have a significant risk of developing multiorgan complications and psychosocial problems (Robinson, 2005). Finally, the chance that a second malignant neoplasia

M.A. Hayat (ed): *Brain Metastases from Primary Tumors, Volume 1*
DOI: http://dx.doi.org/10.1016/B978-0-12-800896-6.00006-1

© 2014 Elsevier Inc. All rights reserved.

(SMN) might develop over time in these individuals has led to great concern (Reulen et al., 2011). Improvement in survival has also involved children affected by neuroblastoma, although it has been less evident compared to other childhood malignancies, particularly leukemias, lymphomas, and nephroblastoma (Smith et al., 2010). In the experience of the Italian Neuroblastoma Group, the cure rate of neuroblastoma patients has increased from 35% in the early 1980s to a remarkable 64% recorded between 2000 and 2005 (Haupt et al., 2010). Even for neuroblastoma survivors, the occurrence of SMNs is no longer considered an exceptional event, although it remains less frequent than for leukemias and lymphomas (Reulen et al., 2011). This may be due in part to the peculiar clinical behavior of neuroblastoma itself, including the ability to undergo spontaneous regression and the chance of being cured by surgery alone. Furthermore, it has to be taken into consideration that treatment for neuroblastoma has considerably changed over time following a number of remarkable discoveries regarding the tumor's clinical and biological features (Øra and Eggert, 2011). However, the correlation between the occurrence of an SMN in children diagnosed with neuroblastoma and the previously administered treatment remains unclear.

We report our personal experience and the results of a search of the literature to describe the incidence and type of SMNs in neuroblastoma as related to the type of treatment, possible genetic implications, clinical implications and survival after the diagnosis of an SMN.

RISK OF SMN IN CHILDREN TREATED FOR NEUROBLASTOMA

The British Childhood Cancer Survivor Study analyzed a large population-based cohort of 5-year survivors of childhood cancer who had been diagnosed before 15 years of age between 1940 and 1981 in Great Britain. Among 17981 such patients who had been followed up for a median of 24.3 years, a total of 1354 developed an SMN. The most frequently observed SMNs were brain tumors, non-melanoma skin cancer, and gastrointestinal, genitourinary and breast carcinomas, as well as bone tumors. The standardized incidence ratio (SIR) for these patients was four times more than expected, while it was 2.8 times higher for neuroblastoma patients (Reulen et al., 2011). A similar investigation was carried out in the USA by the Childhood Cancer Survivor Study (CCSS). Of 14359 5-year survivors of childhood cancer diagnosed between 1970 and 1986 and followed up for a median of 30 years, a total of 1402 developed at least one SMN for a total of 2703 neoplasms with a cumulative incidence of 20.5% at 30 years from the first malignancy and an SIR of 6.0. The highest SIR was found for Hodgkin's lymphoma (8.7; 95% CI, 7.7–8.8) and Ewing's sarcoma (8.5; 95% CI, 6.2–11.7), while it was 6.9 for neuroblastoma (95% CI, 4.9–9.7), (Friedman et al., 2010). The CCSS also reported data on a selected group of 954 neuroblastoma patients who had survived more than 5 years from diagnosis. The cumulative incidence of any relevant chronic health condition for these neuroblastoma patients was 41% with an 8.3-fold increased risk as compared to their siblings. Nearly 6% of these patients died, most often of disease recurrence (n = 43, 5% of all deaths) and SMN (n = 13). Cumulative mortality was associated with older age at diagnosis. The cumulative incidence of SMN after 5 years from diagnosis was 3.5% at 25 years from diagnosis. The most frequent SMN was thyroid cancer (n = 8) followed by renal cell carcinoma (n = 5), (Levardière et al., 2009). The real incidence of secondary leukemias in these reports is likely underestimated, as these studies focused on SMNs that occurred after 5 years of follow up. However, a number of case reports and even large series have described instances of secondary leukemias that occurred within a shorter interval. In a French series of 61 cases of secondary leukemias detected at 0.8–12.8 years (median, 3.4) from an initial diagnosis of solid tumors, nine occurred in patients with neuroblastoma. Three of these nine patients, in whom leukemia occurred at 16, 17 and 27 months from diagnosis, respectively, had intermediate risk factors and had been treated with standard-dose chemotherapy (Allard et al., 2010). In addition, Kushner reported eight cases of secondary leukemia that occurred at 12–50 months (median, 16) from the initial diagnosis in a group of 184 high-risk neuroblastoma patients treated with dose-intensive induction chemotherapy (Kushner et al., 2009). Finally, at least two cases of simultaneous occurrence of neuroblastoma and acute myeloid leukemia have been reported (Di Cataldo et al., 2011).

In the experience of the Italian Neuroblastoma Registry (Garaventa, unpublished), based on more than 3000 children and adolescents diagnosed with neuroblastoma between 1979 and 2011, a total of 27 patients developed an SMN, including one who also developed a third tumor (Table 6.1). SMN or myelodysplasia occurred at a median interval of 10 years from the primary diagnosis. Thyroid carcinoma was the most frequently observed SMN ($n = 11$). A possible explanation for this high incidence may be the aggressive treatment we administered to these patients and, in particular, to the stage 4 patients that were diagnosed after 1985 and who underwent hematopoietic stem cell transplantation (HSCT) and total body irradiation (TBI). A second reason could be related to the different attitudes in the screening policies that were adopted to detect SMNs in these patients. For example, in several Italian centers, the thyroid gland is evaluated by ultrasonography every year and nodules >1 cm in diameter are routinely biopsied thus making it possible to detect some tumors that would otherwise never be detected. Finally, we did not observe any SMNs of the gastrointestinal or genitourinary tracts, likely because a number of patients were lost to follow up after entering adulthood.

INCIDENCE OF SELECTED SMNs

Leukemias and Lymphomas

Our literature search allowed us to identify at least 40 instances of leukemia and lymphoma that developed in children with a history of neuroblastoma. These cases were reported in detail and included type of malignancy and interval between first and second tumor. Most of them occurred less than 5 years after the first tumor and the majority was acute myeloid leukemias (AML). The series includes: (1) eight cases of myelodysplasia which occurred at 17–36 months from diagnosis (median, 26); all of the patients had been treated with chemotherapy, four of them had also undergone radiation therapy and one had received one course of therapeutic ^{131}I-metaiodobenzylguanidine (MIBG); (2) 31 cases of acute myeloid leukemia at 0–136 months from diagnosis (median, 20); all had received chemotherapy, eight had also received local radiation therapy and nine had had at least one course of therapeutic MIBG; (3) two cases of chronic myeloid leukemia detected at 15 and 161 months from diagnosis in patients treated with chemotherapy alone; (4) six cases

TABLE 6.1 Details of the 27 Patients who Developed an SMN

	Diagnosis of Neuroblastoma		Therapy						
Patient Number	**Age (At Diagnosis – Months)**	**Stage**	**CT**	**^{131}I MIBG**	**Ext RT**	**TBI**	**SMN**	**Interval**	**Outcome**
1174	37	1	No	No	No	No	Non-Hodgkin's lymphoma	177	Alive
11	90	2A	Yes	No	Yes	No	Thyroid carcinoma	185	Alive
9	5	2B	Yes	No	No	No	Chronic myeloid leukemia	161	Alive
384	26	3	Yes	Yes	No	No	Schwannoma	179	Dead
701	12	3	Yes	No	No	No	Thyroid carcinoma	201	Alive
852	47	3	Yes	Yes	No	No	Fibrous angiomatoid histiocytoma	87	Alive
878	37	3	Yes	Yes	No	No	Schwannoma	87	Dead[†]
549	41	4	Yes	Yes	No	Yes	Acute myeloid leukemia	136	Dead
592	32	4	Yes	No	No	Yes	Thyroid carcinoma	221	Alive
688	46	4	Yes	No	No	Yes	Acute myeloid leukemia	11	Dead
771	71	4	Yes	No	No	Yes	Thyroid carcinoma	154	Alive
779	70	4	Yes	No	No	Yes	Thyroid carcinoma	104	Alive
798	21	4	Yes	No	No	Yes	Thyroid carcinoma	156	Alive
797	40	4	Yes	No	No	Yes	Thyroid carcinoma	184	Alive

1007	47	4	Yes	No	No	No	Hodgkin's lymphoma – Melanoma	124/140	Alive
1038	54	4	Yes	Yes	No	No	Acute myeloid leukemia	28	Dead
1440	70	4	Yes	Yes	No	No	Myelodysplasia	96	Alive
1664	42	4	Yes	No	No	No	Myelodysplasia	25	Dead
1817	25	4	Yes	No	No	No	Chronic myeloid leukemia	14	Dead
610	10	4S	Yes	No	No	TBI	Thyroid carcinoma	181	Alive
2601	1	4S	Yes	No	No	No	Non-Hodgkin's lymphoma	9	Alive
2613	11	4	Yes	No	Yes*	No	Anaplastic ependymoma	48	Alive
2508	384	3	Yes	No	No	No	Pituitary adenoma	19	Alive
926	164	4	Yes	No	No	No	Thyroid carcinoma	204	Alive
1046	114	3	No	No	No	No	Disgerminoma	120	Alive
2954	24	4	Yes	Yes	No	Yes	Thyroid carcinoma	108	Alive
497	76	2	No	No	No	No	Thyroid carcinoma	100	Alive

**SMN outside the RT field.*
†Died of neuroblastoma progression.
Abbreviations: CT: chemotherapy; MIBG: therapeutic dosage of ^{131}I metaiodobenzylguanidine; Ext RT: external radiotherapy; TBI: total body irradiation.
Note: Interval is the time that elapsed between the diagnosis of neuroblastoma and the second malignant neoplasm.

of acute lymphoblastic leukemia; three of the four cases (that included detailed reports) at 12–60 months (median, 46); all had been pretreated with chemotherapy, four had also undergone radiation therapy, and one had been administered MIBG; (5) two cases of non-Hodgkin's lymphoma (T-cell type in one, ALK-T in the other) at 9 and 177 months from diagnosis, respectively, of whom only one had been pretreated with chemotherapy; and (6) two cases of Hodgkin's lymphoma (Evans et al., 1994; Schiavetti et al., 2001; Weiss et al., 2003; Laverdière et al., 2005; George et al., 2006; Kushner et al., 2009; Baker et al., 2010; Kramer et al., 2010; Di Cataldo et al., 2011; Garaventa, unpublished).

Solid Tumors

There are only two reports of solid tumors (a fibrosarcoma and a clear-cell carcinoma) occurring as SMNs in children who were treated for neuroblastoma after less than 5 years from the initial diagnosis (Evans et al., 1994; Matthay et al., 2009). In a number of other cases that were described in two series, the secondary tumor occurred after an interval of 5–35 years from the initial diagnosis (median, 17.8 and 19.5 years, respectively) (Rubino et al., 2003; Friedman et al., 2010). The majority of these secondary solid tumors were thyroid cancers ($n = 24$), followed by soft tissue sarcomas ($n = 14$, four of which were schwannomas), brain tumors ($n = 10$), non-melanoma skin cancers ($n = 6$), colon carcinomas ($n = 5$), breast carcinomas ($n = 4$), osteogenic sarcomas ($n = 5$), hepatocellular carcinoma following hepatitis B virus infection ($n = 1$) (Perwein et al., 2011) and, in our own experience, one case each of fibrous angiomatoid histiocytoma, ependymoma, pituitary adenoma and disgerminoma (Garaventa, unpublished). Thyroid cancer as an SMN reportedly occurred more often among children with neuroblastoma who had undergone treatment including irradiation compared to other childhood neoplasias treated similarly, thus suggesting an independent association (Rubino et al., 2003). The CCSS also reported five cases of renal cell carcinoma, some of which were observed in patients who had not previously been exposed to chemotherapy, indicating the possible influence of an underlying genetic predisposition (Laverdière et al., 2009). Finally, we should also consider that subsequent secondary cancers have been reported in at least six patients. One of them developed thyroid carcinoma followed by hepatocellular carcinoma (Perwein et al., 2011), another patient developed Hodgkin's lymphoma followed by melanoma (Garaventa, unpublished), a third developed non-Hodgkin's lymphoma followed by myelodysplasia (Garaventa, unpublished), the fourth patient with associated neurofibromatosis 1 had a hypothalamic/optic astrocytoma followed by a malignant peripheral nerve sheet tumor (Laverdière et al., 2005); the fifth patient had a leiomyosarcoma of the uterus followed by a melanoma, and the sixth developed malignant breast carcinoma followed by AML, which was diagnosed 16 years after the first SMN (Rubino et al., 2003).

FACTORS INCREASING THE RISK OF SMNs

The great majority of children diagnosed with neuroblastoma who developed an SMN much later received multiple courses of polychemotherapy often combined with radiation therapy and, less frequently, with radiometabolic therapy (MIBG or F3 monoclonal antibody). Clearly, the combination of these modalities makes it difficult to define the role of the individual treatments and drugs in the eventual occurrence of an SMN. However, some studies suggest that up to 10% of all pediatric cancers could be related to a genetic susceptibility (Garber and Offit, 2005). Were this true, the actual incidence of genetic predisposition for the development of multiple secondary cancers could be higher due to under-recognition and under-reporting. A predisposition may be advocated considering that SMNs have also been reported in stage 4S patients as well as in those with localized disease, representing the majority of *long-term* survivors of this disease who were treated with short-lasting, non-intensive chemotherapy, or had no treatment at all (but surgery). A significantly higher risk of SMN among females was reported in the CCSS Group study (Friedman et al., 2010). A similar, but not significant result was observed in the neuroblastoma cohort studied by the French and British investigators (Rubino et al., 2003).

Genomic Aberrations and Second Malignancies

Very few data have been reported about the genomic study of second malignancies occurring in neuroblastoma patients. Imashuku et al. (1996) observed the 11q23 translocation in a neuroblastoma patient who developed acute lymphoblastic leukemia (ALL) following treatment. Chromosome 11q is often deleted in advanced neuroblastoma without *MYCN* gene amplification. The 11q deletion that is observed in ALL cells overlaps with the region that is deleted in neuroblastoma, thus suggesting that, in this case, common genes may have participated in the development of the second cancer.

Medeiros et al. (1999) reported four cases of renal cell carcinoma after neuroblastoma. Several chromosomal abnormalities were observed in the renal cell carcinoma that included chromosome imbalances of 2p31-32.2, 8p22, 9p22-24, 13q22, 20q13, and 22q11. However, the overall cytogenetic analysis showed distinct types of abnormalities in the tumors, indicating that the origins of neuroblastoma and renal cell carcinomas differ.

Succinate dehydrogenase gene mutations have been observed in a few families with cases of neuroblastoma (NB), pheochromocytoma and renal cell carcinoma (Schimke et al., 2010). The occurrence of neuroblastoma in a patient with gastrointestinal stromal tumor (GIST) was quite interesting. Since the c-kit oncogene is activated in GIST as well as in NB, it could be hypothesized that the c-kit gene played a role in both subsequent tumors (Gonçalves et al., 2010).

A case of Xp11 translocation was reported by Hedgepeth et al. (2009) in a renal cell carcinoma subsequent to NB. Chromosome X is rarely affected in NB, suggesting that the neoplasias derive from different cell clones. Weiss et al. (2003) reported three children with secondary myelodysplasia/leukemia observed after I^{131} MIBG. Cytogenetic analysis of tumor cells revealed chromosome 2q, 5 and 7 abnormalities and, furthermore, monosomy of chromosome 11 and trisomy of 12 were also observed. Chromosome 11q deletion has been found in about 23% of neuroblastoma cases, while a numerical loss of chromosome 11 is less frequently observed. Again, the likelihood that the same chromosome was involved in two different tumors is quite low. All the above reported data suggest that second malignancies arise as a new cancer that does not share the same genetic abnormalities. It must be highlighted that a complete and in-depth genomic study of second malignancies in patients with neuroblastoma is lacking. An extensive genomic analysis of second malignancies in patients treated for neuroblastoma would be useful better to manage patients with a second malignancy.

Chemotherapy

Chemotherapy was administered to the large majority, but not to all patients. We encountered one instance of acute myeloid leukemia that was diagnosed at the same time as neuroblastoma, and one case of T-cell non-Hodgkin's lymphoma that occurred 15 years after the diagnosis of stage 1 neuroblastoma which had been treated by surgery alone (Garaventa, unpublished). Besides these rare instances, treated patients usually received polychemotherapy, often including at least one course of high-dose chemotherapy, followed by hematopoietic stem cell rescue. However, some patients who developed leukemia as an SMN had not undergone aggressive chemotherapy (Baker et al., 2010). Kushner et al. (2009) claim that repeated courses of intensive chemotherapy play a role in the occurrence of an SMN. They described seven cases of secondary leukemia occurring in a series of 108 neuroblastoma patients who had received more than five courses of dose-intensive treatment, while only one case of leukemia occurred in the 76 patients who had received five courses or less (Kushner et al., 2009).

Most publications reporting the occurrence of SMNs did not specify the type of chemotherapy that had been administered. However, etoposide (or teniposide) had been largely employed in neuroblastoma patients, and several instances of leukemia have been reported in patients who were treated with epipodophyllotoxins. Furthermore, some authors have highlighted the risk of secondary leukemia (of myeloid type) in patients treated with prolonged palliative oral etoposide, the incidence of which appears much higher than expected, also considering that most of these patients have a short follow up (Schiavetti et al., 2001). Co-administration of an alkylating agent and/or a topoisomerase II inhibitor occurs frequently in regimens used for neuroblastoma patients and this combination could be more leukemogenic than administering these agents alone. The routine use of repeated courses of G-CSF to overcome excessive myelotoxicity and/or to collect peripheral blood stem cells could have a leukemogenic effect, but it is difficult to draw definitive conclusions in this regard.

High-Dose Chemotherapy

Most neuroblastoma patients who underwent high-dose chemotherapy had poor prognosis features at the time of diagnosis and therefore had little chance of cure. It is therefore difficult to define precisely the role of megatherapy in the occurrence of SMNs. A study by the Children's Oncology Group (COG) reported the long-term results of this type of treatment administered to these children who were enrolled in a randomized trial that included megatherapy followed by 13-cis-retinoic acid. The study was carried out between 1991 and 1996, and the effect of myeloablative chemotherapy associated with TBI plus purged autologous bone marrow transplantation (ABMT) was compared to the effect of continuous intensive chemotherapy without ABMT. An update on the long-term outcome of these patients (more than 8 years after the end of the trial) was published in 2009 (Matthay et al., 2009). The authors reported the occurrence of SMNs in four of 291 patients, more precisely in two of the 137 in the chemotherapy arm (one case of T-acute lymphoblastic leukemia, one of clear cell carcinoma), and in two of the 154 who underwent ABMT (one case of acute myeloid leukemia, one of thyroid carcinoma).

French authors compared the occurrence of late sequelae in two groups of children with stage 4 neuroblastoma who were treated by megatherapy, or megatherapy plus TBI, respectively. The two groups were similar with regard to age, stage of disease, period of treatment, chemotherapy protocol, and disease-free survival. Six SMNs occurred among the 32 patients treated with megatherapy plus TBI (thyroid carcinoma = 3, osteogenic sarcoma = 1; colon carcinoma = 1, malignant schwannoma = 1), while of the 30 children treated with megatherapy alone, one developed acute myeloblastic leukemia, and one a degenerative CNS tumor. All these patients who developed an SMN survived. The French authors underline the importance of a meticulous follow up for these patients to allow early diagnosis and proper treatment of SMNs (Flandin et al., 2006).

Radiotherapy

The most frequent radiation-related SMNs are thyroid carcinomas which usually occur after a latency period of more than 5 years. A study by the CCSS showed that the incidence correlates with the increase in the radiation dose, but that it drops close to zero when the dosage is particularly high. The incidence was higher when treatment was administered to patients younger than 5 years of age at the time of the first diagnosis (Bhatti et al., 2010). In the same study, an excess of secondary thyroid carcinomas was observed in children who had received radiation, suggesting that neuroblastoma patients have a greater risk of developing thyroid cancer, regardless of the exposure to therapeutic irradiation. Similar data have been reported concerning another cohort of childhood cancer survivors (de Vathaire et al., 1999). However, the hypothesis appears limited by the small number of patients that were described, i.e. nine, four of whom were diagnosed with neuroblastoma in the first year of life. Thus, given the strong correlation between type of first cancer, age at exposure and radiation dose, we could hypothesize that the degree of risk of developing thyroid cancer in children treated for neuroblastoma may be related to the young age at exposure.

The role of radiation therapy in inducing sarcoma, thyroid carcinoma and other solid tumors in early childhood is well known. A number of studies have indicated that radiation therapy may be a causative factor in the development of SMNs after treatment for childhood cancer, but it has to be taken into account that not all SMNs occurred in the irradiated field. French authors showed a 5.2-fold increased risk of mortality due to an SMN in patients who received an integral radiation dose exceeding 150 joules, and they suggest that irradiation of small volumes does not significantly increase the risk of developing secondary carcinomas or hematologic malignancies (Tukenova et al., 2011).

Combined modality therapy may increase the risk of leukemia, and the role of epipodophyllotoxins associated with radiotherapy has been underlined as a risk factor in the development of secondary leukemia (Allard et al., 2010). On the other hand, the risk of leukemia following radiation alone is lower than after chemotherapy (Tukenova et al., 2011). However, some cases of osteogenic sarcoma, renal cell carcinoma and also thyroid carcinoma, as well as some lymphoblastic leukemia–lymphomas have been reported in patients who were not treated at all, suggesting a possible genetic predisposition (Friedman et al., 2005).

Metabolic MIBG Radiation Therapy

Targeted radiotherapy to neuroblastoma cells was developed to exploit the ability of tumor cells to take up MIBG. Several trials using this radioelement as treatment have been carried out in poor responders or after relapse, and some institutions have tested it on newly diagnosed patients prior to "traditional" induction chemotherapy. Some cases of SMNs have been reported in trials that included MIBG in the treatment protocol. In particular, Weiss et al. (2003) reported three instances of secondary myelodysplastic syndrome and leukemia. Afterwards, we observed one more case of acute myeloid leukemia (Garaventa, unpublished). An additional case has been described by Incesoy-Ozdemir et al. (2011). Chromosomal studies were carried out on 11 patients reported in the literature, four of whom had monosomy of chromosome 7. Although these patients had all been heavily exposed to alkylating agents, epipodophyllotoxins and radiation therapy, the possible effect of MIBG cannot be ruled out. In fact, irradiation of the hematopoietic precursor in neuroblastoma patients treated with MIBG is due to both the uptake of the radioelement by platelets and megakaryocytes, and to bystander irradiation ("cross-fire" effect) from bone marrow micrometastases (Garaventa et al., 2003). An additional case of acute myeloid leukemia has been reported in a patient who received intrathecal radioimmunotherapy with ^{131}I monoclonal antibody targeting B7H3. However, this patient had also previously received heavy chemotherapy and external irradiation (Kramer et al., 2010).

Our own experience also includes two cases of malignant schwannoma and one of fibrous angiomatoid histiocytoma. These patients received chemotherapy, but not external radiation therapy. In the two patients who developed a schwannoma, the tumor occurred within the residual mass which had lost the initial "aggressive" histological pattern and had evolved into ganglioneuroma. In both cases, the metabolic radiotherapy probably played a role in triggering the malignant transformation of stromal cells within the neuroblastoma mass. In the case of the fibrous histiocytoma, chance alone might explain the occurrence of a borderline second malignant tumor in an area where MIBG likely did not produce a significant effect (Garaventa et al., 2003).

With one single exception, i.e. a patient of ours who also received TBI, instances of secondary thyroid carcinomas have not been reported following ^{131}I metabolic radiotherapy, while a high incidence of this type of SMN has been observed mainly, although not exclusively, in neuroblastoma patients who received external radiotherapy (Bhatti et al., 2010). The length of follow up may be one of the reasons for the almost lack of thyroid malignancies in patients receiving MIBG therapy, since thyroid neoplasms usually occur after a latency period longer than 5 years. Moreover, in patients with thyroid dysfunction, both the high-dose thyroid irradiation of MIBG and the replacement therapy may also have played a protective role. MIBG represents an alternative treatment for patients with relapsed or refractory neuroblastoma. However, the cumulative radiation burden of MIBG treatment with that of alkylating agents has potentially serious late effects, including SMNs. Therefore, all children who receive MIBG therapy require careful, long-term follow up.

SURVIVAL AFTER SMNs

In our experience, out of 27 cases of SMN (see Table 6.1), six died of progression of the secondary tumor (one of the two schwannomas, and five of the seven leukemias), and one died of progression of the initial neuroblastoma (this patient had developed a schwannoma). A similar experience was reported by Paulino and Fowler (2005), who observed 14 instances of SMNs in a series of 492 children diagnosed with a malignant solid tumor treated at a single radiation oncology institution. Of these 14 patients, three (who had developed a breast carcinoma, an osteogenic sarcoma and a chronic myeloid leukemia, respectively) died of progression of the SMN. More than two-thirds of children described in this study who developed a radiation-induced malignancy were alive at least 10 years after the diagnosis of the SMN. However, the two studies with longer follow up show that mortality due to SMN increases as the interval from diagnosis increases (Tukenova et al., 2011; Reulen et al., 2010) and in the CCSG study beyond 4–5 years an excess number of deaths is observed and second primary cancers and circulatory deaths together accounted for 77% of causes of death (Reulen et al., 2011). The poor prognosis of secondary leukemia (both lymphoblastic and myeloid) was previously reported by Shivakumar et al. (2008). These authors clearly state that allogeneic transplantation represents the only chance of cure for these patients.

CLINICAL IMPLICATIONS AND DISCUSSION

A large body of data convincingly supports the hypothesis that radiation therapy plays an important role in the development of an SMN, both for neuroblastoma patients and other childhood cancers. As a consequence, it is conceivable that both reducing the radiation dose and field size may translate into a decrease of SMNs in children treated for neuroblastoma, similar to what has been documented for Hodgkin's lymphoma patients. A similar beneficial effect could be obtained by refining doses and schedules of chemotherapy. This improvement was achieved, for instance, by Kushner, who lowered the number of courses of intensive chemotherapy from seven to five. This led to a significant decrease in the number of secondary leukemias that occurred in a series of high-risk neuroblastoma patients (Kushner et al., 2009). On this basis, it clearly appears that reducing the number of chemotherapy courses is an appealing objective. Carefully tailored treatment for childhood cancers bearing specific risk factors may reduce the risk that these individuals will develop SMNs as well as other late complications.

Finally, patients, their parents and/or guardians, and the physicians in charge of their follow up must be fully aware of the risk of the possible occurrence of SMNs and of the screening strategies that may lead to early detection and management. A recent CCSS study has shown, in fact, that survivors of neuroblastoma receive less information compared to children diagnosed with other malignancies, especially hematologic ones (Kadan-Lottick et al., 2002).

The data that have been collected in the last two decades indicate that particular attention must be paid to following up children diagnosed with tumors who have received aggressive chemotherapy, including alkylating agents, toposomerase II inhibitors and epipodophyllotoxin derivatives, especially when given in association with radiation therapy. The role of radiometabolic therapy is probably relevant, but it has not yet been fully defined, and thus it requires longer patient observation.

Data on familiarity and genetic predisposition are still scarce, but the occurrence of SMNs in subjects who received no antitumor therapy (except for surgery) underlines the importance of the accurate observation of families with children diagnosed with neuroblastoma who develop an SMN. As an example, we mention an instance of paraganglioma that was detected 15 years following diagnosis of neuroblastoma, which showed a familial mutation of the *SDHB* gene (Schimke et al., 2010). Collecting family histories of cancer is important and families must be encouraged to provide updates. If a hereditary cancer syndrome is suspected, mutation-specific testing can determine which family members are at increased risk and should therefore undergo screening, but it can also identify which family members should be reassured.

CONCLUSIONS

On the basis of the published information, the cumulative incidence of SMNs for neuroblastoma patients is in the range of 2% at 20 years from the initial diagnosis. Next to late recurrence, SMNs represent the main cause of death in long-term survivors of neuroblastoma. The most commonly encountered SMNs were thyroid carcinomas, osteogenic and soft tissue sarcomas, breast and colon carcinomas, acute myeloid and lymphoid leukemias, Hodgkin's and non-Hodgkin's lymphomas, and brain tumors. Female survivors seem to be at higher risk of developing an SMN than males. Other predisposing features include young age at the time of diagnosis of the first cancer, high-dose administration of alkylating agents and topoisomerase II inhibitors, high cumulative doses and protracted schedules of epipidophyllotoxins. However, some studies advocate a possible genetic predisposition based on reports of SMNs in patients who received only a few courses of chemotherapy or even none. Longer and more target-specific surveillance should be recommended with specific cancer screening at younger ages compared to the general population.

The risk of the late effects of treatment, especially second cancers, is directly proportional to the treatment exposure. Refinement of the treatments with risk-adapted and response-related regimens, reduction of the doses and changes in schedules, as well as the use of new radiotherapy modalities and of modern instruments, such as proton and photon radiation, together with a reduction of fields and doses may likely reduce the risk of SMNs. Clearly, long-term follow up is mandatory to assess fully the possible benefits of these refinements for survivors of pediatric cancers.

References

Allard, A., Haddy, N., Le Deley, 2010. Role of radiation dose in the risk of secondary leukemia after a solid tumor in childhood treated between 1980 and 1999. Int. J. Radiat. Oncol. Biol. Phys. 78, 1474–1482.

Bhatti, P., Veiga, L.H., Ronckers, C.M., et al., 2010. Risk of second primary thyroid cancer after radiotherapy for a childhood cancer in a large cohort study: an update from the childhood cancer survivor study. Radiat. Res. 174, 741–752.

Baker, D.L., Schmidt, M.L., Cohn, S.L., Children's Oncology Group, 2010. Outcome after reduced chemotherapy for intermediate-risk neuroblastoma. N. Engl. J. Med. 363, 1313–1323.

de Vathaire, F., Hardiman, C., Shamsaldin, A., et al., 1999. Thyroid carcinomas after irradiation for a first cancer during childhood. Arch. Intern. Med. 59, 2713–2719.

Di Cataldo, A., Mazzocco, K., Magro, G., et al., 2011. Simultaneous tumors: acute myeloid leukemia infiltrating mediastinal ganglioneuroblastoma. Pediatr. Blood Cancer 56, 298–300.

Evans, A.E., August, C.S., Kamani, N., et al., 1994. Bone marrow transplantation for high risk neuroblastoma at the Children's Hospital of Philadelphia: an update. Med. Pediatr. Oncol. 23, 323–327.

Flandin, I., Hartmann, O., Michon, J., et al., 2006. Impact of TBI on late effects in children treated by megatherapy for Stage IV euroblastoma. A study of the French Society of Pediatric Oncology. Int. J. Radiat. Oncol. Biol. Phys. 64, 1424–1431.

Friedman, D.L., Kadan-Lottick, N.S., Whitton, J., et al., 2005. Increased risk of cancer among siblings of long-term childhood cancer survivors: a report from the childhood cancer survivor study. Cancer Epidemiol. Biomarkers Prev. 14, 1922–1927.

Friedman, D.L., Whitton, J., Leisenring, W., et al., 2010. Subsequent neoplasms in 5-year survivors of childhood cancer: the Childhood Cancer Survivor Study. J. Natl. Cancer Inst. 102, 1083–1095.

Garaventa, A., Gambini, C., Villavecchia, G., et al., 2003. Second malignancies in children with neuroblastoma after combined treatment with 131I-metaiodobenzylguanidine. Cancer 97, 1332–1338.

Garber, J.E., Offit, K., 2005. Hereditary cancer predisposition syndromes. J. Clin. Oncol. 23, 276–292.

George, R.E., Li, S., Medeiros-Nancarrow, C., et al., 2006. High-risk neuroblastoma treated with tandem autologous peripheral-blood stem cell-supported transplantation: long-term survival update. J. Clin.Oncol. 24, 2891–2896.

Gonçalves, R., Linhares, E., Albagli, R., et al., 2010. Occurrence of other tumors in patients with GIST. Surg. Oncol. 19, e140–e143.

Haupt, R., Garaventa, A., Gambini, C., et al., 2010. Improved survival of children with neuroblastoma between 1979 and 2005: a report of the Italian Neuroblastoma Registry. J. Clin. Oncol. 28, 2331–2338.

Hedgepeth, R.C., Zhou, M., Ross, J., 2009. Rapid development of metastatic Xp11 translocation renal cell carcinoma in a girl treated for neuroblastoma. J. Pediatr. Hematol. Oncol. 31, 602–604.

Imashuku, S., Hibi, S., Kosaka, K., et al., 1996. Secondary lymphoid malignancy in two children with neuroblastoma. Med. Pediatr. Oncol. 27 (1), 54–56.

Incesoy-Ozdemir, S., Bozkurt, C., Yüksek, N., et al., 2011. Secondary childhood acute myeloid leukemia with complex karyotypic anomalies including monosomy 7, monosomy 5 and translocation (1;10) after 131I-metaiodobenzylguanidine therapy for relapsed neuroblastoma. Turk. J. Pediatr. 53, 83–86.

Kadan-Lottick, N.S., Robinson, L.L., Gurney, J.G., et al., 2002. Childhood cancer survivors' knowledge about their past diagnosis and treatment. J. Am. Med. Assoc. 287, 1832–1839.

Kramer, K., Kushner, B.H., Modak, S., et al., 2010. Compartmental intrathecal radioimmunotherapy: results for treatment for metastatic CNS neuroblastoma. J. Neurooncol. 97, 409–418.

Kushner, B.H., Kramer, K., Modak, S., et al., 2009. Reduced risk of secondary leukemia with fewer cycles of dose-intensive induction chemotherapy in patients with neuroblastoma. Pediatr. Blood Cancer 53, 17–22.

Laverdière, C., Cheung, N.K., Kushner, B.H., et al., 2005. Long-term complications in survivors of advanced stage neuroblastoma. Pediatr. Blood Cancer 45, 324–332.

Laverdière, C., Liu, Q., Yasui, Y., et al., 2009. Long-term outcomes in survivors of neuroblastoma: a report from the Childhood Cancer Survivor Study. J. Natl. Cancer Inst. 101, 1131–1140.

Matthay, K.K., Reynolds, C.P., Seeger, R.C., et al., 2009. Long-term results for children with high-risk neuroblastoma treated on a randomized trial of myeloablative therapy followed by 13-cis-retinoic acid: a Children's Oncology Group Study. J. Clin. Oncol. 27, 1007–1013.

Medeiros, L.J., Palmedo, G., Krigman, H.R., et al., 1999. Oncocytoid renal cell carcinoma after neuroblastoma: a report of four cases of a distinct clinicopathologic entity. Am. J. Surg. Pathol. 23 (7), 772–780.

Øra, I., Eggert, A., 2011. Progress in treatment and risk stratification of neuroblastoma: impact on future clinical and basic research. Semin. Cancer Biol. 21, 217–228.

Paulino, A.C., Fowler, B.Z., 2005. Secondary neoplasms after radiotherapy for a childhood solid tumor. Pediatr. Hematol. Oncol. 22 (2), 89–101.

Perwein, T., Lackner, H., Sovinz, P., et al., 2011. Survival and late effects in children with stage 4 neuroblastoma. Pediatr. Blood Cancer 57, 629–635.

Reulen, R.C., Winter, D.L., Frobisher, C., British Childhood Cancer Survivor Study Steering Group, 2010. Long-term cause-specific mortality among survivors of childhood cancer. J. Am. Med. Assoc. 304, 172–179.

Reulen, R.C., Frobisher, C., Winter, D.L., for the British Childhood Cancer Survivor Study Steering Group, 2011. Long-term risks of subsequent primary neoplasms among survivors of childhood cancer. J. Am. Med. Assoc. 305, 2311–2319.

Robinson, L.L., Green, D.M., Hudson, M., et al., 2005. Long-term outcomes of adult survivors of childhood cancer. Cancer 104, 2557–2564.

Rubino, C., Adjadj, E., Guérin, S., et al., 2003. Long-term risk of second malignant neoplasms after neuroblastoma in childhood: role of treatment. Int. J. Cancer 107, 791–796.

Schiavetti, A., Varrasso, G., Maurizi, P., Castello, M.A., 2001. Two secondary leukemias among 15 children given oral etoposide. Med. Pediatr. Oncol. 37, 148–149.

Schimke, R.N., Collins, D.L., Stolle, C.A., 2010. Paraganglioma, neuroblastoma, and a SDHB mutation: Resolution of a 30-year-old mystery. Am. J. Med. Genet. 152A, 1531–1535.

Shivakumar, R., Tan, W., Wilding, G.E., Wang, E.S., Wetzler, M., 2008. Biologic features and treatment outcome of secondary acute lymphoblastic leukemia: a review of 101 cases. Ann. Oncol. 19, 1634–1638.

Smith, M.A., Seibel, N.L., Altekruse, S.F., et al., 2010. Outcomes for children and adolescents with cancer: challenges for the twenty-first century. J. Clin. Oncol. 28, 2625–2634.

Tukenova, M., Guibout, C., Hawkins, M., et al., 2011. Radiation therapy and late mortality from second sarcoma, carcinoma, and hematological malignancies after a solid cancer in childhood. Int. J. Radiat. Oncol. Biol. Phys. 80, 339–346.

Weiss, B., Vora, A., Huberty, J., Hawkins, R.A., Matthay, K.K., 2003. Secondary myelodysplastic syndrome and leukemia following 131I-metaiodobenzylguanidine therapy for relapsed neuroblastoma. J. Pediatr. Hematol. Oncol. 25, 543–547.

CHAPTER

7

The Role of Chemotherapy in Metastatic Brain Tumors

Lynn Mubita and Steven N. Kalkanis

OUTLINE

Introduction	75	Breast Cancer	78
Standard of Care for Brain Metastases	76	Melanoma	78
Current Chemotherapy Options for Brain Metastases	77	Other Tumors	78
Non-Small Cell Lung Cancer	78	Conclusion	79
		References	79

INTRODUCTION

Brain metastases pose a major treatment challenge and typically confer a poor prognosis for patients diagnosed with these secondary tumors. While surgical resection and various forms of radiation therapy play important roles in the multidisciplinary therapy of brain metastases, the role of chemotherapy is less clear. In this chapter we will examine the evidence for and against the use of chemotherapy for brain metastases.

The American Cancer Society Registry data show that ≈1.4 million Americans are diagnosed with cancer every year; 40% of these will develop brain metastases (Kalkanis and Linskey, 2009). However, the exact incidence of brain metastases is often underestimated due to the way information is gathered from epidemiological studies. For example, most epidemiological studies use death certificates, tumor registries, and hospital records to gather information regarding the incidence of brain metastases. These are often incomplete

M.A. Hayat (ed): *Brain Metastases from Primary Tumors, Volume 1*
DOI: http://dx.doi.org/10.1016/B978-0-12-800896-6.00007-3

© 2014 Elsevier Inc. All rights reserved.

as patients with brain metastases are usually coded under their primary tumor, leaving the brain metastases uncoded. A study (Gavrilovic and Posner, 2008) looked at the incidence of brain metastases found at autopsy and estimated the incidence of brain metastases to be more than double the incidence of primary brain tumors. This is as compared to epidemiologic studies which put the incidence of brain metastases to be equal to or no more than double that of primary brain tumors. Another study (Davis and Dolecek, 2012) looked at the rate that brain metastases occurred in a given group of patients diagnosed with cancer and estimated that of 1 497 926 patients diagnosed with cancer in 2007, 70 000, or 4.6% would develop brain metastases over their lifetime. This is approximately three times the incidence of primary brain tumors per year. Even this was regarded as an underestimate by the authors of the study.

There is a tremendous amount of research being done on therapy for brain metastases as well as for primary brain tumors. Most cancers, when found early, can be treated with a combination of surgical resection, chemotherapy and/or radiation. However, by the time a patient develops a metastatic brain tumor, the prognosis is generally poor. The recently published evidence-based guidelines for the treatment of patients with metastatic brain tumors (Mehta et al., 2010) provide an excellent resource as an analysis of the current literature to aid the modern day physician in determining which of several multidisciplinary and multimodality treatment options to use.

STANDARD OF CARE FOR BRAIN METASTASES

Despite the poor prognosis and burden of disease, studies show that patients with brain metastases are surviving longer (Kondziolka et al., 2005). This is primarily due to advances in treatment options as well as more aggressive care. With the advent of computerized tomography in the 1970s, radiation therapy for brain metastases was initially the mainstay of treatment. Outcomes, however, remained poor. A landmark study (Patchell et al., 1990) randomized patients with single brain metastases to either surgical resection followed by radiation or needle biopsy followed by radiation and concluded that patients with single brain metastases who receive both surgical resection and radiation had a longer length of survival and longer functionality compared to treatment with radiation alone. In addition, a follow-up study by the same authors compared outcomes after whole brain radiotherapy with surgical resection to surgical resection alone. Although length of survival and functionality were not statistically significant, patients who received whole brain radiotherapy and surgical resection were less likely to die of neurologic causes. Thus, surgical resection followed by radiation has since been the standard of care for single brain metastatic lesions; more recently, stereotactic radiosurgery has also become an important treatment option.

Therapeutic modalities for most primary cancers and for many metastatic cancers involve chemotherapy. However, cancer that is metastatic to the brain poses a significant challenge due to the presence of the blood–brain barrier. The blood–brain barrier is a specialized layering of cells that effectively separates the systemic circulating blood from the brain, providing a microenvironment that is distinct from the rest of the body. Many substances are therefore excluded from the brain unless they can be actively transported across the blood–brain barrier (Kandel et al., 2000). In addition to the blood–brain barrier, astrocytes provide a second barrier to the movement of foreign substances into the brain – they may absorb and break down certain substances. As such, there is a trend for chemotherapeutic agents to be selected based on their potential to permeate the blood–brain barrier, regardless of whether or not they are effective against brain metastases in treatment. For instance, temozolomide is an alkylating agent that has relatively good central nervous system penetration (Friedman et al., 2000). As such, it has been studied for treatment of metastatic breast cancer to the brain. However, it has limited efficacy in treating breast cancer. On the other hand, capecitabine, which has good efficacy in treating breast cancer, has limited penetration into the blood–brain barrier (Grimm, 2012). Experimental models show that when a metastatic brain tumor grows more than 1–2 mm, there is structural and functional damage to the blood–brain barrier (Eichler et al., 2011). Thus, some chemotherapeutic drugs may potentially be able to permeate a disrupted blood–brain barrier, eventually reaching metastases.

CURRENT CHEMOTHERAPY OPTIONS FOR BRAIN METASTASES

Chemotherapy for brain metastases remains a controversial matter within the literature (Kalkanis and Linskey, 2009). The three most common tumors that metastasize to the brain in order of frequency are non-small cell lung cancer, breast cancer, followed by melanoma. Most of the studies that have looked at outcomes in treating brain metastases with chemotherapy have focused on these three. In addition, because the standard of care for brain metastases involves a multidisciplinary approach including radiation and surgical resection, there are relatively few studies that investigate the effects of chemotherapy alone. One such study (Mornex et al., 2003) compared the response of malignant melanoma to fotemustine with and without whole brain radiation, in a randomized phase III trial. Patients treated with fotemustine had worse baseline performance status compared to those treated with whole brain radiation as well (ECOG 2–3 of 54% compared to 30% in the combination therapy group). The median time interval between primary diagnosis and onset of brain metastases was statistically different (550 days for the fotemustine group and 1131 days for the combination therapy group). In addition, there was a statistical difference in time to cerebral progression (49 days in the fotemustine group and 56 days in the combination therapy group).

Another study (Postmus et al., 2000) looked at teniposide vs teniposide with whole brain radiation in patients with small cell lung cancer metastastic to the brain in a randomized phase III trial. The response rate was higher in the combination therapy group (57%) compared to teniposide alone (22%). In addition, time to progression was longer in the combination therapy group.

A third study (Moscetti et al., 2007) included 110 patients with newly diagnosed non-small cell lung cancer with brain metastases in a retrospective cohort study. One group received chemotherapy alone while the other group received chemotherapy and whole brain radiation. Response rates were 27.3% in the chemotherapy only group compared to 34.8% in the combination therapy group. However, there was no statistical difference in median time to progression of disease.

NON-SMALL CELL LUNG CANCER

Non-small cell lung cancer is the most common cancer to metastasize to the brain. Studies that have examined outcomes of brain metastases treated with chemotherapy have usually done so with multiple agents or in combination with other modes of therapy such as whole brain radiation. For example, one randomized phase III study looked at the effect of motexafin gadolinium as a radiation sensitizing agent for whole brain radiation therapy (Langer and Mehta, 2005). Adding motexafin gadolinium improved the interval to neurologic progression compared to whole brain radiation alone. While this study is favorable for motexafin gadolinium as a chemotherapeutic agent, this does not explore its use as an agent alone.

There is a percentage of non-small cell lung cancers that have mutations in the epidermal growth factor receptor (EGFR) that respond to erlotinib, an EGFR inhibitor. In a study (Porta et al., 2011) of 69 patients with brain metastases from non-small cell lung cancer, 17 of these had mutations in the epidermal growth factor receptor. The response rate to erlotinib was 82.4% in those that had the mutation. In addition, the median time to progression was 11.7 months in patients with the mutation compared to 5.8 months in those whose mutation status was not assessed. Given the small sample size and the rarity of the mutation, this again cannot be generalized to other brain metastases.

BREAST CANCER

Breast cancer is the second most common cancer to metastasize to the brain. Multiple chemotherapeutic agents including cisplatin, etoposide, anthracyclines, cyclophosphamide, high dose methotrexate and 5-fluorouracil have achieved response rates ranging from 50 to 59% but have not significantly impacted survival (Boogerd et al., 1992; Lin et al., 2004).

MELANOMA

Melanoma is relatively uncommon; however, it represents the third most common cause of brain metastases. A phase II study (Mornex et al., 2003) looked at ipilimumab, a T-cell potentiator that works by blocking cytotoxic T-lymphocyte antigen-4. It divided patients into two groups based on whether they required steroids. Of 51 patients in the steroid-free group, there were five with partial response and six with stable disease at week 12, with a response duration of 3 to 12 months. Further studies have shown no additional benefit with chemotherapy (Margolin et al., 2012).

OTHER TUMORS

Certain rare tumors, including germinomas, do not often metastasize to the brain, but when they do, they tend to be more sensitive to chemotherapy (Packer et al., 2000). These, however, have not been studied as much in the literature and therefore have less evidence as to their response to chemotherapy.

CONCLUSION

There is limited evidence to support the efficacy of chemotherapy for brain metastases. In addition, since most of the research has been done on the three most common brain metastases, response to chemotherapy in other more rare tumors has not been as extensively studied. Most of the literature, by virtue of incidence rates, is heavily weighted in the analysis of one of the most common sources of brain metastases, non-small cell lung cancer. It also focuses on multiple modes of therapy including whole brain radiation, stereotactic radiosurgery and surgical resection. Primary endpoints vary from study to study, making head to head comparisons difficult. As such, in deciding on which therapeutic modality to pursue, each patient should be considered on an individual basis, paying attention to age, performance status, chemosensitivity of the tumor and pathology type as well as extent of disease. Future considerations include identification of agents that enhance responses to multiple modes of therapy – for instance, medications that enhance effects of whole brain radiation – as the standard of care for metastatic brain tumors is currently multidisciplinary. In addition, small molecule inhibitors that easily pass through the blood–brain barrier continue to be identified and may play a more prominent role in the near future.

References

Boogerd, W., Dalesio, O., Bais, E.M., 1992. Response of brain metastases from breast cancer to systemic chemotherapy. Cancer 69, 972–980.

Davis, F.G., Dolecek, T.A., 2012. Toward determining the lifetime occurrence of metastatic brain tumors estimated from 2007 United States cancer incidence data. Neuro-Oncology 14 (9), 1171–1177.

Eichler, A.F., Chung, E., Kodack, D.P., 2011. The biology of brain metastases – translation to new therapies. Nat. Rev. Clin. Oncol. 8, 344–356.

Friedman, H., Kerby, T., Calvert, H., 2000. Temozolomide and treatment of malignant glioma. Clin. Cancer Res. 6, 2585–2597.

Gavrilovic, I.T., Posner, J.P., 2008. Brain metastases: epidemiology and pathophysiology. J. Neurooncol. 75, 5–14.

Grimm, S., 2012. Treatment of brain metastases: chemotherapy. Curr. Oncol. Rep. 2012, 85–90.

Kalkanis, S., Linskey, M., 2009. Evidence-based, clinical practice parameter guidelines for the treatment of patients with metastatic brain tumors: introduction. J. Neurooncol. 96, 7–10.

Kandel, E., Schwartz, J., Jessell, T., 2000. Principles of Neural Science. McGraw-Hill, New York.

Kondziolka, D., Martin, J.J., Flickinger, J.C., 2005. Long-term survivors after gamma knife radiosurgery for brain metastases. Cancer 104, 2784–2791.

Langer, C.J., Mehta, M.P., 2005. Current management of brain metastases, with a focus on systemic options. J. Clin. Oncol. 23, 6207–6219.

Lin, N.U., Bellon, J.R., Winer, E.P., 2004. CNS metastases in breast cancer. J. Clin. Oncol. 22, 3608–3617.

Margolin, K., Ernstoff, M.S., et al., 2012. Ipilimumab in patients with melanoma and brain metastases: an open-label, phase 2 trial. Lancet Oncol. 13, 459–465.

Mehta, M.P., Paleologos, N.A., Kalkanis, S.N., et al., 2010. The role of chemotherapy in the management of newly diagnosed brain metastases: a systematic review and evidence-based clinical practice guideline. Neuro-Oncology 96, 71–83.

Mornex, F., Thomas, L., Mohr, P., Hauschild, A., Delaunay, M.M., Lesimple, T., 2003. A prospective randomized multicentre phase III trial of fotemustine plus whole brain irradiation versus fotemustine alone in cerebral metastases of malignant melanoma. Melanoma Res. 13, 97–103.

Moscetti, L., Nelli, F., Felici, A., Rinaldi, M., De Santis, S., D'Auria, G., 2007. Up-front chemotherapy and radiation treatment in newly diagnosed nonsmall cell lung cancer with brain metastases: survey by Outcome Research Network for Evaluation of Treatment Results in Oncology. Cancer 109, 274–281.

Packer, R.J., Cohen, B.H., Cooney, K., 2000. Intracranial germ tumors. Oncologist 5, 312–320.

Patchell, R.A., Tibbs, P.A., Walsh, J.W., 1990. A randomized trial of surgery in the treatment of single metastases to the brain. N. Engl. J. Med. 322, 494–500.

Porta, R., Sanchez-Torres, J.M., Paz-Ares, L., et al., 2011. Brain metastases from lung cancer responding to erlotinib: the importance of EGFR mutation. Eur. Resp. J. 37, 624–631.

Postmus, P.E., Haaxma-Reiche, H., Smit, E.F., Groen, H.J., Karnicka, H., Lewinski, T., 2000. Treatment of brain metastases of small-cell lung cancer: comparing teniposide and teniposide with whole-brain radiotherapy – a phase III study of the European Organization for the Research and Treatment of Cancer Lung Cancer Cooperative Group. J. Clin. Oncol. 18, 3400–3408.

CHAPTER

8

Multiple Metastases to the Brain from Primary Cancers: Whole Brain Radiotherapy

Hany Soliman, Arjun Sahgal and May Tsao

OUTLINE

Introduction 81

Whole Brain Radiation Therapy 82

Whole Brain Radiation Therapy Technique 82

Whole Brain Radiation Therapy Tumor Response 83

Expected Survival after Whole Brain Radiation Therapy 84

Whole Brain Radiation Therapy with Other Therapies 84

Whole Brain Radiation Therapy and Surgery 84

Whole Brain Radiation Therapy and Radiosurgery 85

Whole Brain Radiation Therapy and Radiosensitizers 86

Whole Brain Radiation Therapy Re-Irradiation 88

Side Effects 88

Neurocognition 88

The Future of Whole Brain Radiation Therapy 89

References 90

INTRODUCTION

Brain metastases from primary cancers represent a significant disease burden and common source of morbidity and mortality in the cancer population. Brain metastases, for example, are estimated to occur in 20–40% of all patients with cancer during the course of their illness (Tsao et al., 2012). In diseases such as melanoma, the incidence of brain metastases has been found to be close to 60% in autopsy studies (Patel et al.,1978). Whole brain

M.A. Hayat (ed): Brain Metastases from Primary Tumors, Volume 1
DOI: http://dx.doi.org/10.1016/B978-0-12-800896-6.00008-5

© 2014 Elsevier Inc. All rights reserved.

radiotherapy (WBRT) was historically the only treatment for patients with multiple brain metastases and now, despite many advances in radiation technology, still plays a major role in treatment. In the past couple of decades, advancements in imaging, surgical techniques, and radiation planning and delivery, the options for treatment of brain metastases have expanded. Current management options include: surgical resection, stereotactic radiosurgery (SRS), WBRT, and supportive care measures only.

Beginning in the 1970s, multiple phase III trials assessing different WBRT fractionation schedules were studied, and overall no benefit above standard dose fractionation schedules of 2000 cGy in five daily fractions or 3000 cGy in 10 daily fractions has been observed. The results of trials adding radiosensitizers have been disappointing with no additional benefit to WBRT in either local tumor response or overall survival.

Treatment recommendations for multiple brain metastases are currently in flux. Aggressive local therapy in the form of SRS or, in some cases, surgery should be considered for patients with favorable prognostic factors presenting with up to four brain metastases. These prognostic factors include the presence of symptoms, age, performance status, histology, and status of extracranial disease. The role of WBRT in patients with up to four brain metastases has been questioned as there is no survival benefit and there may be worsening neurocognitive outcomes (Chang et al., 2009). In patients with more than four brain metastases, the standard treatment continues to be WBRT, however, ongoing studies are challenging the role of WBRT in select patients.

WHOLE BRAIN RADIATION THERAPY

The therapeutic effects of WBRT for brain metastasis were appreciated as far back as the 1960s, with symptomatic improvement and prolongation of life noted in a large proportion of treated patients. The RTOG has conducted numerous WBRT randomized trials answering key questions on altered dose and fractionation schedules (Borgelt et al., 1980, 1981; Kurtz et al., 1981; Coia, 1992; Murray et al., 1997). With extended fractionation schedules (50 Gy in 20 fractions daily or 54.4 Gy at 1.6 Gy twice daily) compared to the more commonly prescribed 30 Gy in 10 fractions daily, no differences in survival, symptomatic response or duration of response were observed. Hypofractionated WBRT (10 Gy in one fraction, 12 Gy in two fractions daily, 15 Gy in two fractions over 3 days), showed a possible increased risk of herniation and death within a few days of treatment and are generally avoided. As a result, the most common WBRT fractionation schemes include 20 Gy in five fractions or 30 Gy in 10 fractions, daily (Sahgal et al., 2012).

Whole Brain Radiation Therapy Technique

WBRT simulation, planning and treatment have changed over the past couple of decades with advances in computed tomography (CT) simulation, treatment planning and delivery technology. WBRT in the past was often done as a clinical mark-up without simulation. Typically ≤6 MV photon beams with a right and left lateral parallel opposed field arrangement were used. The inferior border was set below a line that approximates the location of the skull base – connecting the supraorbital ridge with the mastoid tip. The superior border was set up above the cranial apex. This type of a set up, however, often led to underdosage of the middle cranial fossa. Also, the lack of computerized dosimetry would result in variation in the dose within the brain that could be as much as ±20% depending on the cranial anatomy. Presently, with the availability of CT simulation, multileaf collimators (MLCs) and advanced treatment planning software, it is possible to plan and deliver more homogeneous radiation treatments that do not underdose parts of the brain and still limit the dose to organs at risk (such as the eyes).

Whole Brain Radiation Therapy Tumor Response

The few studies that have analyzed tumor response after WBRT suggest poor long-term control. Nieder et al. (1997) analyzed CT scans in 108 patients with 336 measurable lesions following WBRT of 30 Gy in 10 fractions daily. Complete and partial response rates at up to 3 months were 24% and 35%, respectively. Response rates were dependent on histology with, for example, 37% of small cell carcinoma and 35% of breast cancer patients having a complete response while 0% of renal cell carcinoma and melanoma tumors having a complete response. Smaller tumor volume and absence of necrosis were associated with improved complete response rates. Complete response rates were 39% for solid metastases, 15% if less than 50% necrosis, and 11% if 50% or more necrosis. Complete response rates were inversely related to volume, with 52% of metastases <0.5 cm^3 having a complete response versus 0% of tumors >10 cm^3. In a follow-up study, Nieder et al. (1998) analyzed the CT scans of 322 patients treated with different WBRT schedules and calculated the biologically effective dose (BED). Partial remission rates improved with increasing BED. Figure 8.1 illustrates the response in a cerebellar metastases after WBRT in a patient with multiple brain metastases from lung cancer. Data from randomized trials illustrate poor longer-term control. Actuarial 1-year local control following WBRT ranges between 0% and 14% (Patchell et al., 1990; Kondziolka et al., 1999). Overall, WBRT is unlikely to provide long-term control in most

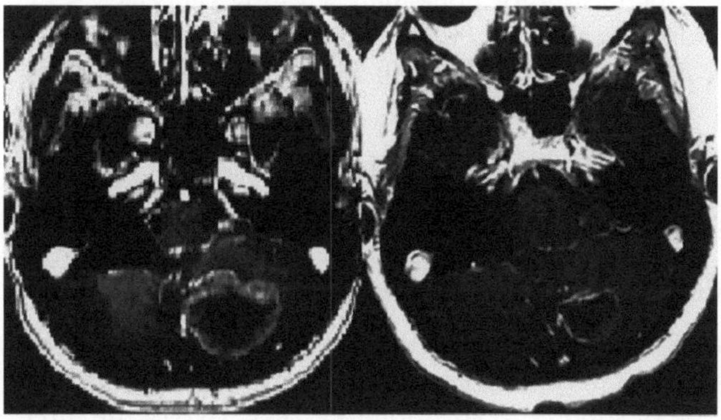

FIGURE 8.1 Response to treatment after WBRT in a patient with multiple brain metastases from lung cancer. (Left) A 3.6 by 3.1 cm left cerebellar tumor is present before treatment. (Right), 2 months post-WBRT of 30 Gy in 10 daily fractions, the tumor shrunk to 2.5 by 2.0 cm. The patient also had an improvement in gait.

TABLE 8.1 Recursive Partitioning Analysis Classification

Class	Factors	Median survival (months)
I	KPS ≥70, age <65, controlled primary tumor, no extracranial mets	7.1
II	All patients not in Class I or III	4.2
III	KPS <70	2.3

KPS: Karnosky performance status.

patients, however, favorable histology, small tumor volume and higher doses may result in improved local control.

Expected Survival after Whole Brain Radiation Therapy

Survival after WBRT varies from a few weeks to a few years. The RTOG has published two widely used and validated indices, the recursive partition analysis (RPA) (Gaspar et al., 1997) and the graded prognostic assessment (GPA) (Sperduto et al., 2008). The RPA (Table 8.1) categorizes patients into three classes based on age, Karnosky performance status (KPS) and control of extracranial disease. Class 1 patients (KPS ≥70, age <65, and controlled primary with no extracranial metastases) have the best median survival of 7.1 months, while Class 3 patients (KPS <70) have the worst median survival of 2.3 months. Class 2 patients (all others) have an intermediate median survival of 4.2 months. The GPA was developed to account for the number of brain metastases and remove the subjective factor of control of systemic disease. The GPA evaluates the factors of age, KPS, presence or absence of extracranial metastases and number of metastases (one, two to three, and more than three), and assigns a score for each and the overall sum predicts for median survival. The diagnosis-specific GPA (DS-GPA) improves on the GPA and utilizes histology as a key factor that predicts survival. For example, the significant prognostic factors for non-small cell lung cancer (NSCLC) and SCLC include the original four factors whereas, for breast and gastrointestinal cancers, the only significant prognostic factor is KPS (Sperduto et al., 2010).

WHOLE BRAIN RADIATION THERAPY WITH OTHER THERAPIES

Whole Brain Radiation Therapy and Surgery

The combination of surgery and WBRT in the treatment of brain metastases, in particular solitary metastases, has been well established. Three prospective randomized trials have evaluated the addition of surgery in addition to WBRT. Two of the three studies support the addition of surgery to WBRT in selected patients with good performance status, controlled extracranial disease, and a single brain metastasis. Patients had improved local control, increased duration of functional independence, and increased median survival. Factors found to be associated with longer survival included younger age, no extracranial disease, surgical resection, and longer interval from primary diagnosis to diagnosis of brain metastasis (Patchell et al., 1990; Noordijk et al., 1994).

The addition of WBRT following surgical resection has been addressed in two randomized trials. The first study by Patchell et al. (1998) had 95 adults with solitary brain metastases treated with complete surgical resection and randomly assigned to observation versus postoperative WBRT (50.4 Gy in 28 fractions). The WBRT arm was found to have a significantly decreased risk of local failure (10% vs 46% for observation), distant brain failure (14% vs 37%), and any brain failure (18% vs 70%), longer median time to local failure (more than 52 vs 27 weeks), and longer median time to any brain failure (more than 70 vs 26). Patients randomized to WBRT were significantly less likely to die neurologic deaths (14% vs 44%), though they had similar median survival and length of functional independence. The second trial by the EORTC randomized patients to WBRT (30 Gy in 10 fractions daily) or observation with one to three brain metastases treated with either surgery or radiosurgery. One-hundred and sixty patients underwent surgery, with 79 patients allocated to observation, and 81 allocated to adjuvant WBRT. WBRT reduced 2-year relapse at initial sites from 59% to 27%, and at new sites from 42% to 23%. WBRT reduced the frequency of salvage treatment, and death from intracranial progression (Kocher et al., 2011).

Whole Brain Radiation Therapy and Radiosurgery

Radiosurgery plays an important role in the treatment of brain metastases and indications for treatment alone or in combination with WBRT have been well established. The first trial by Kondziolka et al. (1999) randomized patients with two to four brain metastases treated with WBRT to radiosurgery boost or observation. WBRT consisted of 30 Gy delivered in 12 fractions. Radiosurgery was delivered at any time within 1 month before or after WBRT and consisted of a single dose of 16 Gy. The radiosurgery arm had a significantly improved time to local failure (median 36 months vs 6 months, $p = 0.0005$) and time to any brain failure (median 34 months vs 5 months, $p = 0.002$). Survival, however, was similar as several patients who failed WBRT alone underwent salvage radiosurgery. The second trial by RTOG randomized 333 patients with one to three brain metastases treated with WBRT (37.5 Gy in 15 fractions daily) to radiosurgery boost versus observation. Radiosurgery doses were based on tumor size according to RTOG 9005 toxicity information (Shaw et al., 2000). No survival benefit was seen in patients with multiple metastases. Univariate analysis demonstrated a significant survival advantage in the WBRT plus SRS group for the following patients: single brain metastases (median survival 6.5 vs 4.9 months, $p = 0.039$), patients with tumor size greater than 2 cm (median survival 6.5 vs 5.3 months, $p = 0.045$), and RPA class 1 patients (median survival 11.6 vs 9.6 months, $p = 0.045$). No differences were noted for time to intracranial tumor progression, neurologic death rate, or mental status, although the risk of developing local recurrence was 43% greater in the WBRT alone arm. The authors concluded that WBRT plus radiosurgery improved functional status for patients with one to three metastases and survival for patients with a single unresectable brain metastasis (Andrews et al., 2004).

Three randomized trials have evaluated the role of WBRT in addition to SRS in patients with less than three or four metastases. Aoyama et al. (2006) randomized 132 patients with one to four brain metastases, each less than 3 cm to WBRT and radiosurgery or radiosurgery alone. The primary endpoint was overall survival, and secondary endpoints included brain tumor recurrence, salvage brain treatment, functional preservation, toxicity, and cause of death. The median survival times were similar at 7.5 months in the WBRT plus SRS group and 8 months for SRS alone group ($p = 0.42$). The 1-year brain tumor recurrence rate was 46.8% in the WBRT plus SRS group and 76.4% for SRS alone group ($p < 0.0001$). Salvage brain treatment was less frequently required in the WBRT plus SRS group. Death from neurologic causes was similar between the groups.

Chang et al. (2009) conducted a randomized trial on patients (stopped early by the data monitoring committee) with one to three brain metastases and used neurocognition assessed through the validated Hopkins Verbal Learning Test (HVLT) as the primary endpoint. After 58 patients were recruited, the trial was stopped by the data monitoring committee as significant differences in learning and memory at 4 months were observed favoring the SRS alone arm. An absolute difference of 18% at 4 months was reported in the probability of neurocognitive decline favoring SRS alone. One-year local control (67% vs 100%) and 1-year distant brain control (45% vs 73%) favored the SRS and WBRT arm. Substantially more salvage procedures in the group treated with SRS alone (83% vs 7%) were observed. Although, this study was not powered to detect differences in overall survival (OS), median OS was 15 months vs 6 months favoring SRS alone. This apparent difference in OS favoring SRS alone, despite higher rates of recurrence, was likely at least in part due to imbalances in the two arms. More patients in the SRS and WBRT arm had liver or adrenal metastases and larger intracranial volume of disease.

The EORTC (Kocher et al., 2011) randomized 199 patients with one to three brain metastases who underwent SRS to observation ($n = 100$) vs WBRT ($n = 99$). The primary endpoint evaluated functional independence by measuring time to WHO performance status (PS) deterioration to more than 2. WBRT reduced the 2-year relapse rate both at initial sites from 31% to 19% ($p = 0.04$) and at new sites from 48% to 33% ($p = 0.023$). Salvage therapies were used more frequently in the observation arm. The median time to WHO PS more than 2 was 10.0 months in the observation arm and 9.5 months in the WBRT arm ($p = 0.71$). From these trials and a Cochrane systematic review (Tsao et al., 2012), there is evidence that the addition of WBRT to radiosurgery in patients with a limited number of brain metastases reduces intracranial relapses (local and distant) but fails to improve the duration of functional independence, likely has no impact on overall survival and is detrimental to neurocognitive function.

Whole Brain Radiation Therapy and Radiosensitizers

Radiosensitizers have been administered with RT to try to improve the efficacy of WBRT. A number of cytotoxic chemotherapeutic drugs (such as cisplatin and vinorelbine) and non-cytotoxic agents (such as temozolomide, metronidazole, misonidazole, bromodeoxyuridine, motexafin gadolinium and efaproxiral) have been used for their radiosensitizing properties, but have shown limited benefit when added to WBRT in clinical practice (Sahgal et al., 2012; Tsao et al., 2012).

One of the drugs studied is an analog of the magnetic resonance imaging (MRI) contrast agent thought to potentiate the effect of radiation. A phase III trial of WBRT with or without motexafin gadolinium was conducted on 401 patients. No significant differences were seen in median survival (5.2 months in the sensitizer arm compared to 4.9 months in the control arm) or median time to neurologic progression (9.5 months compared to 8.3 months). However, among 251 NSCLC patients, motexafin gadolinium was found to improve median time to neurologic progression (not reached compared to 7.4 months, $p = 0.048$) and overall neurologic function (Mehta et al., 2003). A follow-up randomized study of WBRT with or without motexafin gadolinium in NSCLC patients only, revealed a trend to improved time to neurologic progression (15 months in the motexafin gadolinium arm vs 10 months in the WBRT alone arm, $p = 0.12$) (Mehta et al., 2009). A similar selective benefit of the addition of efaproxiral (RSR13, Efraproxyn), a compound with radiosensitizing properties in hypoxic tissues, with WBRT was observed in the subgroup of patients with brain metastases from a breast cancer primary (Suh et al., 2006). A confirmatory trial in only breast cancer patients with brain metastases, however, failed to demonstrate improved survival (8.5 months in the efaproxiral arm compared to 7.5 months in the control arm, $p = 0.233$) (Suh et al., 2008).

Clinical trials with WBRT adding drugs that are known to cross the blood–brain barrier and have documented activity in different malignanices have been disappointing. The RTOG 0320 published in abstract form only after premature closure due to slow accrual, the results of a three-arm phase III trial in patients with one to three brain metastases from NSCLC. Patients received WBRT plus radiosurgery ($n = 126$) and were randomized to one of three arms; no further treatment in arm 1, combined with temozolomide (75 mg/m^2/day) in arm 2, or combined with erlotnib (150 mg/day) in arm 3. Temozolomide is an oral alkylating agent with activity in gliomas and malignant melanoma and readily crosses the blood–brain barrier (BBB) achieving significant concentrations in the central nervous system. Erlotinib is an inhibitor of the epidermal growth factor receptor (EGFR) tyrosine kinase pathway, and also readily crosses the BBB and is active against some NSCLCs. Neither the addition of temozolomide or erlotinib resulted in an improvement in OS, nor time to CNS progression compared to WBRT and SRS alone. In fact, median survival favored WBRT and SRS alone (13.4 months in arm 1, 6.3 months in arm 2, 6.1 months in arm 3). This surprising result was not related to excess toxicity (Sperduto et al., 2012).

In contrast to radiosensitizers, some studies have attempted to use drugs that may have neuroprotective properties. RTOG 0641 has recently presented in abstract form the results of a study on 508 eligible patients treated with WBRT of 37.5 Gy in 15 daily fractions, randomized to memantine 20 mg daily for 28 weeks versus placebo. Memantine is an N-methyl-D-aspartate (NMDA) receptor antagonist, and is approved for the treatment of moderate to severe Alzheimer's disease. The primary objective was assessment of memory on the Hopkins Verbal Learning Test-Revised (HVLT-R) at 24 weeks. The secondary endpoints were time to cognitive decline, overall survival and progression-free survival. Memantine resulted in less decline in delayed recognition at 24 weeks ($p = 0.015$), cognitive function failure at 24 weeks ($p = 0.01$) and increased the time to cognitive decline (HR 0.78, $p = 0.015$). Memantine also resulted in fewer declines in executive and global function. There were no differences in overall or progression-free survival (Brown et al., 2012).

WHOLE BRAIN RADIATION THERAPY RE-IRRADIATION

WBRT re-irradiation is usually avoided especially in patients who are expected to live more than 6 months. However, in poor prognosis patients, it may be repeated as radiation injury is less likely to happen during their lifetime. The most frequent retreatment doses are 25 Gy in 10 daily fractions, 20 Gy in 10 daily fractions, 15 Gy in five daily fractions, 20 Gy in eight daily fractions and 30 Gy in 30 twice daily fractions. Response rates are similar to initial WBRT treatment and median survival ranges between 3 and 6 months (Cooper et al., 1990; Wong et al., 1996; Abdel-Wahab et al., 1997; Sadikov et al., 2007). The risk of serious radiation toxicity following repeat WBRT is thought to be low in patients who are unlikely to survive beyond 6 months (Sahgal et al., 2012).

SIDE EFFECTS

Acute side effects of WBRT begin shortly after treatment and typically include hair loss, mild skin reaction, and fatigue. In patients with significant tumor-related edema, WBRT may lead to temporary worsening neurologic symptoms including increasing headaches, nausea or vomiting. Acute disruption of the BBB and subsequent brain edema are generally believed to be the underlying mechanisms of these acute symptoms after WBRT and patients are often treated with dexamethasone with symptomatic relief. Hair begins to regrow starting at 3 months post-treatment and skin reactions resolve after a few weeks. Fatigue in some patients may persist for several months but, in most patients, will improve in about 1 month. Slotman et al. (2007) reported on quality of life using the EORTC QLQ-C30 instrument in patients undergoing prophylactic cranial radiation (PCI) versus observation in patients with extensive stage SCLC. At 6 weeks and 3 months, patients receiving PCI had significantly higher rates and intensity of toxicities of hair loss, fatigue, appetite loss, nausea and vomiting and leg weakness. However, the impact of PCI was not clinically significant for global health status and role, emotional, and patient-reported cognitive functioning at 6 weeks and 3 months.

Late effects of WBRT usually include changes in memory and neurocognition. WBRT may lead to radiologic changes on CT and MRI that are associated with cognitive impairment. Leukoencephalopathy is a radiologic diagnosis with features of periventricular white matter abnormalities (hyper-intensity on T2 and fluid-attenuated inversion recovery sequences), ventricular dilatation and cortical atrophy (Figure 8.2). Radiation-induced leukoencephalopathy can lead to significant cognitive impairment and even dementia. In patients with pre-existing leukoaraiosis (a radiological finding of bilateral patchy or diffuse areas of hyperintensity on T2-weighted MRI), or impaired baseline cognition, it may be prudent to withhold WBRT, particularly, if extended survival is anticipated (Sahgal et al., 2012). Rates of leukoencephalopathy and dementia range between 2 and 10% after WBRT with conventional fractionation doses (DeAngelis et al., 1989; Conill et al., 2007).

Neurocognition

WBRT has an adverse effect on memory and neurocognition. Aoyama et al. (2007) utilized the mini-mental status exam (MMSE) as a tool to assess the impact of WBRT in

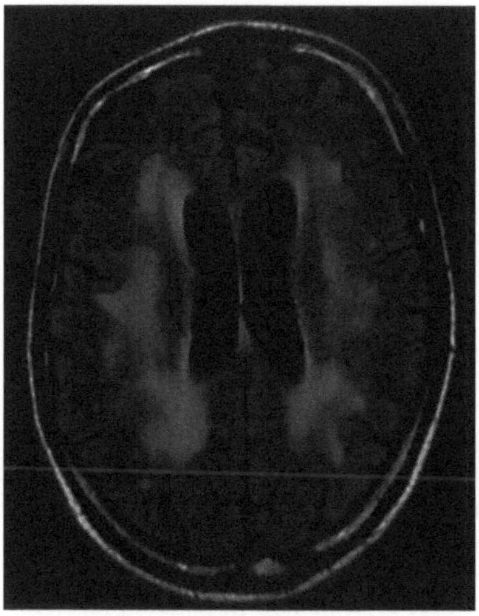

FIGURE 8.2 MRI of a patient with changes suggestive of leukoencephalopathy after retreatment with WBRT. Note the hyperintense T2-weighted signal changes and mild atrophy.

patients with up to four brain metastases. Although no significant differences were reported in MMSE between the two arms, they report the rate of decline in MMSE scores to be accelerated in patients treated with SRS alone due to more brain failures. They concluded that brain tumor control is the key to the preservation of neurocognition as opposed to the treatment effects of WBRT. The criticism of this study is that they used the MMSE, which is a screening test for dementia and is an insensitive tool to smaller changes in neurocognition (Meyers et al., 2004). In contrast, Chang et al. (2009) demonstrated that memory and neurocognition were adversely affected by the addition of WBRT using a validated tool for assessing neurocognition, the HVLT-R. Many centers have removed upfront WBRT treatment and do SRS for patients with up to four brain metastases, because of the increased risk of neurocognitive decline without improvement in survival.

THE FUTURE OF WHOLE BRAIN RADIATION THERAPY

Despite the significant advances in radiation technology, WBRT still remains the standard treatment for patients with multiple brain metastases particularly in patients with greater than four brain tumors. The role of WBRT in the setting of up to and even sometimes greater than 10 brain metastases is being challenged, with studies showing safety and efficacy of SRS alone. Attempts at decreasing the late effects of WBRT have yielded some promise with, for example, neuroprotectors such as memantine. However, confirmatory studies are needed before adoption into clinical practice. Another approach that is under investigation involves WBRT sparing of the hippocampus, the part of the brain that plays a critical role in the acquisition and consolidation of new memory and a central role in learning (Squire, 1993). The cognitive sequelae of WBRT may be related to irradiation of these structures. The RTOG has recently closed a phase II trial evaluating the role of hippocampal sparing WBRT and, as yet, no conclusion can be drawn as to the benefits or risks of this approach.

References

Abdel-Wahab, M.M., Wolfson, A.H., et al., 1997. The role of hyperfractionated re-irradiation in metastatic brain disease: a single institutional trial. Am. J. Clin. Oncol. 20, 158–160.

Andrews, D.W., Scott, C.B., et al., 2004. Whole brain radiation therapy with or without stereotactic radiosurgery boost for patients with one to three brain metastases: phase III results of the RTOG 9508 randomised trial. Lancet 363, 1665–1672.

Aoyama, H., Shirato, H., et al., 2006. Stereotactic radiosurgery plus whole-brain radiation therapy vs stereotactic radiosurgery alone for treatment of brain metastases: a randomized controlled trial. J. Am. Med. Assoc. 295, 2483–2491.

Aoyama, H., Tago, M., et al., 2007. Neurocognitive function of patients with brain metastasis who received either whole brain radiotherapy plus stereotactic radiosurgery or radiosurgery alone. Int. J. Radiat. Oncol. Biol. Phys. 68, 1388–1395.

Borgelt, B., Gelber, R., et al., 1980. The palliation of brain metastases: final results of the first two studies by the Radiation Therapy Oncology Group. Int. J. Radiat. Oncol. Biol. Phys. 6, 1–9.

Borgelt, B., Gelber, R., et al., 1981. Ultra-rapid high dose irradiation schedules for the palliation of brain metastases: final results of the first two studies by the Radiation Therapy Oncology Group. Int. J. Radiat. Oncol. Biol. Phys. 7, 1633–1638.

Brown, P.D., Shook, S., et al., 2012. Memantine for the prevention of cognitive dysfunction in patients receiving whole-brain radiation therapy (WBRT): first report of RTOG 0614, a placebo-controlled, double-blind, randomized trial. Int. J. Radiat. Oncol. Biol. Phys. 84, S1–S2.

Chang, E.L., Wefel, J.S., et al., 2009. Neurocognition in patients with brain metastases treated with radiosurgery or radiosurgery plus whole-brain irradiation: a randomised controlled trial. Lancet Oncol. 10, 1037–1044.

Coia, L.R., 1992. The role of radiation therapy in the treatment of brain metastases. Int. J. Radiat. Oncol. Biol. Phys. 23, 229–238.

Conill, C., Berenguer, J., et al., 2007. Incidence of radiation-induced leukoencephalopathy after whole brain radiotherapy in patients with brain metastases. Clin. Transl. Oncol. 9, 590–595.

Cooper, J.S., Steinfeld, A.D., et al., 1990. Cerebral metastases: value of reirradiation in selected patients. Radiology 174, 883–885.

DeAngelis, L.M., Delattre, J.Y., et al., 1989. Radiation-induced dementia in patients cured of brain metastases. Neurology 39, 789–796.

Gaspar, L., Scott, C., et al., 1997. Recursive partitioning analysis (RPA) of prognostic factors in three Radiation Therapy Oncology Group (RTOG) brain metastases trials. Int. J. Radiat. Oncol. Biol. Phys. 37, 745–751.

Kocher, M., Soffietti, R., et al., 2011. Adjuvant whole-brain radiotherapy versus observation after radiosurgery or surgical resection of one to three cerebral metastases: results of the EORTC 22952-26001 study. J. Clin. Oncol. 29, 134–141.

Kondziolka, D., Patel, A., et al., 1999. Stereotactic radiosurgery plus whole brain radiotherapy versus radiotherapy alone for patients with multiple brain metastases. Int. J. Radiat. Oncol. Biol. Phys. 45, 427–434.

Kurtz, J.M., Gelber, R., et al., 1981. The palliation of brain metastases in a favorable patient population: a randomized clinical trial by the Radiation Therapy Oncology Group. Int. J. Radiat. Oncol. Biol. Phys. 7, 891–895.

Mehta, M.P., Rodrigus, P., et al., 2003. Survival and neurologic outcomes in a randomized trial of motexafin gadolinium and whole-brain radiation therapy in brain metastases. J. Clin. Oncol. 21, 2529–2536.

Mehta, M.P., Shapiro, W.R., et al., 2009. Motexafin gadolinium combined with prompt whole brain radiotherapy prolongs time to neurologic progression in non-small-cell lung cancer patients with brain metastases: results of a phase III trial. Int. J. Radiat. Oncol. Biol. Phys. 73, 1069–1076.

Meyers, C.A., Smith, J.A., et al., 2004. Neurocognitive function and progression in patients with brain metastases treated with whole-brain radiation and motexafin gadolinium: results of a randomized phase III trial. J. Clin. Oncol. 22, 157–165.

Murray, K.J., Scott, C., et al., 1997. A randomized phase III study of accelerated hyperfractionation versus standard in patients with unresected brain metastases: a report of the Radiation Therapy Oncology Group (RTOG) 9104. Int. J. Radiat. Oncol. Biol. Phys. 39, 571–574.

Nieder, C., Berberich, W., et al., 1997. Tumor-related prognostic factors for remission of brain metastases after radiotherapy. Int. J. Radiat. Oncol. Biol. Phys. 39, 25–30.

Nieder, C., Nestle, U., et al., 1998. Dose/effect relationships for brain metastases. J. Cancer. Res. Clin. Oncol. 124, 346–350.

Noordijk, E.M., Vecht, C.J., et al., 1994. The choice of treatment of single brain metastasis should be based on extracranial tumor activity and age. Int. J. Radiat. Oncol. Biol. Phys. 29, 711–717.

Patchell, R.A., Tibbs, P.A., et al., 1990. A randomized trial of surgery in the treatment of single metastases to the brain. N. Engl. J. Med. 322, 494–500.

Patchell, R.A., Tibbs, P.A., et al., 1998. Postoperative radiotherapy in the treatment of single metastases to the brain: a randomized trial. J. Am. Med. Assoc. 280, 1485–1489.

Patel, J.K., Didolkar, M.S., et al., 1978. Metastatic pattern of malignant melanoma. A study of 216 autopsy cases. Am. J. Surg. 135, 807–810.

Sadikov, E., Bezjak, A., et al., 2007. Value of whole brain re-irradiation for brain metastases – single centre experience. Clin. Oncol. 19, 532–538.

Sahgal, A., Soliman, H., et al., 2012. Whole-brain radiation therapy of brain metastasis. Prog. Neurol. Surg. 25, 82–95.

Shaw, E., Scott, C., et al., 2000. Single dose radiosurgical treatment of recurrent previously irradiated primary brain tumors and brain metastases: final report of RTOG protocol 90-05. Int. J. Radiat. Oncol. Biol. Phys. 47, 291–298.

Slotman, B., Faivre-Finn, C., et al., 2007. Prophylactic cranial irradiation in extensive small-cell lung cancer. N. Engl. J. Med. 357, 664–672.

Sperduto, P.W., Berkey, B., et al., 2008. A new prognostic index and comparison to three other indices for patients with brain metastases: an analysis of 1,960 patients in the RTOG database. Int. J. Radiat. Oncol. Biol. Phys. 70, 510–514.

Sperduto, P.W., Chao, S.T., et al., 2010. Diagnosis-specific prognostic factors, indexes, and treatment outcomes for patients with newly diagnosed brain metastases: a multi-institutional analysis of 4,259 patients. Int. J. Radiat. Oncol. Biol. Phys. 77, 655–661.

Sperduto, P.W., Wang, M., et al., 2012. Abstract 736: RTOG 0320:A phase III trial comparing whole brain radiation therapy (WBRT) and stereotactic radiosurgery (SRS) alone versus WBRT with temozolomide (TMZ) or erlotinib for non-small cell lung cancer (NSCLC) and 1-3 brain metastases. Cancer Res. 72, 1538.

Squire, L.R., 1993. The hippocampus and spatial memory. Trends Neurosci. 16, 56–57.

Suh, J.H., Stea, B., et al., 2006. Phase III study of efaproxiral as an adjunct to whole-brain radiation therapy for brain metastases. J. Clin. Oncol. 24, 106–114.

Suh, J.H., Stea, B., et al., 2008. Results of the phase III ENRICH (RT-016) study of efaproxiral administered concurrent with whole brain radiation therapy (WBRT) in women with brain metastases from breast cancer. Int. J. Radiat. Oncol. Biol. Phys. 72, S50.

Tsao, M.N., Lloyd, N., et al., 2012. Whole brain radiotherapy for the treatment of newly diagnosed multiple brain metastases. Cochrane Database Syst. Rev. 4, CD003869.

Wong, W.W., Schild, S.E., et al., 1996. Analysis of outcome in patients reirradiated for brain metastases. Int. J. Radiat. Oncol. Biol. Phys. 34, 585–590.

CHAPTER

9

Synovial Sarcoma Metastasized to the Brain

Nikolaos Sakellaridis and Lygeri Sakellaridi

OUTLINE

Introduction	93
Brain Synovial Sarcomas	93
Synovial Sarcoma	94
Epidemiology	94
Clinical Features	94
Radiology	95
Pathology	95
Genetics	96
Treatment	96
Future Treatment Issues	97
Prognosis	97
Head and Neck Synovial Sarcomas	98
Does a Primary Brain Synovial Sarcoma Exist?	98
Metastases in Continuity Through the Skull Base	98
Hematogenous Metastases to the Brain	99
Brain Synovial Sarcoma Classification	99
Treatment of Intracranial Synovial Sarcomas	99
References	100

INTRODUCTION

Synovial sarcoma is a distinct mesenchymal spindle cell tumor, which displays variable epithelial differentiation and has a characteristic chromosomal translocation t(X; 18) (p11; q11). It can rarely metastasize to the brain.

BRAIN SYNOVIAL SARCOMAS

By searching Pubmed for synovial sarcoma and brain, we could find 38 references.

M.A. *Hayat (ed): Brain Metastases from Primary Tumors, Volume 1*
DOI: http://dx.doi.org/10.1016/B978-0-12-800896-6.00009-7

© 2014 Elsevier Inc. All rights reserved.

Nine of them described nine cases of brain synovial sarcoma. One of these patients was the same in two papers, thus leaving eight patients. Three cases were described as primary brain synovial sarcoma. They were dura based. All were treated surgically (Kleinschmidt-DeMasters et al., 1998; Horbinski et al., 2008; Lin et al., 2012). Another five cases were described as metastases: one of them was treated surgically, due to cerebral hemorrhage (Przkora et al., 2003), one with biopsy and conservative treatment and three conservatively (Kaufman and Tsukada, 1976; Singh et al., 2011).

Another 33 cases of synovial sarcoma of the brain were found by looking at the references of the previous articles and mainly by using the first 200 references of Google Scholar for synovial sarcoma and brain. These patients were usually described as part of large series of synovial sarcomas, soft tissue sarcomas or sarcomas in general. Their description was consequently not as detailed as in the previous cases. One of these patients has a dural-based primary synovial sarcoma of the brain.

All these 41 patients were the material of our present paper. We could not find any systematic review of brain synovial sarcoma in the literature.

In order to classify properly brain synovial sarcoma, we must first review synovial sarcoma in general.

SYNOVIAL SARCOMA

Epidemiology

Synovial sarcomas constitute ≈8% of soft tissue sarcomas. They can occur at any age, but almost 90% occur in young adults before the age of 50 and most between the ages of 15 and 35 years. There is a slight male preponderance (ratio ≈1.2:1).

Clinical Features

There is usually a mass of 3–10 cm, with or without pain. Location is mainly 71% in the lower and 16% in the upper extremities (Palmerini et al., 2009). Local symptoms in specific sites can also be observed. Growth is often slow, with a mean history of 2–4 years; 20-year histories have been described. Within the soft tissues, the neoplasm is typically situated in deeper structures, such as tendon or muscle rather than the subcutis. General symptoms related to malignancies can be reported, such as fatigue. At the time of diagnosis, ≈10% of cases present with metastases.

The natural course of the disease is such that many patients will experience recurrence of the primary tumor and/or metastatic disease. Up to 50% can recur locally. Metastatic disease occurs in around 50% of patients. The most common sites of metastasis are the lungs, occurring in 74–81% of patients with metastatic disease, lymph nodes, occurring in 3–23%, and bone, occurring in 10–20%.

Among the different grading systems available, the French system, FNCLCC (French Federation of Cancer Centers Sarcoma Group), is the most often used for adult-type soft tissue sarcomas (Guillou et al., 1997). It is a score system in which the sum of D (differentiation; 'D3' by default in synovial sarcoma), M (mitoses: below 10/10 high power fields (HPF); between 10 and 19/10 HPF; more than 19/10 HPF) and N (necrosis: absent; less than 50%; more than 50%) gives the grade 1, 2 or 3. Even if in therapeutic protocols synovial sarcoma is considered among high-grade sarcomas by definition, the FNCLCC grade is reported as its most predictive histological factor. The NCI grading system is more common in the USA (Costa et al., 1984).

Radiology

In the case of synovial sarcoma, a computed tomography (CT) scan will identify calcifications in approximately one-third of cases. Only a minority are bone destructive.

The magnetic resonance imaging (MRI) appearance most indicative of the tumor is an inhomogeneous septated mass with well-defined margins in the majority of cases, located close to a joint, a tendon, or bursa. In soft tissue lesions, MRI shows variation in intensity and enhancement. Most tumors are relatively iso- or hypointense compared to muscle and iso- or slightly hyperintense compared to fat and, in cystic areas, show a high fluid signal. Hyperintense lesions in both T1- and T2-weighted images suggest hemorrhage. Such lesions are generally uncommon in most soft-tissue sarcomas other than synovial sarcoma. Triple signal intensity and fluid–fluid levels have been described (O' Sullivan et al., 2008).

Pathology

Many synovial sarcomas arise near joints. It was initially thought that areas of epithelial differentiation were of synovial origin and hence the name. We now know that synovial sarcoma is unrelated to synovium. It is now thought to arise from primitive undifferentiated mesenchymal cells (Enzinger and Weiss, 1993). Epithelial and some spindle cells of the tumor express cytokeratins and epithelial membrane antigen (EMA), antigens not expressed by synovial cells. Its epithelial cells have ultrastructural features identical to those of normal epithelial cells, such as desmosomes, microvilli, tight junctions and basal lamina. Less than 5% of cases originate within a joint or bursa. Over 80% originate in deep soft tissue of the extremities. Approximately 5% arise in the head and neck region. Any site can be affected. The tumor is usually 3–10cm in diameter. It can be circumscribed or infiltrative. It is yellow-tan or gray. It can be multinodular, multicystic and can have gross calcification and areas of necrosis.

Histologically, it can be biphasic or monophasic. Biphasic synovial sarcoma has distinct epithelial and spindle cell components, which can merge in some areas. The epithelial cells have ovoid nuclei and abundant cytoplasm. They can form solid nests, glands with lumina or papillary structures. The spindle cells are small, uniform, with sparse cytoplasm and indistinct cell borders. The spindle cell component can exhibit thick collagen bundles, calcification or a hemangiopericytoma-like vascular network, which, when present, is distinctive for the tumor. Monophasic synovial sarcoma resembles the spindle cell component of the biphasic variety. Purely glandular monophasic synovial sarcoma can theoretically exist, but it is indistinguishable from adenocarcinoma without cytogenetics. Poorly differentiated synovial sarcomas constitute up to 20% of cases and exhibit a predominance of areas with high cellularity, closely packed cells, numerous mitoses and often necrosis.

Distant metastases of biphasic synovial sarcoma may contain either component alone or both. In the first case, it is usually the spindle cell component that is solely present. Metastases of monophasic synovial sarcoma almost always remain monophasic.

Approximately, 90% of all synovial sarcomas express cytokeratins, mainly in their epithelial component but also in about 50% of the spindle cells of the monophasic and 70% of the biphasic tumors. Cytokeratins 7 and 19, expressed in synovial sarcoma, are absent in malignant peripheral nerve sheath tumor and Ewing sarcoma, thus helping in the differential diagnosis. Epithelial membrane antigen is also usually expressed and can be especially helpful in the poorly differentiated subtype where 95% of cases are positive. S-100 is detectable in 30% of cases and CD-99 in 60%. BCL2 is diffusely expressed in all cases, especially in spindle cells. CD34 is usually negative. Carcinoembryonic antigen (CEA) is expressed focally in a few cases, mainly in the epithelial cells. Among muscle markers, calponin is usually found, desmin is absent. Vimentin is present in 85% of the spindle and 15–30% of the epithelial component.

Genetics

The t(X; 18) (p11; q11) translocation is present in more than 90% of the reported cases. This translocation probably arises exclusively in synovial sarcomas. Variant, more complex translocations have also been described. The genes affected by the translocation have been described: SS18 (a.k.a. SYT) from chromosome 18 and SSX1, SSX2 and SSX4 from the X chromosome.

The SS18 gene is expressed ubiquitously and codes for a 418 amino acid protein. The SSX gene family encompasses at least five members of 188 amino acid proteins with high sequence homologies. After the translocation, SS18–SSX fusion proteins are identified. During this fusion, the QPGY domain of SS18 is interrupted and may lose its function. The CRAB domain of SSX is also lost during the fusion process.

Biphasic tumors appear uniformly to contain the SS18–SSX1 fusion transcript, whereas equal numbers of monophasic tumor contain the SS18–SSX1 and SS18–SSX2 fusion transcripts.

Patients with SYT–SSX2 expressing tumors have a significantly better prognosis when compared to those with SYT–SSX1 tumors in terms of rates of metastasis and overall survival (Kawai et al., 1998). There is some debate about whether the molecular observation itself is definitional of synovial sarcoma. Molecular testing is not required if the diagnosis of synovial sarcoma is certain or probable on the basis of clinical, histologic, and immunohistochemical evaluation. However, it proved to be very helpful or necessary when its diagnosis was only possible and was challenged by other tumor types, mainly other spindle cell sarcomas, round cell sarcomas, carcinomas, myoepitheliomas, and epithelioid fibrosarcomas (Coindre et al., 2003).

Treatment

The main treatment of synovial sarcoma is en bloc surgical resection and radiotherapy. Adequate margins are >1 cm in all directions around the tumor.

At surgery, a positive margin at excision and larger tumor size independently predict adverse local control. In cases of unresected tumor, delayed tumor resection and radiotherapy should be offered. Any influence of delayed definitive surgery in cases of unplanned soft-tissue sarcoma surgery is likely to be of minor clinical importance (Ilkyu et al., 2011).

Radiotherapy is offered, especially in adults, and when no negative margin at surgical excision can be obtained. In children, radiotherapy is not standard treatment and must be individualized. It has been shown that postoperative radiotherapy significantly improves local recurrence-free survival, but there is no proof of effectiveness for distant recurrence-free or overall survival (Italiano et al., 2009).

Evidence for a well-defined role of chemotherapy to improve survival in localized synovial sarcoma remains elusive (Al-Hussaini et al., 2011). Synovial sarcomas are considered to be of medium sensitivity to chemotherapy, between the chemosensitive rhabdomyosarcoma and various non-chemosensitive sarcomas. Chemotherapy is more readily offered to children. The standard first-line therapy is doxorubicin. Compared to doxorubicin alone, combination chemotherapy including ifosfamide significantly improves response rate but not 1-year survival, due to higher rates of adverse effects. Response rates of approximately 50% can be expected.

In cases of advanced disease, surgical removal of metastases is not associated with improved prognosis (Spurrell et al., 2005). Palliative chemotherapy is the mainstay of treatment in the advanced disease setting of locally advanced, inoperable or metastatic cases. In a small subset this treatment can be curative or a response may be observed that may render the disease resectable. More than 20% of soft-tissue sarcoma patients treated with second-line chemotherapy can obtain prolonged benefit for over 6 months (Minchom et al., 2010).

Future Treatment Issues

As with other soft tissue sarcomas, in the coming years we expect to improve our understanding of synovial sarcoma, and we particularly need novel therapeutic approaches. The specific chromosomal translocation occurring in synovial sarcoma, as well as the tyrosine kinases' receptors identified, epidermal growth factor receptors (EGFR) and HER-2/neu, may become the targets of new molecular agents specifically designed to influence the tumor's biology. Clinical investigative trials on targeted therapy are ongoing. Similarly, further studies are needed to investigate the role of the Bcl-2 antisense oligonucleotide therapy, as most tumors overexpress the anti-apoptotic protein Bcl-2 that correlates with tumor growth, chemoresistance and poor outcome in various cancers. Anti-angiogenic agents have also been tried with promising results (Do et al., 2012).

Prognosis

Five-year survival is 36–76% and 10-year survival is 20–63%. Up to 50% of synovial sarcomas recur, usually within 2 years, but sometimes up to 30 years after diagnosis.

About 50% metastasize, mainly to lungs, bone and regional lymph nodes.

A better outcome is obtained when the tumor is totally removed, with postoperative radiotherapy, in childhood patients and younger age, in tumors <5cm in diameter, in those having <10 mitoses per 10 HPF and in the calcifying variant. It has been suggested that cases of the SS18–SSX2 variant, which is found in monophasic synovial sarcomas, have a better prognosis. A worse prognosis is expected in cases presenting with metastases, in patients with poorly differentiated synovial sarcoma, as well as in cases with extended necrosis. In a major clinical study with 213 children and adolescents and 1055 adults, no major differences in stage distribution (localized, regional, and distant stage) were observed comparing the two age groups. The estimated 5-year cancer-specific survival was 83% for children/adolescents and 62% for adults. Female sex, non-black race, tumors located in the extremities, localized tumors, and tumors

<5 cm in size were associated with better survival. In multivariate analysis, adult patients had statistically significantly higher mortality rates than children after adjusting for other variables (Sultan et al., 2009).

HEAD AND NECK SYNOVIAL SARCOMAS

Theses constitute around 5% of the total cases. They can arise in the orofacial area, tongue, tonsils, larynx, trachea, parapharynx, nasal cavity, maxilla, frontal sinus, orbit, sellar area and cavernous sinus (Eeles et al., 1993; Scheithauer et al., 2007).

Synovial sarcomas of the head and neck have comparable imaging features to their counterparts at the extremities; however, well-defined homogeneous tumors may be difficult to distinguish from benign lesions such as neurofibromas. They can cause intracranial metastases by continuity through the skull base. Five-year survival is ≈40–55%.

DOES A PRIMARY BRAIN SYNOVIAL SARCOMA EXIST?

Its existence is not certain and anyhow it is distinctly rare. Only four cases have been described in the literature and all of them were dura based. One could suppose that primary intracranial synovial sarcomas do not exist. If so, we must assume that an unknown primary tumor has been missed or that the pathological diagnosis was not correct. On the other hand, at least one case had a long history almost precluding the existence of a primary in another location and two more were verified by the characteristic translocation in molecular analysis. We believe that dura-based primary synovial sarcoma of the brain should be accepted as a very rare entity, because this tumor can appear in any location. We do not know its exact cell of provenance, but we must remark that the dura-based origin of the described cases is compatible with the theory that synovial sarcomas arise from primitive undifferentiated mesenchymal cells, because dura mater is derived from mesoderm.

We also want to emphasize that many cases have been described arising from neural tissue, especially peripheral nerves. At least 12 cases of intraneural synovial sarcoma have been described in the literature. Four intraneural synovial sarcomas have been reported arising from the median nerve, along with one apiece from the radial, common digital, posterior tibialis, peroneal, and facial nerves and one from each of the S1 root, C7 root, and brachial plexus (Lipira et al., 2010).

METASTASES IN CONTINUITY THROUGH THE SKULL BASE

About 10% of patients with synovial sarcoma involving the skull base present with intracranial tumor extension (Ji et al., 2011). Even if these cases are metastases in continuity to the brain, in such cases, there only exists one primary synovial sarcoma without hematogenous metastases. In these patients, radical surgery should be offered early, if possible. En bloc resection and even more wide clean margins are not easily obtained in brain surgery. Perineural and brain invasion can have an adverse impact on overall survival.

Modern techniques of skull base surgery and neurosurgery can help improve our results. Further treatment with radiotherapy and/or chemotherapy should be readily offered to these surgically treated patients for local control, because surgical margins are likely to be close, in order to preserve important neurovascular structures.

Sometimes surgery does not have any possibility of leading to cure, as for example when we observe leptomeningeal spread of the tumor. A relevant case of leptomeningeal spread from a paraspinal tumor has been described (Puffer et al., 2011). Other patients with invasion of eloquent brain, nerve or vessel areas are also usually treated only with radiotherapy, radiosurgery and/or chemotherapy. The same is obviously true when skull base invasion is due to hematogenous metastases. Prognosis for the whole group is generally grave, with more than half of the patients dying from local recurrence or metastasis within a year.

HEMATOGENOUS METASTASES TO THE BRAIN

These should generally be treated like hematogenous metastases to other body areas, with radiotherapy and chemotherapy. Some patients have been surgically treated, for example when the tumor has hemorrhaged and hematoma removal is necessary. In some patients without a clear diagnosis, biopsy should be offered. Some authors believe that sarcoma's metastases to the brain should be operated if the neurologic state of the patient is good (Yoshida et al., 2000). Prognosis is generally not good.

BRAIN SYNOVIAL SARCOMA CLASSIFICATION

We can conclude that the main distinction in patients with intracranial synovial sarcoma is between those with a primary tumor and those with terminal hematogenous metastases. Primary synovial sarcoma is treated with surgery, radiotherapy and/or chemotherapy, as already described, with the aim of obtaining cure. Its hematogenous metastases are mostly treated with a palliative aim. We consequently propose the following classification scheme for brain synovial sarcoma:

Primary brain synovial sarcoma. All four described cases were dura based.

Metastases in continuity from head and neck synovial sarcoma. In these cases, it is as if there exists only one primary tumor and radical treatment can offer possible cure. These cases should be considered equivalent to primary synovial sarcoma, even if in reality they are metastases in continuity. If possible, they should be radically removed.

Hematogenous metastases from remote areas. In these cases treatment is nowadays almost always palliative.

TREATMENT OF INTRACRANIAL SYNOVIAL SARCOMAS

All four cases described as primary intracranial synovial sarcoma were described as case reports. They were dura based and surgical treatment was offered. Surgical series with total surgical resection of sarcomas of the skull base and good results have been published (Shotton et al., 1992). Orbital involvement, perineural and cranial invasion along with other factors were statistically significant for their adverse impact on overall survival in these cases. Local recurrence was associated with tumors located in the infratemporal space, perineural invasion, pathological grade 3, and tumor size >5 cm (Ji et al., 2011).

Gamma knife radiosurgery can also be used for intracranial sarcomatous metastases. A local tumor control rate of 88% was achieved. New remote brain metastases developed in one-third of patients. The median survival after diagnosis of intracranial metastasis was 16 months, and the 1-year survival rate was 61% (Flannery et al., 2010).

References

Al-Hussaini, H., Hogg, D., Blackstein, M.E., et al., 2011. Clinical features, treatment, and outcome in 102 adult and pediatric patients with localized high-grade synovial sarcoma. Sarcoma 2011, 231789.

Coindre, J.M., Pelmus, M., Hostein, I., Lussan, C., Bui, B.N., Guillou, L., 2003. Should molecular testing be required for diagnosing synovial sarcoma? A prospective study of 204 cases. Cancer 98, 2700–2707.

Costa, J., Wesley, R.A., Glatstein, E., Rosenberg, S., 1984. The grading of soft tissue sarcomas. Cancer 53, 530–541.

Do, K., Doroshow, J.H., Kummar, S., 2012. Antiangiogenic approaches for the treatment of advanced synovial sarcomas. Curr. Opin. Oncol. 24, 425–430.

Eeles, R.A., Fisher, C., A'Hern, R.P., et al., 1993. Head and neck sarcomas: prognostic factors and implications for treatment. Br. J. Cancer 68, 201–207.

Enzinger, F.M., Weiss, S.W., 1993. Soft tissue tumors. Synovial Sarcoma. Mosby, St Louis, pp. 757–786.

Flannery, T., Kano, H., Niranjan, A., et al., 2010. Gamma knife radiosurgery as a therapeutic strategy for intracranial sarcomatous metastases. Int. J. Radiat. Oncol. Biol. Phys. 76, 513–519.

Guillou, L., Coindre, J.M., Bonichon, F., et al., 1997. Comparative study of the National Cancer Institute and French Federation of Cancer Centers Sarcoma Group grading systems in a population of 410 adults patients with soft tissue sarcoma. J. Clin. Oncol. 15, 350–362.

Horbinski, C., Cieply, K., Bejjani, G.K., McFadden, K., 2008. Primary intracranial dural-based synovial sarcoma with an unusual SYT fluorescence in situ hybridization pattern. J. Neurosurg. 109, 897–903.

Ilkyu, H., Hyun, G.K., Seung, C.K., Jay, R.C., Han-Soo, K., 2011. Does delayed reexcision affect outcome after unplanned excision for soft tissue sarcoma? Clin. Orthop. Relat. Res. 469, 877–883.

Italiano, A., Penel, N., Robin, Y.M., et al., 2009. Neo/adjuvant chemotherapy does not improve outcome in resected primary synovial sarcoma: a study of the French Sarcoma Group. Ann. Oncol. 20, 425–430.

Ji, T., Ma, C.Y., Ow, A., Wang, L.Z., Sun, J., Zhang, C.P., 2011. Synovial sarcoma involving skull base – a retrospective analysis of diagnosis and treatment of 21 cases in one institution. Oral Oncol. 47, 671–676.

Kaufman, J., Tsukada, Y., 1976. Synovial sarcoma with brain metastases. Report of a case responding to supervoltage irradiation and review of the literature. Cancer 38, 96–99.

Kawai, A., Woodruff, J., Healey, J.H., Brennan, M.F., Antonescu, C.R., Ladanyi, M., 1998. SYT-SSX gene fusion as a determinant of morphology and prognosis in synovial sarcoma. N. Engl. J. Med. 338, 153–160.

Kleinschmidt-DeMasters, B.K., Mierau, G.W., Sze, C.I., et al., 1998. Unusual dural and skull-based mesenchymal neoplasms: a report of four cases. Hum. Pathol. 29, 240–245.

Lin, Y.J., Yang, Q.X., Tian, X.Y., Li, B., Li, Z., 2012. Unusual primary intracranial dural-based poorly differentiated synovial sarcoma with t(X; 18)(p11; q11). Neuropathology doi: 10.1111/j.1440-1789.2012.01320.x.

Lipira, A.B., Kasukurthi, R., Ray, W.Z., Pruzansky, M.E., Mackinnon, S.E., 2010. Intraneural synovial sarcoma of the median nerve. Rare Tumors 2, e32.

Minchom, A., Jones, R.L., Fisher, C., et al., 2010. Clinical benefit of second-line palliative chemotherapy in advanced soft-tissue sarcoma. Sarcoma 2010, 264360.

O' Sullivan, P.J., Harris, A.C., Munk, P.L., 2008. Radiological features of synovial cell sarcoma. Br. J. Radiol. 81, 346–356.

Palmerini, E., Staals, E.L., Alberghini, M., et al., 2009. Synovial sarcoma. Cancer 115, 2988–2998.

Przkora, R., Vogel, P., Ullrich, O.W., Knüchel, R., Jauch, K.W., Bolder, U., 2003. Synovial sarcoma – unusual presentation with cerebral hemorrhage. Arch. Orthop. Trauma Surg. 123, 376–378.
Puffer, R.C., Daniels, D.J., Giannini, C., Pichelmann, M.A., Rose, P.S., Clarke, M.J., 2011. Synovial sarcoma of the spine: A report of three cases and review of the literature. Surg. Neurol. Int. 2, 18.
Scheithauer, B.W., Silva, A.I., Kattner, K., Seibly, J., Oliveira, A.M., Kovacs, K., 2007. Synovial sarcoma of the sellar region. Neuro. Oncol. 9, 454–459.
Shotton, J.C., Kuhwoede, R., Fisch, U., 1992. Mesenchymal tumors of the skull base with particular reference to surgical management and outcome. Skull Base Surg. 2, 112–117.
Singh, A., Kate, M.P., Nair, M.D., Kesavadas, C., Kapilamoorthy, T.R., 2011. Bilateral perisylvian infarct: a rare cause and a rare occurrence. Singapore Med. J. 52, e62–e65.
Spurrell, E.L., Fisher, C., Thomas, J.M., Judson, I.R., 2005. Prognostic factors in advanced synovial sarcoma: an analysis of 104 patients treated at the Royal Marsden Hospital. Ann. Oncol. 16, 437–444.
Sultan, I., Rodriguez-Galindo, C., Saab, R., Yasir, S., Casanova, M., Ferrari, A., 2009. Comparing children and adults with synovial sarcoma in the Surveillance, Epidemiology, and End Results program, 1983 to 2005: an analysis of 1268 patients. Cancer 115, 3537–3547.
Yoshida, S., Morii, K., Watanabe, M., Saito, T., 2000. Brain metastasis in patients with sarcoma. Surg. Neurol. 54, 160–164.

PART II

BRAIN METASTASES FROM NON-SMALL CELL LUNG CARCINOMA

10 *Multiple Small Brain Metastases with Limited Focal Brain Edema from Non-Small Cell Lung Cancer with Epidermal Growth Factor Receptor Mutations* 105

11 *Brain Metastasis of Patients with Lung Adenocarcinoma: Epidermal Growth Factor Receptor Mutations and Response to Whole-Brain Radiation Therapy* 113

12 *Metastatic Spread of Lung Cancer to Brain and Liver: Role of CX3CR1* 123

13 *Solitary Brain Metastasis from Non-Small Cell Lung Cancer: Treatment with Linac-Based Stereotactic Radiosurgery* 131

14 *Brain Metastases from Non-Small Cell Lung Cancer: Clinical Benefits of Erlotinib and Gefitinib* 141

15 *Bispecific Targeted Toxin DTATEGF Against Metastatic NSCLC Brain Tumors* 157

16 *Intracranial Disease in Patients with Non-Small Cell Lung Cancer: Treatment with Erlotinib* 169

17 *Radiation Management of Synchronous Brain Metastases from Non-Small Cell Lung Cancer* 181

CHAPTER

10

Multiple Small Brain Metastases with Limited Focal Brain Edema from Non-Small Cell Lung Cancer with Epidermal Growth Factor Receptor Mutations

Akimasa Sekine

OUTLINE

Introduction 106

Epidermal Growth Factor Receptor Mutations 106

Multiple Brain Metastases and EGFR Mutations: Influence of the Exon 19 Deletion on Radiographical Features 107

Miliary Brain Metastases and EGFR Mutations 108

Management of Brain Metastases from NSCLC with EGFR Mutations 108

Management of Neurologically Asymptomatic NSCLC Patients with EGFR Mutations 109

Management of Neurologically Symptomatic NSCLC Patients with EGFR Mutations 109

Treatment of Multiple Brain Metastases from NSCLC with EGFR Mutations 109

Acknowledgment 110

References 110

M.A. Hayat (ed): *Brain Metastases from Primary Tumors, Volume 1*
DOI: http://dx.doi.org/10.1016/B978-0-12-800896-6.00010-3

© 2014 Elsevier Inc. All rights reserved.

INTRODUCTION

Lung cancer remains the leading cause of cancer-related death worldwide. Non-small cell lung cancer (NSCLC) accounts for approximately 80% of cases of primary lung cancer (Jemal et al., 2009). Lung cancer is also the most frequent origin of metastatic brain tumors and accounts for 50% of cases. In addition, more than 25% of patients with lung cancer develop brain metastases (BM) during the clinical course of their illness (Langer and Mehta, 2005; Burel-Vandenbos et al., 2013). Despite treatment with systemic chemotherapy and/or local radiotherapy, the prognosis of NSCLC patients with BM remains extremely poor. Most cases of BM are characterized by the presence of multiple tumors, up to four in number (Weisberg, 1979). Although stereotactic radiosurgery is a treatment option for BM with up to four tumors (Aoyama et al., 2006), the standard therapy for multiple BM is still whole brain radiotherapy (WBRT). Since the results of treatment with WBRT are not satisfactory, an alternative promising therapeutic option for multiple BM is needed (Langer and Mehta, 2005).

Recently, epidermal growth factor receptor tyrosine-kinase inhibitors (EGFR-TKIs), including gefitinib and erlotinib, have been developed as molecular-targeted drugs for use in the treatment of lung and other cancers. Dramatic effects of EGFR-TKIs have been reported with regard to the treatment of NSCLC with EGFR mutations (Lynch et al., 2004; Paez et al., 2004). In addition, a positive effect of these molecular-targeted drugs on multiple BM from NSCLC with EGFR mutations has also been demonstrated in comparison with the effects of conventional systemic chemotherapy (Park et al., 2012). Therefore, EGFR-TKIs have become an efficient therapeutic option for multiple BM. This chapter discusses the clinical characteristics, management, and treatment of BM in NSCLC patients with EGFR mutations.

EPIDERMAL GROWTH FACTOR RECEPTOR MUTATIONS

EGFR is a member of the ErbB receptor tyrosine kinase (TK) family, and its dysregulation leads to the development and progression of NSCLC (Nicholson et al., 2001; Onn et al., 2004). EGFR-TKI blocks this signaling pathway and has proved effective for NSCLC with EGFR mutations within the TK domain (Lynch et al., 2004; Paez et al., 2004). Ninety percent of EGFR mutations are an exon 19 deletion and exon 21 point mutation, which are called major EGFR mutations (Kosaka et al., 2004). These mutations are commonly associated with Asian ethnicity, female gender, and a never or former light smoking history. EGFR mutations are identified in approximately 60–70% of Asian NSCLC patients with a never or former light smoking history (Mok et al., 2009; Takano et al., 2005). On the other hand, 6–11% non-Asian current smokers possess EGFR mutations. To date, the assessment of EGFR mutation status is generally considered necessary for all NSCLC patients if possible (Rosell et al., 2009; D'Angelo et al., 2011). Since the advent of EGFR-TKIs, the overall survival of NSCLC patients with EGFR mutations ranges from 24 to 30 months compared with a 10–15 month overall survival of NSCLC patients with EGFR wild-type (Brugger and Thomas, 2012). The presence of EGFR mutations has been reported as a better prognostic factor, regardless of the presence or absence of BM (Eichler et al., 2010; Wu et al., 2010).

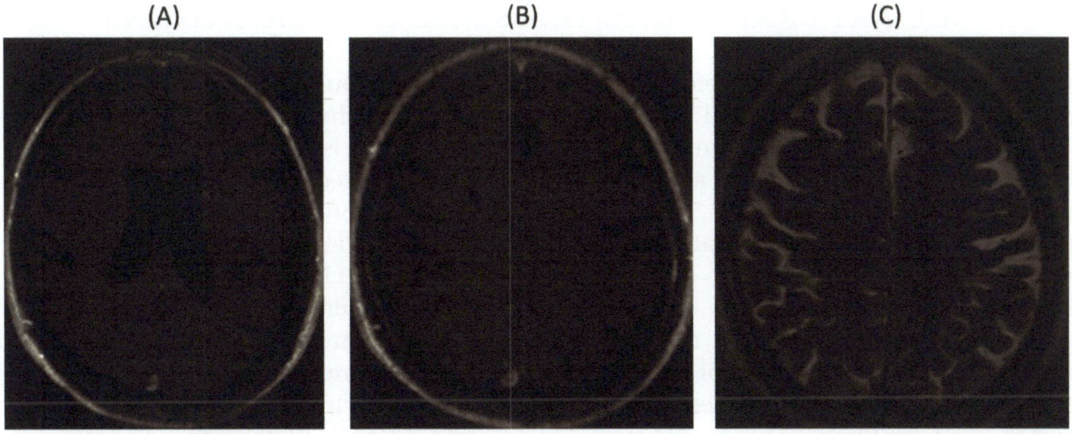

FIGURE 10.1 Typical case of brain metastasis from non-small lung cancer with exon 19 deletion. (A)(B) T1-weighted Gd enhanced image demonstrates poor-defined multiple small nodules in the cerebrum (short arrow). (C) T2-weighted image shows no obvious focal brain edema.

MULTIPLE BRAIN METASTASES AND EGFR MUTATIONS: INFLUENCE OF THE EXON 19 DELETION ON RADIOGRAPHICAL FEATURES

Eichler et al. (2010) first reported that EGFR mutations were frequently identified in NSCLC patients with multiple BM. Laack et al. (2011) demonstrated the association of an exon 19 deletion with miliary lung metastases. With reference to these two reports, we investigated the radiographical characteristics of synchronous BM from NSCLC with major EGFR mutations at the time of NSCLC diagnosis and found that NSCLC patients with the exon 19 deletion possessed multiple small BM with limited focal edema, unlike the features of NSCLC patients with EGFR wild-type (Sekine et al., 2012). A typical case of BM from NSCLC with the exon 19 deletion is presented in Figure 10.1. The mechanism to explain these results remains unclear. Although very few reports have examined the clinical characteristics of NSCLC patients with the exon 19 deletion, we propose the following three mechanisms. First, NSCLC with the exon 19 deletion may metastasize more easily to other organs, including the brain. In fact, EGFR mutations have been frequently identified in NSCLC patients with multiple brain and lung metastases (Eichler et al., 2010; Wu et al., 2013). Second, NSCLC with the exon 19 deletion may be related to smaller tumor diameter compared with NSCLC with EGFR wild-type. In primary site tumors, a correlation has been reported between EGFR mutations and smaller tumor diameter (Lee et al., 2009). Finally, NSCLC with the exon 19 deletion may have less ability to produce edemagenic factors and destroy the blood–brain barrier. Previous reports have demonstrated that brain edema is generally caused by the production of edemagenic factors such as vascular endothelial growth factor and aquaporin, and by destruction of the blood–brain barrier (Huang et al., 2005; Langer and Mehta, 2005; Saadoun and Papadopoulos, 2009). In addition, our results may indicate that BM from NSCLC with the exon 19 deletion has some features in common with miliary BM. This possibility is discussed below.

MILIARY BRAIN METASTASES AND EGFR MUTATIONS

Miliary BM is a rarity and refers to the presence of numerous small tumors in a perivascular distribution without focal brain edema and intraparenchymal invasion. The primary site of miliary BM is mostly lung. Histologically, miliary BM is mainly identified as papillary adenocarcinoma (Iguchi et al., 2007), which is frequently recognized in NSCLC patients with EGFR mutations (Li et al., 2013). These characteristics of miliary BM may be similar to those of BM from NSCLC patients with the exon 19 deletion (Sekine et al., 2012). In our study, evaluation was limited to synchronous BM at the time of NSCLC diagnosis; therefore, it remains unclear whether the characteristics of metachronous BM may differ from those of synchronous BM. However, miliary BM in most reports are metachronous. Mochizuki et al. (2012) reported the cases of two patients who developed miliary BM during the clinical course of their illness and possessed the exon 19 deletion. Taking into account these results and those of our previous study, BM from NSCLC with the exon 19 deletion may have some features in common with miliary BM, regardless of the time of BM diagnosis.

To the best of our knowledge, detailed clinical characteristics of NSCLC with other EGFR mutations, including an exon 21 point mutation, have not been reported. However, two cases of NSCLC patients with miliary BM accompanied by an exon 20 deletion and exon 21 point mutation, respectively, have been reported (Ruppert et al., 2010; Inomata et al., 2012). In addition, our study showed that NSCLC patients with an exon 21 point mutation tended to have smaller BM with limited focal edema compared with NSCLC patients with EGFR wild-type, although the difference was not significant (Sekine et al., 2012). Therefore, BM from NSCLC with other EGFR mutations may share some features with those with the exon 19 deletion to some extent. Further studies on BM from NSCLC with each EGFR mutation are required to clarify this issue.

MANAGEMENT OF BRAIN METASTASES FROM NSCLC WITH EGFR MUTATIONS

EGFR-TKIs improve the prognosis of NSCLC patients with EGFR mutations. However, this improved prognosis would result in a new problem: long-term survival is associated with a higher risk of developing BM. The incidence of BM in one report was 40% in 2-year survivors and 52% in 3-year survivors (Sorensen et al., 1988). Particularly in EGFR-TKIs responders, isolated central nervous system progression has been reported to develop frequently without other systemic progression (Lee et al., 2010). BM sometimes cause seizures and decreased quality of life. Therefore, early tumor detection is important to facilitate the appropriate treatment before the development of neurological symptoms (Langer and Mehta, 2005; van Breemen et al., 2007). However, the optimal management of NSCLC patients at the point of BM diagnosis remains to be determined. With consideration of the results of previous reports, the following management measures may be necessary.

Management of Neurologically Asymptomatic NSCLC Patients with EGFR Mutations

Importantly, numerous small BM resembling miliary BM do not always cause neurological symptoms (Kahveci et al., 2012; Mochizuki et al., 2012). Patients with BM from NSCLC with the exon 19 deletion tend to be neurologically asymptomatic compared with NSCLC patients with EGFR wild-type because of smaller tumor size and limited focal brain edema (Sekine et al., 2012). However, even in NSCLC patients with asymptomatic BM, multiple BM like miliary BM might develop during their clinical courses, unless an appropriate treatment can be provided. In fact, most reported cases of miliary BM were those of metachronous BM (Iguchi et al., 2007; Mochizuki et al., 2012). Considering the similarity between BM from NSCLC with the exon 19 deletion and miliary BM, regular evaluation should be performed, particularly in NSCLC patients with the exon 19 deletion, regardless of the presence or absence of neurologic symptoms.

Management of Neurologically Symptomatic NSCLC Patients with EGFR Mutations

Although radiographical evaluation should be performed in neurologically symptomatic patients, the presence of BM cannot be denied even in the absence of radiological abnormalities. Some reports showed the inability of enhanced computed tomography and magnetic resonance imaging to detect BM in a certain number of NSCLC patients (Nakamura et al., 2001; McGuigan et al., 2005; Iguchi et al., 2007). Micrometastatic tumors are generally so avascular that their detection requires a certain amount of time. When the tumors become vascular and expand in size, detection becomes easier (Zetter, 1998). Considering the characteristics of BM in NSCLC patients with the exon 19 deletion, the presence of micrometastatic BM may be more likely. Therefore, repeated radiographical evaluation should be considered, particularly in NSCLC patients with the exon 19 deletion, if progressive neurological symptoms develop.

TREATMENT OF MULTIPLE BRAIN METASTASES FROM NSCLC WITH EGFR MUTATIONS

The optimal treatment for multiple BM remains to be determined. Although stereotactic radiosurgery is considered a therapeutic option for cases with fewer than five small brain tumors (<3 cm) (Aoyama et al., 2006), the standard therapy for multiple BM is still WBRT (Langer and Mehta, 2005).WBRT is reported to be more effective in NSCLC patients with EGFR mutations than in NSCLC patients with EGFR wild-type; however, WBRT generally plays only a limited role in controlling multiple BM (Gow et al., 2008). The effect of systemic chemotherapy is considered insufficient because of limited drug delivery through the blood–brain barrier (Langer and Mehta, 2005).

EGFR-TKIs have revolutionized the treatment of BM. These molecular-targeted drugs are effective against BM in NSCLC patients with EGFR mutations, and response rates of up to 83% have been reported (Park et al., 2012). EGFR-TKIs offer a promising therapeutic option, especially in cases with multiple BM. Among EGFR-TKIs, the maximum tolerated dose of erlotinib is higher than that of gefitinib. Therefore, erlotinib may be more effective for the treatment of BM, especially in NSCLC patients with the development of progressive disease only in the brain during gefitinib treatment (Hata et al., 2011). However, most NSCLC patients (80.9%) treated with any EGFR-TKI developed progressive disease in the brain and required radiotherapy during the clinical course of their illness (Park et al., 2012). Therefore, monotherapy with either radiotherapy or EGFR-TKIs may be insufficient to control multiple BM, particularly miliary-like BM. Recently, combination therapy with EGFR-TKIs and WBRT was reported to be more effective for multiple (miliary-like) BM in NSCLC patients with EGFR mutations compared with monotherapy alone (Gow et al., 2008; Mochizuki et al., 2012). Although the optimal combination of EGFR-TKIs, WBRT, and stereotactic radiosurgery remains to be determined, the concurrent use of EGFR-TKIs and WBRT may be preferable in patients with multiple BM, especially miliary-like BM, from NSCLC with EGFR mutations. Future studies to establish the optimal strategy for treatment of such BM are necessary.

In conclusion, although WBRT is considered as a standard therapy, EGFR-TKIs have become an important therapeutic option for the treatment of BM from NSCLC with EGFR mutations. Accumulation of knowledge about the clinical characteristics of BM from NSCLC with EGFR mutations will aid in the management and treatment of this disease.

Acknowledgment

We thank Dr Hiroaki Satoh and Dr Eri Hagiwara for their special contributions to this paper.

References

Aoyama, H., Shirato, H., Tago, M., et al., 2006. Stereotactic radiosurgery plus whole-brain radiation therapy vs stereotactic radiosurgery alone for treatment of brain metastases: a randomized controlled trial. J. Am. Med. Assoc. 295, 2483–2491.

Brugger, W., Thomas, M., 2012. EGFR-TKI resistant non-small cell lung cancer (NSCLC): new developments and implications for future treatment. Lung Cancer 77, 2–8.

Burel-Vandenbos, F., Ambrosetti, D., Coutts, M., Pedeutour, F., 2013. EGFR mutation status in brain metastases of non-small cell lung carcinoma. J. Neurooncol. 111, 1–10.

D'Angelo, S.P., Pietanza, M.C., Johnson, M.L., et al., 2011. Incidence of EGFR exon 19 deletions and L858R in tumor specimens from men and cigarette smokers with lung adenocarcinomas. J. Clin. Oncol. 29, 2066–2070.

Eichler, A.F., Kahle, K.T., Wang, D.L., et al., 2010. EGFR mutation status and survival after diagnosis of brain metastasis in nonsmall cell lung cancer. Neuro. Oncol. 12, 1193–1199.

Gow, C.H., Chien, C.R., Chang, Y.L., et al., 2008. Radiotherapy in lung adenocarcinoma with brain metastases: effects of activating epidermal growth factor receptor mutations on clinical response. Clin. Cancer Res. 14, 162–168.

Hata, A., Katakami, N., Yoshioka, H., et al., 2011. Erlotinib after gefitinib failure in relapsed non-small cell lung cancer: clinical benefit with optimal patient selection. Lung Cancer 74, 268–273.

Huang, H., Held-Feindt, J., Buhl, R., Mehdorn, H.M., Mentlein, R., 2005. Expression of VEGF and its receptors in different brain tumors. Neurol. Res. 27, 371–377.

Iguchi, Y., Mano, K., Goto, Y., et al., 2007. Miliary brain metastases from adenocarcinoma of the lung: MR imaging findings with clinical and post-mortem histopathologic correlation. Neuroradiology 49, 35–39.

Inomata, M., Hayashi, R., Kambara, K., et al., 2012. Miliary brain metastasis presenting with calcification in a patient with lung cancer: a case report. J. Med. Case Rep. 6, 279.

Jemal, A., Siegel, R., Ward, E., Hao, Y., Xu, J., Thun, M.J., 2009. Cancer statistics. CA Cancer J. Clin. 59, 225–249.

Kahveci, R., Gurer, B., Kaygusuz, G., Sekerci, Z., 2012. Miliary brain metastases from occult lung adenocarcinoma: radiologic and histopathologic confirmation. J. Neurosci. Rural Pract. 3, 386–389.

Kosaka, T., Yatabe, Y., Endoh, H., Kuwano, H., Takahashi, T., Mitsudomi, T., 2004. Mutations of the epidermal growth factor receptor gene in lung cancer: biological and clinical implications. Cancer Res. 64, 8919–8923.

Laack, E., Simon, R., Regier, M., et al., 2011. Miliary never-smoking adenocarcinoma of the lung: strong association with epidermal growth factor receptor exon 19 deletion. J. Thorac. Oncol. 6, 199–202.

Langer, C.J., Mehta, M.P., 2005. Current management of brain metastases, with a focus on systemic options. J. Clin. Oncol. 23, 6207–6219.

Lee, Y.J., Park, I.K., Park, M.S., et al., 2009. Activating mutations within the EGFR kinase domain: a molecular predictor of disease-free survival in resected pulmonary adenocarcinoma. J. Cancer Res. Clin. Oncol. 135, 1647–1654.

Lee, Y.J., Choi, H.J., Kim, S.K., et al., 2010. Frequent central nervous system failure after clinical benefit with epidermal growth factor receptor tyrosine kinase inhibitors in Korean patients with nonsmall-cell lung cancer. Cancer 116, 1336–1343.

Li, H., Pan, Y., Li, Y., et al., 2013. Frequency of well-identified oncogenic driver mutations in lung adenocarcinoma of smokers varies with histological subtypes and graduated smoking dose. Lung Cancer 79, 8–13.

Lynch, T.J., Bell, D.W., Sordella, R., et al., 2004. Activating mutations in the epidermal growth factor receptor underlying responsiveness of non-small-cell lung cancer to gefitinib. N. Engl. J. Med. 350, 2129–2139.

McGuigan, C., Bigham, S., Johnston, D., Hart, P.E., 2005. Encephalopathy in a patient with previous malignancy but normal brain imaging. Neurology 65, 165.

Mochizuki, S., Nishimura, N., Inoue, A., Murakami, K., Nukiwa, T., Chohnabayashi, N., 2012. Miliary brain metastases in 2 cases with advanced non-small cell lung cancer harboring EGFR mutation during gefitinib treatment. Respir. Investig. 50, 117–121.

Mok, T.S., Wu, Y.L., Thongprasert, S., et al., 2009. Gefitinib or carboplatin-paclitaxel in pulmonary adenocarcinoma. N. Engl. J. Med. 361, 947–957.

Nakamura, H., Toyama, M., Uezu, K., Nakamoto, A., Toda, T., Saito, A., 2001. Diagnostic dilemmas in oncology: case 1. Lung cancer with miliary brain metastases undetected by imaging studies. J. Clin. Oncol. 19, 4340–4341.

Nicholson, R.I., Gee, J.M., Harper, M.E., 2001. EGFR and cancer prognosis. Eur. J. Cancer 37 (Suppl. 4), S9–15.

Onn, A., Correa, A.M., Gilcrease, M., et al., 2004. Synchronous overexpression of epidermal growth factor receptor and HER2-neu protein is a predictor of poor outcome in patients with stage I non-small cell lung cancer. Clin. Cancer Res. 10, 136–143.

Paez, J.G., Janne, P.A., Lee, J.C., et al., 2004. EGFR mutations in lung cancer: correlation with clinical response to gefitinib therapy. Science 304, 1497–1500.

Park, S.J., Kim, H.T., Lee, D.H., et al., 2012. Efficacy of epidermal growth factor receptor tyrosine kinase inhibitors for brain metastasis in non-small cell lung cancer patients harboring either exon 19 or 21 mutation. Lung Cancer 77, 556–560.

Rosell, R., Moran, T., Queralt, C., et al., 2009. Screening for epidermal growth factor receptor mutations in lung cancer. N. Engl. J. Med. 361, 958–967.

Ruppert, A.M., Stankoff, B., Lavole, A., Gounant, V., Milleron, B., Seilhean, D., 2010. Miliary brain metastases in lung cancer. J. Clin. Oncol. 28, e714–e716.

Saadoun, S., Papadopoulos, M.C., 2009. Aquaporin-4 in brain and spinal cord oedema. Neuroscience 168, 1036–1046.

Sekine, A., Kato, T., Hagiwara, E., et al., 2012. Metastatic brain tumors from non-small cell lung cancer with EGFR mutations: distinguishing influence of exon 19 deletion on radiographic features. Lung Cancer 77, 64–69.

Sorensen, J.B., Hansen, H.H., Hansen, M., Dombernowsky, P., 1988. Brain metastases in adenocarcinoma of the lung: frequency, risk groups, and prognosis. J. Clin. Oncol. 6, 1474–1480.

Takano, T., Ohe, Y., Sakamoto, H., et al., 2005. Epidermal growth factor receptor gene mutations and increased copy numbers predict gefitinib sensitivity in patients with recurrent non-small-cell lung cancer. J. Clin. Oncol. 23, 6829–6837.

van Breemen, M.S., Wilms, E.B., Vecht, C.J., 2007. Epilepsy in patients with brain tumours: epidemiology, mechanisms, and management. Lancet Neurol. 6, 421–430.

Weisberg, L.A., 1979. Computerized tomography in intracranial metastases. Arch. Neurol. 36, 630–634.

Wu, M., Zhao, J., Song, S.W., et al., 2010. EGFR mutations are associated with prognosis but not with the response to front-line chemotherapy in the Chinese patients with advanced non-small cell lung cancer. Lung Cancer 67, 343–347.

Wu, S.G., Hu, F.C., Chang, Y.L., et al., 2013. Frequent EGFR Mutations in NSCLC presenting with miliary intrapulmonary carcinomatosis. Eur. Respir. J. 41, 417–424.

Zetter, B.R., 1998. Angiogenesis and tumor metastasis. Annu. Rev. Med. 49, 407–424.

CHAPTER

11

Brain Metastasis of Patients with Lung Adenocarcinoma: Epidermal Growth Factor Receptor Mutations and Response to Whole-Brain Radiation Therapy

Shang-Gin Wu and Jin-Yuan Shih

OUTLINE

Introduction	**114**
Brain Metastasis and EGFR Mutation	**114**
Preclinical Study and Mechanism	**115**
EGFR and Radiation-Induced DNA Damage	*115*
EGFR Mutation and Radiotherapy	*115*
EGFR-TKIs Combined with Radiotherapy	*116*
Clinical study (Table 11.1)	**116**
EGFR Mutation and Radiotherapy	*116*
EGFR-TKIs Treatment for Brain Metastasis	*118*
EGFR-TKIs Combined with Radiotherapy	*118*
Conclusion	**119**
References	**119**

M.A. *Hayat (ed): Brain Metastases from Primary Tumors, Volume 1*
DOI: http://dx.doi.org/10.1016/B978-0-12-800896-6.00011-5

© 2014 Elsevier Inc. All rights reserved.

INTRODUCTION

Approximately 1.2 million new cases of lung cancer occur worldwide every year (Siegel et al., 2011). Most patients with non-small cell lung cancer (NSCLC) are diagnosed at an advanced stage (Siegel et al., 2011). Brain metastases develop during the course of the disease in ≈30–50% of the NSCLC patients, especially in those with adenocarcinoma (Sorensen et al., 1988). Brain metastasis results in significant morbidity and mortality in NSCLC patients, so the prognoses of these patients are very poor. The overall survival after brain metastasis has occurred is around 1–4 months (Nussbaum et al., 1996).

Whole brain radiotherapy (WBRT) plays an important role in the treatment of NSCLC patients with brain metastasis (Khuntia et al., 2006). The recently used regimen for WBRT is usually 30 Gy delivered in 10 fractions over 2 weeks. The effect of WBRT includes improvement of neurologic symptoms, such as headache, nausea or other neurologic deficits, and quality of life (Khuntia et al., 2006). NSCLC patients with brain metastasis who received WBRT had median overall survival ranging from 3 to 6 months (Berk, 1995). It is uncommon for WBRT to produce complications, particularly acute toxicity. When acute toxicities occur, they are often self-limited. Dementia is the most common late-delayed complication, and it was noted 4–36 months after treatment in approximately 10–15% of the patients who received WBRT (DeAngelis et al., 1989; Chang et al., 2009).

Epidermal growth factor receptor (EGFR), a transmembrane glycoprotein of the ErbB receptor family, controls cell proliferation, differentiation, anti-apoptosis, angiogenesis, and invasion (Scagliotti et al., 2004). After ligand binding, dimerization develops between HER receptors, which triggers tyrosine phosphorylation. Then, several intracellular signaling cascades are activated by EGFR, including: Ras/Raf/MEK/ERK, phophotidylinositol 3-kinase (PI3K)/AKT, Src tyrosine kinases, PLCγ, PKC, and STAT activation and downstream signaling (Marmor et al., 2004). NSCLC patients with tumors harboring EGFR mutations have a dramatic treatment response to the epidermal growth factor receptor tyrosine kinase inhibitors (EGFR-TKI), gefitinib and erlotinib (Lynch et al., 2004). EGFR mutations are frequently associated with lung adenocarcinoma, females, never smokers, and East-Asian ethnicity. L858R mutation and a deletion in exon-19 (del-19) account for 90% of the EGFR mutations (Sharma et al., 2007).

Because lung adenocarcinoma frequently metastasizes to the brain and has a high EGFR mutation rate, interaction between brain metastasis, radiotherapy and EGFR mutation has been reported in preclinical and clinical studies. This may provide a new clinical treatment concept and modality. The more we understand the issue, the better care we can provide for our patients.

BRAIN METASTASIS AND EGFR MUTATION

The brain is a frequent metastatic site of lung cancer, especially adenocarcinoma (Sorensen et al., 1988). However, the mechanism by which lung cancer metastasizes to the brain is still unknown. For breast cancer, ErbB2 overexpression is associated with brain metastases and poor prognosis, and ErbB2 amplification is an important risk factor for brain metastasis in breast cancer patients (Gabos et al., 2006). Overexpression of ErbB2, specifically in lung adenocarcinoma, is correlated with poor prognosis and intrinsic chemoresistance (Tsai et al., 1993). ErbB2 may phosphorylate downstream molecules and activate PI-3 kinase/AKT pathways. These pathways are also activated in NSCLC with EGFR mutations and inhibited by EGFR-TKIs (Sharma et al., 2007). Matsumoto et al. (2006) report that EGFR mutations were detected in 12 of 19 metastatic lung adenocarcinomas to the brain (63%) and 10 patients had del-19. The authors concluded that EGFR mutations frequently present in brain metastases (Matsumoto et al., 2006). EGFR mutations may play an important role in brain metastasis of lung cancer.

PRECLINICAL STUDY AND MECHANISM

EGFR and Radiation-Induced DNA Damage

Radiation produces free radicals which cause DNA damage. The most lethal damage is a double-strand break (DSB), which produces chromosomal deletion, translocation, or disorganization (Sancar et al., 2004), and results in cell cycle arrest, apoptosis, or gene inactivation (Sancar et al., 2004). For radiation-induced DSB of DNA, there are two mechanisms for repair – homologous recombination and non-homologous end-joining (NHEJ) (Wyman et al., 2004; Hefferin and Tomkinson, 2005). NHEJ is pivotal in DSB repair, while homologous recombination is the supportive pathway (Blunt et al., 1995). Proteins necessary for NHEJ include DNA-PK, DNA IV ligase IV, XRCC4 and Artemis. Among them, DNA-PK is a nuclear kinase, and contains three subunits, a DNA-PK catalytic subunit (DNA-PKc) and two regulatory subunits, Ku70 (70 kDa) and Ku80 (80 kDa). NHEJ is initiated from the binding of Ku70 and Ku80 to DNA breaken ends after radiation damage. They translocate inward along the DNA molecule by one helical turn. Then, DNA-PKcs are recruited and form a stable DNA-PKcs–DSB complex to prevent premature processing and ligation of the DNA ends. DNA-PKcs are phosphorylated and recruit several end-processing enzymes, for example, ligase IV, Rad50 Nbs1and Mre11 (Chen and Nirodi, 2007). The complex then repairs radiation-induced DNA damage by joining the DNA ends.

EGFR plays an important role in determining radioresponse, and overexpression of EGFR has radioprotective activity. EGFR-mediated radioprotection could be divided into three phases. First, an immediate early phase of DNA repair involves EGFR internalization, phosphorylation and nuclear translocation (Lin et al., 2001); then, suppression of DNA damage by induction of apoptosis and cell cycle arrest through the activation of phophotidylinositol 3-kinase and protein kinase B/AKT kinase (Zhan and Han, 2004). Finally, activation of Ras/Raf/MEK/ERK and STAT pathways promotes cell proliferation and rapid repopulation (Schmidt-Ullrich et al., 1997).

EGFR Mutation and Radiotherapy

Although a tumor with EGFR overexpression shows radioresistance, the EGFR mutation has been associated with enhanced radiosensitivity in cell lines and clinical practice (Das et al., 2006, 2007; Gow et al., 2008). NSCLC cell lines harboring deletions of E746 to A750 or L858R mutations present with a marked radiosensitive response to 1/500 to 1/1000 compared with wild-type EGFR NSCLCs. NSCLCs with the EGFR mutation show delayed DSB repair kinetics, and lack the ability to block DNA synthesis through the G1 cell cycle checkpoint after ionic radiation. Then, radiation to NSCLC cell lines with the EGFR mutation induces obvious apoptosis and development of micronuclei. Exogenous expression of L858R and deletion in E746-A750 in wild-type cell lines also significantly reduces clonogenic survival after radiation (Das et al., 2006).

In comparison with wild-type EGFR, NSCLC cell lines with EGFR mutations have defects in radiation-induced EGFR nuclear translocation, although the cell lines show high level of tyrosine phosphorylation after ionic radiation. Mutant EGFR fails to bind catalytic subunits (DNA-PKcs) and regulatory factors (Ku70 and Ku 80) of DNA-PK, which are the key enzymes of NHEJ. As a result, NSCLC cell lines with EGFR mutations lack the radioprotective function normally present (Das et al., 2007).

EGFR-TKIs Combined with Radiotherapy

Chemotherapy was considered to have a limited effect in the treatment of brain metastasis in NSCLC patients due to the blood–brain barrier (BBB) (Eichler and Loeffler, 2007). Recently, some animal studies suggest that the BBB is disrupted in brain metastasis because the brain metastatic lesions showed obvious enhancement on computed tomography (CT) or magnetic resonance imaging (MRI). However, intracranial drug concentration is still insufficient (Mehta et al., 2010). EGFR-TKI has low molecular weight and excellent cell penetration (Barker et al., 2001). In addition, radiotherapy treatment may also disrupt the BBB (van Vulpen et al., 2002). Together, combination treatment with EGFR-TKI and WBRT may have a synergistic effect.

Bianco et al. (2002) reported that gefitinib could enhance the antitumor activity of ionizing radiation. Huang et al. (2002) showed that combination treatment with gefitinib and radiation inhibited not only cell proliferative growth but also tumor angiogenesis. This is associated with cell cycle arrest and enhancement of radiation-induced apoptosis. Gefitinib radiosensitizes NSCLC cells by inhibiting ataxia telangiectasia mutated (ATM) activity and therefore inducing mitotic cell death (Park et al., 2010). Thus, combination treatment with EGFR-TKIs and WBRT may be the treatment of choice for NSCLC patients with brain metastasis.

CLINICAL STUDY (TABLE 11.1)

EGFR Mutation and Radiotherapy

In clinical observation, Gow et al. (2008) retrospectively collected 63 NSCLC patients with brain metastasis who all received WBRT. Patients with EGFR mutations had higher response rates to WBRT compared with those with the wild-type (54% versus 24%; $p = 0.045$). Both the administration of EGFR tyrosine kinase inhibitor ($p = 0.034$) and harboring the EGFR mutation ($p = 0.029$) were independently associated with response to WBRT. WBRT produces a significantly good response in NSCLC patients with brain metastasis harboring EGFR mutations. This is consistent with *in vitro* study of relative radiosensitivity in activating EGFR mutations (Das et al., 2006, 2007).

TABLE 11.1 Summary of Clinical Studies about WBRT and/or EGFR-TKIs for NSCLC Patients with Brain Metastasis

Study	Study Design	Treatment (NSCLC patient number)	Race	AdenoCa (mutation patients)	Brain Tumor Response (%)	PFS	Median Survival
Ceresoli et al. (2004)	Phase II trial	Gefitinib ($n = 41$)	European	27[#]	10	3	5
Hotta et al. (2004)	Retrospective	Gefitinib ($n = 14$)[¶]	East-Asian	12[¶]	43		
Wu et al. (2007)	Phase II trial	Gefitinib ($n = 40$)	East-Asian	40	32	9	15
Gow et al. (2008)	Retrospective	WBRT ($n = 18$)	East-Asian	18 (13)	39	—	11.7
		TKI+WBRT (n=45)		45 (33)	67	—	22.3
				mutation(+):	54		17.3
Ma et al. (2009)	Phase II trial	Gefitinib + WBRT ($n = 21$)	East-Asian	14	81	10	13
Porta et al. (2011)	Retrospective	Erlotinib ($n = 69$)	European	47 (14)	26.4	2.9	4.3
				mutation(+):	82.4	11.7	12.9
Park et al. (2012)	Phase II trial	Gefitinib/erlotinib ($n = 23$)[µ]	East-Asian	23 (23)[µ]	83	6.6	15.9
Zeng et al. (2012)	Retrospective	Gefitinib ($n = 45$)	East-Asian	45 (5)*	26.7	4.17	23.4
		Gefitinib+WBRT ($n = 45$)		45 (7)*	64.4	7.12	14.83
						($p = 0.001$)	($p = 0.002$)

*Not all patients received EGFR mutation analysis.
[#]Adenocarcinoma and bronchiolar-alveolar carcinoma.
[¶]Only enrolled patients with brain metastasis.
[µ]Only enrolled patients with tumor harboring either exon 19 or 21 mutation.
NSCLC: non-small cell lung cancer; TKI: EGFR tyrosine kinase inhibitor; WBRT: whole brain radiotherapy; AdenoCa: adenocarcinoma; PFS: progression-free survival.

Eichler et al. (2010) retrospectively analyzed a cohort of NSCLC patients tested for EGFR mutations. There were 93 patients who developed brain metastasis (BM) during the course of their disease, including 41 (44%) patients with EGFR mutations. Median survival from diagnosis of BM was 11.7 months and was longer for patients with EGFR mutations (14.5 versus 7.6 months, $p = 0.09$). On multivariable analysis, harboring an EGFR mutation (HR: 0.50, 95% CI: 0.30 0.82) and age (HR: 1.03, 95% CI. 1.00–1.05) were independently associated with survival. In NSCLC patients with brain metastasis, EGFR mutation status is associated with improved survival, independent of age, functional status, extracranial disease status, and number of brain metastases.

Mak et al. (2011) show that EGFR-mutant patients with locally advanced NSCLC treated with RT had a lower locoregional recurrence rate than wild-type EGFR patients. So, EGFR mutations may also confer sensitivity to radiotherapy and/or chemotherapy in addition to EGFR-TKIs (Eichler et al., 2010). Therefore, planned prospective studies to identify useful treatment modalities for patients with EGFR-mutations NSCLC would be important.

EGFR-TKIs Treatment for Brain Metastasis

For patients with symptomatic brain metastasis, chemotherapy alone usually has poor effect on intracranial disease control; WBRT has proven to be beneficial in prolonging patient survival. EGFR-TKIs, gefitinib or erlotinib, have low molecular weight and excellent cell penetration, and may play an important role in the treatment of brain metastasis.

Initially, some case reports have demonstrated the activity of EGFR-TKIs in NSCLC patients with brain metastasis (Cappuzzo et al., 2003; Fujiwara et al., 2003). In a 2004 report of a phase II trial that enrolled 41 NSCLC patients with brain metastasis, Ceresoli et al. (2004) prescribed gefitinib as second- or third-line treatment. They found that 30% of patients had a partial response and 25% had stable disease. Park et al. (2012) reported that EGFR-TKI treatment showed promising antitumor activity against both intracranial and extracranial tumors in NSCLC patients with exon 19 or exon 21 mutations of EGFR, and the intracranial response reached 83% (23 of 28). Porta et al. (2011) retrospectively collected 69 NSCLC patients with brain metastases (47 adenocarcinoma + 1 bronchioloalveolar carcinoma), 17 of whom had EGFR mutation-positive tumors. EGFR-TKI, erlotinib, is active in patients with brain metastases from NSCLC. Patients harboring tumors with EGFR mutations had an objective response rate of 82.4%; some cases even had highly complete responses (47.1%). EGFR-TKIs may be equally effective as radiotherapy to the brain, and may also delay the development of disease within the brain (Jamal-Hanjani and Spicer, 2012).

EGFR-TKIs Combined with Radiotherapy

For combination treatment with EGFR-TKI and WBRT, only a few reports of retrospective and phase II studies are available. Ceresoli et al. (2004) showed that consecutive NSCLC patients with measurable brain metastases were treated with gefitinib. The disease control rate was higher in patients pretreated with WBRT. Gow et al. (2008) reported that both EGFR mutations and EGFR-TKI use during WBRT were predictive factors for a response to WBRT in patients with brain metastases from lung adenocarcinoma; the highest responsive rate of 84% (11 of 13) was noted in patients with EGFR mutations who received EGFR-TKI during WBRT. Ma et al. (2009) conducted a phase II prospective study administering EGFR-TKI and WBRT concurrently for adenocarcinoma patients with brain metastasis. In this study, the response rate was 81% and median overall survival was 13 months. The effects of combination therapy need to be confirmed by phase III trials.

CONCLUSION

In conclusion, brain metastasis is still a critical problem in NSCLC patients, and standard treatment has a disappointing response. Modern and more effective treatment of lung cancer is necessary to prolong patient survival. More importantly, it is necessary to reduce neurologic dysfunction and decelerate neurocognitive deterioration. With advances of brain imaging providing the means for early detection of small metastatic lesions, more and more patients are diagnosed with brain metastases. Although treatment modalities for brain metastases have progressed substantially during the past decades, WBRT remains the standard management. Systemic treatments, chemotherapy, EGFR-TKI also play an important role in the treatment of brain metastasis, especially when EGFR-TKI combined with WBRT may provide a synergistic effect on the management of NSCLC patients with brain metastases. However, patients with EGFR mutations respond dramatically to EGFR-TKI, so EGFR mutation analysis has become more and more important. It is essential to select suitable patients to receive EGFR-TKI treatment. This is also the new challenge in personalizing cancer therapy in the future.

References

Barker, A.J., Gibson, K.H., Grundy, W., et al., 2001. Studies leading to the identification of ZD1839 (IRESSA): an orally active, selective epidermal growth factor receptor tyrosine kinase inhibitor targeted to the treatment of cancer. Bioorg. Med. Chem. Lett. 11, 1911–1914.

Berk, L., 1995. An overview of radiotherapy trials for the treatment of brain metastases. Oncology (Williston Park) 9, 1205–1212. discussion 1212–16, 1219.

Bianco, C., Tortora, G., Bianco, R., et al., 2002. Enhancement of antitumor activity of ionizing radiation by combined treatment with the selective epidermal growth factor receptor-tyrosine kinase inhibitor ZD1839 (Iressa). Clin. Cancer Res. 8, 3250–3258.

Blunt, T., Finnie, N.J., Taccioli, G.E., et al., 1995. Defective DNA-dependent protein kinase activity is linked to V(D)J recombination and DNA repair defects associated with the murine scid mutation. Cell 80, 813–823.

Cappuzzo, F., Calandri, C., Bartolini, S., Crino, L., 2003. ZD 1839 in patients with brain metastases from non-small-cell lung cancer (NSCLC): report of four cases. Br. J. Cancer 89, 246–247.

Ceresoli, G.L., Cappuzzo, F., Gregorc, V., Bartolini, S., Crino, L., Villa, E., 2004. Gefitinib in patients with brain metastases from non-small-cell lung cancer: a prospective trial. Ann. Oncol. 15, 1042–1047.

Chang, E.L., Wefel, J.S., Hess, K.R., et al., 2009. Neurocognition in patients with brain metastases treated with radiosurgery or radiosurgery plus whole-brain irradiation: a randomised controlled trial. Lancet Oncol. 10, 1037–1044.

Chen, D.J., Nirodi, C.S., 2007. The epidermal growth factor receptor: a role in repair of radiation-induced DNA damage. Clin. Cancer Res. 13, 6555–6560.

Das, A.K., Chen, B.P., Story, M.D., et al., 2007. Somatic mutations in the tyrosine kinase domain of epidermal growth factor receptor (EGFR) abrogate EGFR-mediated radioprotection in non-small cell lung carcinoma. Cancer Res. 67, 5267–5274.

Das, A.K., Sato, M., Story, M.D., et al., 2006. Non-small-cell lung cancers with kinase domain mutations in the epidermal growth factor receptor are sensitive to ionizing radiation. Cancer Res. 66, 9601–9608.

DeAngelis, L.M., Delattre, J.Y., Posner, J.B., 1989. Radiation-induced dementia in patients cured of brain metastases. Neurology 39, 789–796.

Eichler, A.F., Loeffler, J.S., 2007. Multidisciplinary management of brain metastases. Oncologist 12, 884–898.

Eichler, A.F., Kahle, K.T., Wang, D.L., et al., 2010. EGFR mutation status and survival after diagnosis of brain metastasis in nonsmall cell lung cancer. Neuro. Oncol. 12, 1193–1199.

Fujiwara, K., Kiura, K., Ueoka, H., Tabata, M., Hamasaki, S., Tanimoto, M., 2003. Dramatic effect of ZD1839 ('Iressa') in a patient with advanced non-small-cell lung cancer and poor performance status. Lung Cancer 40, 73–76.

Gabos, Z., Sinha, R., Hanson, J., et al., 2006. Prognostic significance of human epidermal growth factor receptor positivity for the development of brain metastasis after newly diagnosed breast cancer. J. Clin. Oncol. 24, 5658–5663.

Gow, C.H., Chien, C.R., Chang, Y.L., et al., 2008. Radiotherapy in lung adenocarcinoma with brain metastases: effects of activating epidermal growth factor receptor mutations on clinical response. Clin. Cancer Res. 14, 162–168.

Hefferin, M.L., Tomkinson, A.E., 2005. Mechanism of DNA double-strand break repair by non-homologous end joining. DNA Repair (Amst) 4, 639–648.

Hotta, K., Kiura, K., Ueoka, H., et al., 2004. Effect of gefitinib ('Iressa', ZD1839) on brain metastases in patients with advanced non-small-cell lung cancer. Lung Cancer 46, 255–261.

Huang, S.M., Li, J., Armstrong, E.A., Harari, P.M., 2002. Modulation of radiation response and tumor-induced angiogenesis after epidermal growth factor receptor inhibition by ZD1839 (Iressa). Cancer Res. 62, 4300–4306.

Jamal-Hanjani, M., Spicer, J., 2012. Epidermal growth factor receptor tyrosine kinase inhibitors in the treatment of epidermal growth factor receptor-mutant non-small cell lung cancer metastatic to the brain. Clin. Cancer Res. 18, 938–944.

Khuntia, D., Brown, P., Li, J., Mehta, M.P., 2006. Whole-brain radiotherapy in the management of brain metastasis. J. Clin. Oncol. 24, 1295–1304.

Lin, S.Y., Makino, K., Xia, W., et al., 2001. Nuclear localization of EGF receptor and its potential new role as a transcription factor. Nat. Cell Biol. 3, 802–808.

Lynch, T.J., Bell, D.W., Sordella, R., et al., 2004. Activating mutations in the epidermal growth factor receptor underlying responsiveness of non-small-cell lung cancer to gefitinib. N. Engl. J. Med. 350, 2129–2139.

Ma, S., Xu, Y., Deng, Q., Yu, X., 2009. Treatment of brain metastasis from non-small cell lung cancer with whole brain radiotherapy and Gefitinib in a Chinese population. Lung Cancer 65, 198–203.

Mak, R.H., Doran, E., Muzikansky, A., et al., 2011. Outcomes after combined modality therapy for EGFR-mutant and wild-type locally advanced NSCLC. Oncologist 16, 886–895.

Marmor, M.D., Skaria, K.B., Yarden, Y., 2004. Signal transduction and oncogenesis by ErbB/HER receptors. Int. J. Radiat. Oncol. Biol. Phys. 58, 903–913.

Matsumoto, S., Takahashi, K., Iwakawa, R., et al., 2006. Frequent EGFR mutations in brain metastases of lung adenocarcinoma. Int. J. Cancer 119, 1491–1494.

Mehta, M.P., Paleologos, N.A., Mikkelsen, T., et al., 2010. The role of chemotherapy in the management of newly diagnosed brain metastases: a systematic review and evidence-based clinical practice guideline. J. Neurooncol. 96, 71–83.

Nussbaum, E.S., Djalilian, H.R., Cho, K.H., Hall, W.A., 1996. Brain metastases. Histology, multiplicity, surgery, and survival. Cancer 78, 1781–1788.

Park, S.J., Kim, H.T., Lee, D.H., et al., 2012. Efficacy of epidermal growth factor receptor tyrosine kinase inhibitors for brain metastasis in non-small cell lung cancer patients harboring either exon 19 or 21 mutation. Lung Cancer 77, 556–560.

Park, S.Y., Kim, Y.M., Pyo, H., 2010. Gefitinib radiosensitizes non-small cell lung cancer cells through inhibition of ataxia telangiectasia mutated. Mol. Cancer 9, 222.

Porta, R., Sanchez-Torres, J.M., Paz-Ares, L., et al., 2011. Brain metastases from lung cancer responding to erlotinib: the importance of EGFR mutation. Eur. Respir. J. 37, 624–631.

Sancar, A., Lindsey-Boltz, L.A., Unsal-Kacmaz, K., Linn, S., 2004. Molecular mechanisms of mammalian DNA repair and the DNA damage checkpoints. Annu. Rev. Biochem. 73, 39–85.

Scagliotti, G.V., Selvaggi, G., Novello, S., Hirsch, F.R., 2004. The biology of epidermal growth factor receptor in lung cancer. Clin. Cancer Res. 10, 4227s–4232s.

Schmidt-Ullrich, R.K., Mikkelsen, R.B., Dent, P., et al., 1997. Radiation-induced proliferation of the human A431 squamous carcinoma cells is dependent on EGFR tyrosine phosphorylation. Oncogene 15, 1191–1197.

Sharma, S.V., Bell, D.W., Settleman, J., Haber, D.A., 2007. Epidermal growth factor receptor mutations in lung cancer. Nat. Rev. Cancer 7, 169–181.

Siegel, R., Ward, E., Brawley, O., Jemal, A., 2011. Cancer statistics, 2011: the impact of eliminating socioeconomic and racial disparities on premature cancer deaths. CA Cancer J. Clin. 61, 212–236.

Sorensen, J.B., Hansen, H.H., Hansen, M., Dombernowsky, P., 1988. Brain metastases in adenocarcinoma of the lung: frequency, risk groups, and prognosis. J. Clin. Oncol. 6, 1474–1480.

Tsai, C.M., Chang, K.T., Perng, R.P., et al., 1993. Correlation of intrinsic chemoresistance of non-small-cell lung cancer cell lines with HER-2/neu gene expression but not with ras gene mutations. J. Natl. Cancer Inst. 85, 897–901.

van Vulpen, M., Kal, H.B., Taphoorn, M.J., El-Sharouni, S.Y., 2002. Changes in blood-brain barrier permeability induced by radiotherapy: implications for timing of chemotherapy? (Review). Oncol. Rep. 9, 683–688.

Wu, C., Li, Y.L., Wang, Z.M., Li, Z., Zhang, T.X., Wei, Z., 2007. Gefitinib as palliative therapy for lung adenocarcinoma metastatic to the brain. Lung Cancer 57, 359–364.

Wyman, C., Ristic, D., Kanaar, R., 2004. Homologous recombination-mediated double-strand break repair. DNA Repair (Amst) 3, 827–833.

Zeng, Y.D., Zhang, L., Liao, H., et al., 2012. Gefitinib alone or with concomitant whole brain radiotherapy for patients with brain metastasis from non-small-cell lung cancer: a retrospective study. Asian Pac. J. Cancer Prev. 13, 909–914.

Zhan, M., Han, Z.C., 2004. Phosphatidylinositide 3-kinase/AKT in radiation responses. Histol. Histopathol. 19, 915–923.

CHAPTER

12

Metastatic Spread of Lung Cancer to Brain and Liver: Role of CX3CR1

David J. Pinato and Francesco A. Mauri

OUTLINE

Introduction 123

Organotropic Spread of Lung Carcinoma: Role of Chemokine Signaling Pathways 124

CX3CR1 As a Molecular Determinant of Organotropic Diffusion of Lung Cancer 126

References 128

INTRODUCTION

Lung cancer leads the ranking of cancer-related mortality in both the USA and Europe (Jemal et al., 2008). Non-small cell lung cancer (NSCLC) shows predominance over small cell histology (SCLC), which accounts for only 15–20% of the incident cases (Govindan et al., 2006). The biologic behavior of the two histological subgroups is inherently different, with SCLC being characterized by intense proliferative activity, higher propensity to early dissemination and intrinsic chemosensitivity (Jackman and Johnson, 2005). Approximately 70% of newly diagnosed cases of SCLC present with extensive disease and, despite the generally favorable response rates to frontline chemotherapy, the life expectancy for these patients does not normally exceed 12 months (Chute et al., 1999).

NSCLC represents a heterogeneous aggregate of histologies including squamous cell, adenocarcinoma and large cell carcinoma. Recent advances in the genetic characterization of NSCLC have enriched such classification introducing molecularly defined tumor phenotypes. The presence of epithelial growth factor receptor (EGFR) activating mutations, for

M.A. Hayat (ed): *Brain Metastases from Primary Tumors, Volume 1*
DOI: http://dx.doi.org/10.1016/B978-0-12-800896-6.00012-7

© 2014 Elsevier Inc. All rights reserved.

example, defines a subgroup of NSCLC affecting approximately 50% of Asian patients and 10% of non-Asians, that are more likely to respond to EGFR tyrosine kinase inhibitors. More recent work on novel targets such as anaplastic lymphoma kinase (ALK) rearrangements, which identify 2–7% of adenocarcinomas with favorable response rates to ALK inhibitors, has further strengthened the concept of molecular classification of NSCLC (Nevins, 2011).

In the context of such a molecularly composite disease, Tumor Node Metastasis (TNM) staging remains a solid guide to treatment allocation and holds prognostic significance. In fact, while patients presenting with either surgically unresectable (stage IIIB) or metastatic tumors (stage IV) will inevitably succumb from their disease, those with operable NSCLC may potentially hope for a cure, with 5-year survival probabilities ranging from 80% for stage IA, to 30% for stage IIIA (Sakurai et al., 2010).

Regardless of histology, metastatic diffusion is viewed as the main factor that influences treatment failure in the curative setting (Nesbitt et al., 1995), reduces the chances of long-term survival as a result of organ failure and determines the symptomatic burden typically affecting patients with advanced cancer. Metastatic dissemination to the liver and the central nervous system (CNS) is fairly common in the evolution of bronchogenic carcinoma. However, the development of metastatic spread to these districts remains difficult to predict in the individual patient.

Intracranial diffusion is the most common pattern of treatment failure in patients who present with potentially curable NSCLC (Mamon et al., 2005), and eventually affects up to 55% of the patients with locally advanced disease (Chen et al., 2007). Cerebral metastases have an invariably fatal clinical course and represent the direct cause of death in these patients (Oh et al., 2009). Although a number of clinical predictors of metastatic spread to the CNS including nodal status and non-squamous histology have been identified, the precise molecular mechanisms contributing to the neurotropic potential of lung cancer cells have not been fully elucidated.

ORGANOTROPIC SPREAD OF LUNG CARCINOMA: ROLE OF CHEMOKINE SIGNALING PATHWAYS

Metastatic spread is viewed as a multistep process involving the adaptive selection of a genetically unstable cancer cell clone towards the acquirement of an invasive phenotype capable of overcoming the intrinsic biological and physical barriers to cell diffusion. The presence of a positive selective pressure to overcome the presence of extracellular matrix components, elude the surveillance of the immune system, secure survival in the bloodstream is fundamental in driving the metastatic phenotype. Similarly, the ability to arrest and extravasate into the target organ and display independent growth capacity are equally important traits that the metastasizing cell is specifically selected to display (Langley and Fidler, 2007).

The concept of cancer cell metastatization as a programmed, multifactorial cascade of events is not novel in oncology, having been first hypothesized by Stephen Paget in 1889, who compared the predisposition of certain organs to become colonized by secondary growths to a "fertile soil" that can actively promote tumor dissemination and growth.

In the context of lung cancer, mechanistic research has started elucidating the laborious genetic reprogramming underlying metastatic spread, that is now known to involve the activation of discrete molecular pathways such as epithelial-to-mesenchymal transition (EMT), a complex signaling cascade by which epithelial cells progressively lose cell–cell adhesion, apical-basal polarity and increase their motility and invasive properties (Nurwidya et al., 2012).

Unequivocal evidence has shown that chemokine signaling pathways, originally discovered as mediators of directional migration of immune cells following tissue injury and inflammation, may participate in systemic diffusion of cancer by modulating the site-specific homing of metastasizing tumor cells (Koizumi et al., 2007).

Chemokines constitute a superfamily of small cytokines with molecular weight ranging from 6 to 14 kD. Historically subclassified as C, CC, CXC or CX3C according to the structure of repeated cystein residue-rich motifs within the N-terminal region of the protein, chemokines were first characterized as mediators of the innate immunity, being secreted by a wide variety of cells paricipating in the acute phase reaction including endothelial cells, monocytes/macrophages and leukocytes (Blanchet et al., 2012). Besides inducing chemotaxis in responsive cells following insult, chemokine subgroups are secreted either phasically or constitutively to participate in tissue homeostatic processes such as organ development, angiogenesis, and wound repair (Le et al., 2004).

More than 50 different chemokines have been identified, all of which mediate their biological functions by binding to a G-protein coupled trans-membrane receptor. Each receptor is characterized by seven hydrophobic trans-membrane domains, an N-terminus extracellular chemokine binding region and an intracellular, serine and threonine rich domain which mediates intracellular signaling by ligand-controlled phosphorylation (Singh et al., 2007). Among the downstream molecular events triggered by chemokine receptor activation, conformational changes in the cytoskeleton and in cell adhesion molecules, such as integrins, facilitate cell motility and chemotaxis (Murdoch and Finn, 2000).

Chemokine signaling pathways can act at various levels in the context of metastatic spread. Recent evidence suggests that the chemokine secretion signature of a given tissue combined with the selective expression of the matched receptors by tumor cell clones might explain the site-specific spread of metastatic foci observed in solid tumors (Zlotnik et al., 2011). Pioneer work in breast cancer demonstrated an elevated expression of chemokine receptors CXCR4 and CCR7 in human breast cancer cell lines and in both primary and secondary specimens and that – more interestingly – the expression of their respective ligands CXCL12 and CCL21 peaks in those organs that are more frequently colonized by secondary deposits (Muller et al., 2001).

In lung cancer, elevated mRNA levels of the chemokine receptor CCR7 measured in primary NSCLC specimens were found to correlate with more advanced stage and predict for a significant lymphotropic behavior (Takanami, 2003). Similarly, the expression of chemokine receptor CXCR4, a highly prevalent molecular trait in NSCLC specimens and immortalized cell lines, guides chemotaxis and metastatic diffusion to those tissues where levels of its ligand CXCL12 are more abundant (Phillips et al., 2003).

Taking advantage of the notoriously pleiotropic and redundant nature of chemokine signaling, additional biological actions that are inherent to the establishment of metastatic cancer growth are at least in part sustained by an intricate network of interactions between chemokines and their receptors, including the acquisition of invasive properties as well as the promotion of neoangiogenesis (Strieter et al., 2004).

CX3CR1 AS A MOLECULAR DETERMINANT OF ORGANOTROPIC DIFFUSION OF LUNG CANCER

An increasing scientific interest has been devoted to the study of the chemokine receptor CX3CR1, a transmembrane protein that uniquely interacts with CX3CL1 or fractalkine, a large, 373 amino acid-long chemokine that exists as a membrane bound protein or in a soluble form (Bazan et al., 1997). The soluble pool of fractalkine is maintained by cleavage of the membrane-bound reservoir, which is operated constitutively by the protease ADAM10 and can be enhanced following tissue injury by ADAM17 (Garton et al., 2001). Fractalkine expression is mainly distributed on endothelial cells, lymphocytes, neurons, microglial cells, and osteoblasts. Besides its established role in chemotaxis, fractalkine promotes neuroprotective effects during brain injury, regulates endothelial cells and tissue homeostasis by exerting anti-apoptotic effects (White and Greaves, 2012).

In solid malignancies, the expression of fractalkine and its receptor CX3CR1 modulates the biologic behavior of the disease in a histotype-dependent manner. With the exception of colorectal and hepatocellular carcinoma, where elevated expression of fractalkine (Ohta et al., 2005) and CX3CR1 (Matsubara et al., 2007) exerts a protective effect on patients' prognosis, possibly through a direct enhancement of antitumor cytotoxic immune response, the effects of fractalkine/CX3CR1 signaling seem to mediate predominantly pro-tumoral effects in most other tumor types. The production of fractalkine by mature osteoblasts and bone marrow endothelial cells has been identified as a major determinant of skeletal diffusion of CX3CR1-bearing prostate adenocarcinoma cells (Jamieson et al., 2008).

A similar molecular interplay guides the neurotropic potential of human pancreatic ductal adenocarcinoma, where malignant cells but not their normal exocrine epithelial counterparts largely express CX3CR1. The interaction between CX3CR1-positive cell clones and fractalkine enhances adhesion and migration through nerve sheaths via conformational changes in β-integrins and activation of focal adhesion kinase. In clinical samples, CX3CR1 positivity was associated with worse disease-free survival and increased rates of perineural invasion, a recognized adverse prognostic factor in early-stage pancreatic carcinoma (Marchesi et al., 2010).

In epithelial ovarian carcinoma, the CX3CR1/fractalkine axis guides transcelomic diffusion by favoring migration of cancer cells in ascitic fluid and modulating their adhesion to mesothelial surfaces (Kim et al., 2012), whereas in breast cancer, CX3CR1 overexpression in the primary tumor confers a 10-fold risk increase for the development of brain metastases in a group of 142 patients with node-positive breast carcinoma undergoing radical treatment (Andre et al., 2006).

Based on the increasing body of evidence supporting the role of CX3CR1 and its ligand as molecular determinants of metastatic diffusion in a wide range of solid tumors, our interest in CX3CR1 was focused on understanding its role in the malignant progression of lung cancer and investigating whether CX3CR1 may represent a molecular factor involved in the metastatic spread of both SCLC and NSCLC.

To test this hypothesis we assembled a large isogeneic collection of primary lung cancer specimens and matching metastatic deposits by reviewing post-mortem examination records of 499 patients with a definitive histological diagnosis of lung cancer and absence of active anticancer treatment prior to the patient's death. Original paraffin embedded samples were reviewed and only 98 cases with satisfactory preservation of the tissue were sampled to construct a tissue microarray block. CX3CR1 expression was assayed using immunohistochemistry.

Our results show that the CX3CR1 expression in the primary lung tumors was significantly higher in NSCLC (63%) compared to SCLC (7%). Histological subclassification revealed large cell neuroendocrine carcinoma (100%) and squamous cell carcinomas (93%) as being most predominant in CX3CR1 expression when compared to adenocarcinomas (50%).

The disproportion of CX3CR1 immunopositivity seen in the primary tumors was preserved in metastatic deposits, where NSCLC yielded a significantly higher proportion of CX3CR1 immunopositivity (65%) compared to SCLC (29%). Interestingly, the distribution of CX3CR1 expression across the sampled metastatic sites of NSCLC showed that atypical sites of metastatic spread including thyroid, heart, small bowel and skin were entirely positive to CX3CR1, followed by more than 75% of the kidney, liver, bone and brain deposits. All the sampled splenic metastases from NSCLC primaries were negative.

In SCLC cases, 83% of the CNS metastatic sites were positive to CX3CR1, whereas only a minority of the other sites, including locoregional lymph nodes (14%) and liver (28%), expressed the receptor. Adrenal gland metastases arising from SCLC were all negative.

While metastatic disease was predominantly CX3CR1 positive, the subset of primary tumors lacking CX3CR1 expression displayed a significantly higher proportion of liver and brain metastatic deposits, with a predominance of lung adenocarcinoma, a histotype with peculiar neurotropic and hepatotropic potential.

Because fractalkine is expressed in the normal CNS including activated brain endothelial cells, we hypothesize that its constitutive expression may provide a chemoattracting gradient promoting trans-endothelial migration of metastasizing tumor cells (Hurst et al., 2009). Similarly, the abundant expression of fractalkine by hepatic sinusoidal cells may explain the significant association between CX3CR1 status in the primary tumor and the concurrent presence of liver metastatic diffusion (Matsubara et al., 2007).

The high expression rates observed in liver and the central nervous system (CNS) metastatic sites support the hypothesis that the acquisition of CX3CR1 positivity is not a random event, but may represent a site-selective molecular event conferring growth advantage to the metastasized cell clone.

In view of the recognized role of fractalkine in the promotion of angiogenesis, it is also reasonable to presume that the increased proportion of CX3CR1 positivity observed within the brain deposits may reflect a locally enhanced pro-angiogenic environment. As previously shown, brain metastases do not share the same angiogenic phenotype of the corresponding primary NSCLC. In particular, the high production of vascular endothelial growth factor (VEGF) observed in the brain secondary tumors may be mirrored by the consistent and potentially angiogenesis-driven upregulation of CX3CR1 (Jubb et al., 2011). Expression of CX3CR1 receptor in metastatic sites is also relevant to ensure sustained survival of disseminated cancer cells through the activation of discrete intracellular pathways such as AKT and ERK1/2 (Nevo et al., 2009).

Evidence emerging from the study of lung cancer specimens suggests that CX3CR1 is involved in the clinical progression of NSCLC, being expressed in the majority of NSCLC metastatic deposits as well as in a predominant proportion of SCLC brain metastases. Expression of CX3CR1 is differentially distributed across the diverse histological subgroups of primary lung cancer, with almost three-quarters of brain metastatic counterparts spread from both SCLC and NSCLC primaries expressing CX3CR1.

The vast proportion of CX3CR1 positivity observed in metastatic disease provides preliminary, although convincing evidence supporting a potential role for specific inhibitors of the fractalkine/CX3CR1 axis in the setting of advanced lung carcinoma and possibly, as an adjuvant strategy to treat micrometastatic disease. Moreover, pending confirmation in independent, recruited patient cohorts, routine assessment of CX3CR1 status by immunohistochemistry could prove useful in stratifying patients who are more at risk of CNS or hepatic relapse following radical treatment.

References

Andre, F., Cabioglu, N., Assi, H., et al., 2006. Expression of chemokine receptors predicts the site of metastatic relapse in patients with axillary node positive primary breast cancer. Ann. Oncol. 17, 945–951.

Bazan, J.F., Bacon, K.B., Hardiman, G., et al., 1997. A new class of membrane-bound chemokine with a CX3C motif. Nature 385, 640–644.

Blanchet, X., Langer, M., Weber, C., Koenen, R.R., von Hundelshausen, P., 2012. Touch of chemokines. Front Immunol. 3, 175.

Chen, A.M., Jahan, T.M., Jablons, D.M., Garcia, J., Larson, D.A., 2007. Risk of cerebral metastases and neurological death after pathological complete response to neoadjuvant therapy for locally advanced nonsmall-cell lung cancer: clinical implications for the subsequent management of the brain. Cancer 109, 1668–1675.

Chute, J.P., Chen, T., Feigal, E., Simon, R., Johnson, B.E., 1999. Twenty years of phase III trials for patients with extensive-stage small-cell lung cancer: perceptible progress. J. Clin. Oncol. 17, 1794–1801.

Garton, K.J., Gough, P.J., Blobel, C.P., et al., 2001. Tumor necrosis factor-alpha-converting enzyme (ADAM17) mediates the cleavage and shedding of fractalkine (CX3CL1). J. Biol. Chem. 276, 37993–38001.

Govindan, R., Page, N., Morgensztern, D., et al., 2006. Changing epidemiology of small-cell lung cancer in the United States over the last 30 years: analysis of the surveillance, epidemiologic, and end results database. J. Clin. Oncol. 24, 4539–4544.

Hurst, L.A., Bunning, R.A., Couraud, P.O., et al., 2009. Expression of ADAM-17, TIMP-3 and fractalkine in the human adult brain endothelial cell line, hCMEC/D3, following pro-inflammatory cytokine treatment. J. Neuroimmunol. 210, 108–112.

Jackman, D.M., Johnson, B.E., 2005. Small-cell lung cancer. Lancet 366, 1385–1396.

Jamieson, W.L., Shimizu, S., D'Ambrosio, J.A., Meucci, O., Fatatis, A., 2008. CX3CR1 is expressed by prostate epithelial cells and androgens regulate the levels of CX3CL1/fractalkine in the bone marrow: potential role in prostate cancer bone tropism. Cancer Res. 68, 1715–1722.

Jemal, A., Siegel, R., Ward, E., et al., 2008. Cancer statistics, 2008. CA Cancer J. Clin. 58, 71–96.

Jubb, A.M., Cesario, A., Ferguson, M., et al., 2011. Vascular phenotypes in primary non-small cell lung carcinomas and matched brain metastases. Br. J. Cancer 104, 1877–1881.

Kim, M., Rooper, L., Xie, J., Kajdacsy-Balla, A.A., Barbolina, M.V., 2012. Fractalkine receptor CX(3)CR1 is expressed in epithelial ovarian carcinoma cells and required for motility and adhesion to peritoneal mesothelial cells. Mol. Cancer Res. 10, 11–24.

Koizumi, K., Hojo, S., Akashi, T., Yasumoto, K., Saiki, I., 2007. Chemokine receptors in cancer metastasis and cancer cell-derived chemokines in host immune response. Cancer Sci. 98, 1652–1658.

Langley, R.R., Fidler, I.J., 2007. Tumor cell-organ microenvironment interactions in the pathogenesis of cancer metastasis. Endocr. Rev. 28, 297–321.

Le, Y., Zhou, Y., Iribarren, P., Wang, J., 2004. Chemokines and chemokine receptors: their manifold roles in homeostasis and disease. Cell Mol. Immunol. 1, 95–104.

Mamon, H.J., Yeap, B.Y., Janne, P.A., et al., 2005. High risk of brain metastases in surgically staged IIIA non-small-cell lung cancer patients treated with surgery, chemotherapy, and radiation. J. Clin. Oncol 23, 1530–1537.

Marchesi, F., Locatelli, M., Solinas, G., Erreni, M., Allavena, P., Mantovani, A., 2010. Role of CX3CR1/CX3CL1 axis in primary and secondary involvement of the nervous system by cancer. J. Neuroimmunol. 224, 39–44.

Matsubara, T., Ono, T., Yamanoi, A., Tachibana, M., Nagasue, N., 2007. Fractalkine-CX3CR1 axis regulates tumor cell cycle and deteriorates prognosis after radical resection for hepatocellular carcinoma. J. Surg. Oncol 95, 241–249.

Muller, A., Homey, B., Soto, H., et al., 2001. Involvement of chemokine receptors in breast cancer metastasis. Nature 410, 50–56.

Murdoch, C., Finn, A., 2000. Chemokine receptors and their role in inflammation and infectious diseases. Blood 95, 3032–3043.

Nesbitt, J.C., Putnam Jr, J.B., Walsh, G.L., Roth, J.A., Mountain, C.F., 1995. Survival in early-stage non-small cell lung cancer. Ann. Thorac. Surg. 60, 466–472.

Nevins, J.R., 2011. Pathway-based classification of lung cancer: a strategy to guide therapeutic selection. Proc. Am. Thorac. Soc. 8, 180–182.

Nevo, I., Sagi-Assif, O., Meshel, T., et al., 2009. The involvement of the fractalkine receptor in the transmigration of neuroblastoma cells through bone-marrow endothelial cells. Cancer Lett. 273, 127–139.

Nurwidya, F., Takahashi, F., Murakami, A., Takahashi, K., 2012. Epithelial mesenchymal transition in drug resistance and metastasis of lung cancer. Cancer Res. Treat. 44, 151–156.

Oh, Y., Taylor, S., Bekele, B.N., et al., 2009. Number of metastatic sites is a strong predictor of survival in patients with nonsmall cell lung cancer with or without brain metastases. Cancer 115, 2930–2938.

Ohta, M., Tanaka, F., Yamaguchi, H., Sadanaga, N., Inoue, H., Mori, M., 2005. The high expression of Fractalkine results in a better prognosis for colorectal cancer patients. Int. J. Oncol. 26, 41–47.

Phillips, R.J., Burdick, M.D., Lutz, M., Belperio, J.A., Keane, M.P., Strieter, R.M., 2003. The stromal derived factor-1/CXCL12-CXC chemokine receptor 4 biological axis in non-small cell lung cancer metastases. Am. J. Respir. Crit. Care Med. 167, 1676–1686.

Sakurai, H., Asamura, H., Goya, T., et al., 2010. Survival differences by gender for resected non-small cell lung cancer: a retrospective analysis of 12,509 cases in a Japanese Lung Cancer Registry study. J. Thorac. Oncol. 5, 1594–1601.

Singh, S., Sadanandam, A., Singh, R.K., 2007. Chemokines in tumor angiogenesis and metastasis. Cancer Metastasis Rev. 26, 453–467.

Strieter, R.M., Belperio, J.A., Burdick, M.D., Sharma, S., Dubinett, S.M., Keane, M.P., 2004. CXC chemokines: angiogenesis, immunoangiostasis, and metastases in lung cancer. Ann. NY Acad. Sci. 1028, 351–360.

Takanami, I., 2003. Overexpression of CCR7 mRNA in nonsmall cell lung cancer: correlation with lymph node metastasis. Int. J. Cancer 105, 186–189.

White, G.E., Greaves, D.R., 2012. Fractalkine: a survivor's guide: chemokines as antiapoptotic mediators. Arterioscler. Thromb. Vasc. Biol. 32, 589–594.

Zlotnik, A., Burkhardt, A.M., Homey, B., 2011. Homeostatic chemokine receptors and organ-specific metastasis. Nat. Rev. Immunol. 11, 597–606.

CHAPTER

13

Solitary Brain Metastasis from Non-Small Cell Lung Cancer: Treatment with Linac-Based Stereotactic Radiosurgery

Filippo Alongi, Umberto Ricardi and Marta Scorsetti

OUTLINE

Introduction 131

Technical and Technological Aspects 132

Radiobiological Issues and Clinical Data 134

Whole-Brain Radiation Therapy 135

Surgery 135

Surgery and Whole-Brain Radiation Therapy 135

Radiosurgery alone or with Whole-Brain Radiation Therapy 136

Patient Selection 136

Conclusion 137

References 137

INTRODUCTION

Stage IV metastatic disease will be found in approximately 30–40% of patients with non-small cell lung cancer (NSCLC). The brain represents the most common metastatic site for primary lung. The presence of a solitary brain metastasis is a common neurological situation in lung cancer patients (Schouten et al., 2002). The best treatment approach for solitary brain metastasis is still not well defined. Whether a single brain metastasis should be submitted

M.A. Hayat (ed): *Brain Metastases from Primary Tumors, Volume 1*
DOI: http://dx.doi.org/10.1016/B978-0-12-800896-6.00013-9

© 2014 Elsevier Inc. All rights reserved.

to surgical resection or stereotactic radiosurgery (SRS), and which patients should receive whole brain adjuvant radiotherapy (WBRT), are still debated issues (Mintz et al., 2007).

SRS is an effective and non-invasive approach for oligometastatic disease to the brain, usually one to four brain metastases. The size of the lesion is another crucial factor influencing the possibility to use SRS. When a single, small brain lesion is the only site of systemic disease progression, SRS can achieve high uncomplicated local control rates (80–90% local control rates), with median survival improving from 2 to 9–12 months in patients with single or multiple metastatic brain lesions (Kaal et al., 2005). The most commonly available radiosurgery technology uses high-energy X-rays generated from a clinical linear accelerator, or "LINAC". Here we analyze and discuss technical, radiobiological and clinical aspects of LINAC-based radiosurgery for isolated brain metastasis from NSCLC.

TECHNICAL AND TECHNOLOGICAL ASPECTS

The term "stereotactic radiosurgery" was introduced in 1951, when Lars Leksell talked about a method for "the non-invasive destruction of intracranial lesions". The second step was the introduction of his first stereotactic frame, developing a few years later the definitive concept of radiosurgery (Leksell et al., 1968). Thanks to the possibility of localizing, with a high grade of accuracy, a target in three-dimensional space, Leksell affirmed that narrow beams of radiation intersecting at a common point could allow neurosurgeons to concentrate high doses of radiation to a target volume in the brain (Leskell et al, 1983). With this system of delivery, lesions located deeply within the brain or at the base of the skull could be treated with minimal damage to surrounding healthy critical structures. Further research on this field by his group culminated in the development of the Gamma knife (Dinka et al., 2005). In the late 1980s, at the University of Florida, a multidisciplinary team of neurosurgeons, radiation physicists and engineers studied the development of the first LINAC-based radiosurgery system (Friedman and Bova, 1989). From this date, with this LINAC system, more than 2000 patients have been treated with radiosurgery at the University of Florida. From the beginning of the 1990s, several other types of LINAC-based radiosurgery systems are currently available in the commercial market and, to date, it is the most common approach for SRS delivery worldwide.

SRS is a radiation technique able to deliver, in a single fraction, an extremely high dose of ionizing radiation to an intracranial target; the lesion is usually identified using stereotactic parameters on various types of imaging, performed before and during the procedure. The radiation tolerance of normal tissue is volume-dependent, and SRS exploits this concept delivering high conformal doses to small targets (Hoppe et al., 2008). With stereotactic delivery modality, the expected side effects depending on radiation dose delivered to critical structures are reduced, minimizing or eliminating the margins of normal tissue surrounding the lesion usually included in the planning treatment volume with conventional radiotherapy techniques (Halperin et al., 2008). The most commonly available SRS systems are based on high-energy X-rays generated from a clinical LINAC. The intersection of the axis of rotation of the gantry and the treatment couch and the central axis of the photon beam is a point defined as the LINAC isocenter. Planning Target Volumes could be treated using single or multiple isocenter plans. Classic stereotactic LINAC technology uses circular collimators of various diameters (from 5 mm to 50 mm) to reduce the beam penumbra, minimizing irradiation of healthy tissues surrounding the target. More recently, the level of dose conformation to the target can be further increased using micromultileaf collimators that can adapt isodoses to the shape of the target; this is certainly true and quite useful for irregularly-shaped (non-spherical) target volumes. With the intent to increase the performance to conform as better the dose to the target as possible, multiple fixed fields or dynamic-arc radiosurgery systems have been developed and applied in clinical practice. With this technology, LINAC-based SRS systems could be able to generate dose distributions with a conformity level similar to those reported for multiple isocenters Gamma knife plans (Halperin et al., 2008). With the same "philosophy" of the multiple beam Gamma knife, Cyber knife uses multiple fixed-beam positions and multiple isocenters for planning. The Cyber knife System is a LINAC-based system for SRS and stereotactic body radiotherapy: it combines a miniaturized LINAC equipped on a robotic arm with a system for target tracking with two orthogonal diagnostic X-ray generators; subsequently, the beam realignment is performed with a software for correction. Cyber knife is a 6-MeV LINAC and uses circular collimators of various diameters attached to a six-axis robotic arm. Stereotactic frames are not normally useful for target position definition.

Intensity Modulated Radiation delivery (IMRT) can also be used as an SRS treatment delivery technique, further to improve conformity indices, when compared with conventional stereotactic delivery systems. IMRT treatment must be carefully performed using three-dimensional images of the patient in conjunction with complex dose calculation algorithms to create the dose intensity pattern for the best conformity to the treatment volume shape. Usually, various combinations of several intensity-modulated fields with different beam directions generate a custom tailored radiation dose. The result is that dose distribution maximizes target coverage, while better sparing adjacent healthy tissues exposed to higher radiation doses.

Treatment positioning is crucial for precision delivery of SRS: the patient's head is aligned to the LINAC beam and immobilized with a personalized thermoplastic mask. In modern LINAC systems dedicated to SRS, a robotic couch is provided to reduce uncertainties of patient positioning compared to planned parameters, and volumetric Image Guidance systems (IGRT) are used to improve set-up error corrections before and after treatment. To guarantee high accuracy in the SRS treatment, diagnostic three-dimensional images and highly conformal delivery are combined in the same treatment unit. Modern imaging systems integrated on modern LINAC represent a further evolution step for treatment units in terms of technological advances. Because patient position uncertainties, due to movement between image acquisition and dose delivery, is a critical reason for imprecision of the entire treatment, IGRT methods are based on non-invasive immobilization devices and patient position tracking systems. IGRT is available in the market of LINAC as various types of integrated imaging on board systems: very high quality of images, as well as KV cone beam CT or MeV CT and/or electronic portal images, are commonly available on LINACs for SRS and precise treatments. Due to the possibility to correct set up errors with a very high resolution quality of images, more comfortable frameless immobilization devices are used even more for SRS patients when combined with IMRT-IGRT delivery.

Volumetric IMRT techniques (VMAT: Volumetric Modulation Arc Therapy) and other rotational delivery systems have also significantly reduced delivery treatment time compared to the previous classical forms of IMRT delivery (static or dynamic). Flattening Filter Free (FFF) modality for LINAC is currently under evaluation as a new tool to deliver high doses combined with Volumetric Modulation Arc Therapy: it was recently shown that very high dose per fraction (more than 20 Gy) can be delivered in a few minutes with FFF beams. With FFF beams, it was possible to increase the dose/rate by a factor of four, having more dose on the central axis and less peripheral doses (Mancosu et al., 2012; Reggiori et al., 2012). For a particular type of tumor diameter, it could be the perfect approach to reduce normal tissue exposure, to reduce treatment time and potentially to guarantee an improved tumoricidal intensity of the dose, due to the increased dose rate. FFF technical aspects could represent a possible revolution in SRS, allowing clinicians to use LINAC as a safe, effective and extremely rapid arm to treat brain as well as extracranial lesions. Even if promising data regarding feasibility of stereotactic radiotherapy and FFF mode have been recently published, further studies on FFF delivery are still ongoing and warranted (Scorsetti et al., 2011). However, definitive data of clinical results are awaited to consolidate the safety of such an approach for each type of tumor site and size.

RADIOBIOLOGICAL ISSUES AND CLINICAL DATA

SRS is a powerful arm in the radiation treatment of brain tumors. The biological effectiveness of a single high radiation dose provides excellent results in terms of tumor control. Crucial conditions for treatment success are: small tumor size and appropriate location. In the case of a large lesion, the risk of healthy brain parenchyma damage and necrosis is high, regardless of dose conformation due to the steep dose gradient. In the case of specific critical organs, such as optic nerves or brainstem, close to or inside the planning target volumes, the technical ability to deliver an effective dose to the tumor is clearly limited by normal tissue tolerance of such specific normal structures. Thus, to optimize the clinical use of SRS, radiobiologic knowledge is essential fully to understand the potential tumoricidal effect of high single doses and to avoid potential side effects on normal tissues.

From its first applications, stereotactic radiotherapy, especially with Gamma kinfe, was used in a single fraction by clinicians. Thus, its powerful potential was strictly correlated to its ability to irradiate brain lesions with excellent dose distributions. From a radiobiologic point of view, it is recognized that a single-dose fraction could be unable to sterilize even a small tumor that contains hypoxic malignant cells. Based on the "hypoxic" rationale, a single-fraction delivered in radiosurgery is considered a suboptimal modality in the case of malignant tumors (Hall and Brenner, 1993). Thus, a multifractionated stereotactic radiotherapy schedule for a large intracranial malignancy is better advocated to treat this kind of lesion. On the other hand,, even for malignancies, in the case of a small treatment volume that contains little functioning brain tissue, the need for fractionation may not apply (Loeffler et al., 1990; Hall, 2000). Moreover, one of the potential advantages of radiosurgery, compared to multiple sessions, is that it may be able to overcome the radioresistance of a hypoxic tumor with a radiologic ablative effect when very high doses are delivered (Larson et al., 1993).

From a radiobiologic point of view, brain metastases are considered a category of target with early-responding tissue surrounded by late-responding normal tissue. Starting from the consideration that tumor cells are all inside the target, a high therapeutic index, based on the steep dose gradient performed by SRS, would be expected using this technique. Unlike surgery, SRS has also the potential to sterilize cells that may not be contained within the high-dose region (Larson et al., 1993).

Reviewing the past literature on solitary brain metastases in NSCLC patients, no clear consensus on the treatment of choice was found (Kaal et al., 2005). In the case of single brain metastasis from NSCLC, the life expectancy is mainly influenced by the general condition of the patient and the definitive treatment of the primary lung tumor (Flannery et al., 2008). Prognostic factors, besides specific local considerations (site and size of the brain tumor, number of brain metastases), can guide clinicians towards a more accurate treatment decision between surgery, WBRT and SRS (Linskey et al., 2010). Although the presence of brain metastases is often considered as an end-stage of disease, the majority of patients with controlled intracranial metastases will die from systemic disease rather than from recurrence and progression of these metastases.

WHOLE-BRAIN RADIATION THERAPY

Historically, in the 1950s and early 1960s, the first radiation treatment of brain metastasis was represented by whole brain radiation therapy. WBRT obtained the best response in patients with small cell lung cancer, lymphoma, and germ cell tumors. Several schedules of doses have been tested by The Radiation Therapy Oncology Group (RTOG) (Borgelt et al., 1980, 1981; Gelber et al., 1981; Kurtz et al., 1981; Sause et al., 1993; Komarnicky et al., 1991; Sneed et al., 1996; Murray et al, 1997; Phillips et al., 1995).

When a single brain metastasis is not suitable for complete resection, radiation is the treatment of choice. WBRT is the most widely used palliative therapeutic option to treat multiple brain metastases, although treated patients have an expected survival of only a few months. Unfortunately, in long-term survivors, WBRT can cause late radiological and clinical neurological side effects, similar to those of Alzheimer's disease.

SURGERY

In cases of solitary brain metastases, because local treatment is considered non-curative, surgery must be chosen only in selected cases (Flannery et al., 2008). Surgical resection was considered the gold standard treatment of a single metastasis to non-eloquent brain areas. Surgery has the advantage to establish or confirm the diagnosis in patients, especially those without primary tumor identification. Surgery can also determine a fast and effective palliation of neurologic symptoms due to mass effect (Hoppe et al., 2008). To enhance local control, various combinations of local approaches have been proposed in brain metastases.

Surgery and Whole-Brain Radiation Therapy

The combination of surgery and WBRT seems to be more effective than WBRT alone for the treatment of a single brain metastasis in patients with limited or no systemic disease and in good neurologic condition. With the intent to demonstrate that improved local control of a single brain metastasis would result in improved survival, three randomized trials compared WBRT with surgery followed by WBRT for patients with a single metastasis (Patchell et al., 1990; Noordijk et al., 1994; Mintz et al., 1996). Two out of three trials demonstrated an advantage of adding surgery to WBRT.

Radiosurgery alone or with Whole-Brain Radiation Therapy

Radiosurgery has been recognized as the first-line treatment approach for isolated brain metastases smaller than 3–4 cm in diameter, especially in eloquent areas, when edema surrounding the lesion is minimal (Flickinger et al., 1994). Compared to surgery, SRS has the clear advantage that the entire extent of metastasis can usually be encompassed within the planning treatment volume because treatment is linked directly to three-dimensional visualization of the tumor. Moreover, radiosurgery avoids the well-known risks of surgery: hemorrhage, infection, tumor seeding. From a psychological standpoint, physicians and patients are now selecting more often to treat isolated brain metastasis with SRS (Hoppe et al., 2008). Because of its non-invasive nature, radiosurgery provides significant comfort and reassurance. SRS requires also minimal or no hospitalization reducing significantly the costs of therapy.

Brain metastases represent an ideal target for accurate target delineation, planning, and treatment delivery with SRS. Usually the isolated metastasis is: (1) pseudospherical in shape; (2) located at the gray–white junction; (3) with a diameter of less than 4 cm; (3) with non-infiltrative behavior; and (5) surrounded by perilesional edema, displacing the normal brain parenchyma.

With SRS, the local control rates are in the range between 73% and 98%. Single-dose SRS alone appears to be superior to WBRT alone (level of evidence: 3) in terms of patient survival advantage for up to three metastases (Kocher et al., 2004).

SRS and WBRT compared to WBRT alone for patients with a single lesion provided level 1 evidence of a survival benefit (Andrews et al., 2004).

SRS, alone or in conjunction with WBRT, yields results comparable to those reported after surgery followed by WBRT (Soffietti et al 2002; Linskey et al., 2010). The addition of WBRT decreases tumor recurrence rate, both at the original site and in other new deposits, but has not been correlated with better survival (Goyal et al., 2000). When a limited number of brain metastases (one to three) are found, adjuvant WBRT after radiosurgery or surgery reduces intracranial relapses (at the original site and at new metastatic sites) and neurologic deaths, but fails to improve the duration of functional independence and overall survival. At the same time, it is argued that WBRT may be omitted without compromising patient survival or control of intracranial disease with close follow up, limiting salvage therapy only to relapsing patients. Using this approach, more than 70% of patients initially managed with SRS alone may be spared WBRT.

PATIENT SELECTION

In the case of a single brain metastasis and symptoms due to a mass effect, there is a dispute regarding the necessity surgically to remove the lesion. When general conditions are too poor to consider the patient eligible for surgery, or if patients refuse surgical intervention, or if metastasis is located in eloquent areas, SRS represents a logical treatment alternative to surgery. On the other hand, when the lesion is larger than 3–4 cm, the risk of SRS-induced damage of healthy tissues surrounding the metastasis is increased, and also the efficacy is significantly reduced. Particularly for single fraction SRS, the effective impact radiotherapy falls off dramatically as the tumor size increases. Metha et al. clearly demonstrated that the rate of complete response on the magnetic resonance images after SRS is proportionally reduced with tumor volume diameter increase (Mehta et al., 1992).

A clinical situation frequently an object of debate between surgeons and radiation oncologists is represented by patients with a single metastasis smaller than 3 cm, where surgery could be technically performed (Chang et al., 2003; Shehata et al., 2004).

It has to be noted that an NSCLC patient with a brain metastasis is a stage IV "cancer patient". Although the isolated brain lesion frequently represents the unique site of metastatic spread in some steps of the cancer history, this event has to be contextualized in the complex clinical mosaic of stage IV cancer disease, when several variables, including status of tumor at primary site, can influence general conditions and results of SRS. Thus, the decision of the therapeutic strategy should be multidisciplinary to guarantee the best approach for each patient.

CONCLUSION

Although many data have been published and analyzed, no consensus on the subject of isolated brain metastases has yet been reached. The debate continues whether surgery or SRS is better for this kind of patient. Stereotactic radiosurgery has progressively achieved an important role in the management of brain metastases, and LINAC-based SRS availability in most radiation therapy departments has widened the possibility of access to brain radiosurgery wordwide. Retrospective studies and several randomized trials have shown the benefits of SRS as sole treatment, and as an adjunct to WBRT. Undoubted, compared to surgery for isolated brain metastasis, radiosurgery avoids the interventional risks of hemorrhage, infection, and tumor seeding, requiring minimal or no hospitalization, reducing the risks and costs of surgical therapy. Thus, LINAC-based radiosurgery represents a non-invasive, safe and effective treatment option for isolated brain metastasis in lung cancer patients.

References

Andrews, D.W., Scott, C.B., Sperduto, P.W., et al., 2004. Whole brain radiation therapy with or without stereotactic radiosurgery boost for patients with one to three brain metastases: phase III results of the RTOG 9508 randomised trial. Lancet 363, 1665–1672.

Borgelt, B., Gelber, R., Kramer, S., et al., 1980. The palliation of brain metastasis: final results of the first two studies by the Radiation Therapy Oncology Group. Int. J. Radiat. Oncol. Biol. Phys. 6, 1–9.

Borgelt, B., Gelber, R., Larson, M., et al., 1981. Ultra-rapid high-dose irradiation schedules for the palliation of brain metastasis: final result of the first two studies by the Radiation Therapy Oncology Group. Int. J. Radiat. Oncol. Biol. Phys. 7, 1633–1638.

Chang, E.L., Hassenbusch 3rd, S.J., Shiu, A.S., et al., 2003. The role of tumor size in the radiosurgical management of patients with ambiguous brain metastases. Neurosurgery 53, 272–280.

Dinka, D., Nyce, J.M., Timpka, T., 2005. GammaKnife surgery: safety and the identity of users. Technol. Health Care 13, 485–495.

Flannery, T.W., Suntharalingam, M., Regine, W.F., et al., 2008. Long-term survival in patients with synchronous, solitary brain metastasis from non-small-cell lung cancer treated with radiosurgery. Int. J. Radiat. Oncol. Biol. Phys. 72, 1.

Flickinger, J.C., Kondziolka, D., Lunsford, L.D., et al., 1994. A multi-institutional experience with stereotactic radiosurgery for solitary brainmetastasis. Int. J. Radiat. Oncol. Biol. Phys. 28, 777–780.

Friedman, W.A., Bova, F.J., 1989. The University of Florida radiosurgery system. Surg. Neurol. 32, 334–342.

Gelber, R.D., Larson, M., Borgelt, B.B., et al., 1981. Equivalence of radiation schedules for the palliative treatment of brain metastases in patients with favorable prognosis. Cancer 48, 1749–1753.

Goyal, L.K., Suh, J.H., Reddy, C.A., et al., 2000. The role of whole brain radiotherapy and stereotactic radiosurgery on brain metastasis from renal cell carcinoma. Int. J. Radiat. Oncol. Biol. Phys. 47, 1007–1012.

Hall, E.J., 2000. Radiobiology for the Radiologist. Lippincott Williams & Wilkins, Philadelphia.

Hall, E.J., Brenner, D.J., 1993. The radiobiology of radiosurgery: rationale for different treatment regimes for AVMs and malignancies. Int. J. Radiat. Oncol. Biol. Phys. 25, 381–385.

Halperin, E.C., Perez, C.A., Brady, L.W., 2008. Perez and Brady's Principles and Practice of Radiation Oncology, Fifth ed. Lippincott Williams & Wilkins.

Hoppe, R.T., Phillips, T.L., Roach, M., 2008. Leibel and Phillips Textbook of Radiation Oncology. Elsevier Saunders.

Kaal, E.C., Niël, G.C., Vecht, C.J., 2005. Therapeutic management of brain metastasis. Lancet Neurol. 4, 289–298.

Kocher, M., Maarouf, M., Bendel, M., et al., 2004. Linac radiosurgery versus whole brain radiotherapy for brain metastases. A survival comparison based on the RTOG recursive partitioning analysis. Strahlenther. Onkol. 180, 263–267.

Komarnicky, L.T., Philips, T.L., Martz, K., et al., 1991. A randomized phase III protocol for the evaluation of misonidazole combined with radiation in the treatment of patients with brain metastases (RTOG 7916). Int. J. Radiat. Oncol. Biol. Phys. 20, 53–58.

Kurtz, J.M., Gelber, R., Brady, L.W., et al., 1981. The palliation of brain metastasis in a favorable patient population: a randomized clinical trial by the Radiation Therapy Oncology Group. Int. J. Radiat. Oncol. Biol. Phys. 7, 891–895.

Larson, D.A., Flickinger, J.C., Loeffler, J.S., et al., 1993. The radiobiology of radiosurgery. Int. J. Radiat. Oncol. Biol. Phys. 25, 557–561.

Leksell, L., 1968. Cerebral radiosurgery. I. Gammathalanotomy in two cases of intractable pain. Acta Chir. Scand. 134, 585–595.

Linskey, M.E., Andrews, D.W., Asher, A.L., et al., 2010. The role of stereotactic radiosurgery in the management of patients with newly diagnosed brain metastases: a systematic review and evidence-based clinical practice guideline. J. Neurooncol. 96, 45–68.

Loeffler, J.S., Kooy, H.M., Wen, P.Y., et al., 1990. The treatment of recurrent brain metastases with stereotactic radiosurgery. J. Clin. Oncol. 8, 576–582.

Mancosu, P., Castiglioni, S., Reggiori, G., et al., 2012. Stereotactic body radiation therapy for liver tumours using flattening filter free beam: dosimetric and technical considerations. Radiat. Oncol. 7, 16.

Mehta, M.P., Rozental, J.M., Levin, A.B., et al., 1992. Defining the role of radiosurgery in the management of brain metastases. Int. J. Radiat. Oncol. Biol. Phys. 24, 619–625.

Mintz, A.H., Kestle, J., Rathbone, M.P., et al., 1996. A randomized trial to assess the efficacy of surgery in addition to radiotherapy in patients with a single cerebral metastasis. Cancer 78, 1470–1476.

Mintz, A., Perry, J., Spithoff, K., Chambers, A., Laperriere, N., 2007. Management of single brain metastasis: a practice guideline. Curr. Oncol. 14, 131–143.

Murray, K.J., Scott, C., Greenberg, H.M., et al., 1997. A randomized phase III study of accelerated hyperfractionated versus standard in patients with unresected brain metastasis: a report of the Radiation Therapy Oncology Group (RTOG) 9104. Int. J. Radiat. Oncol. Biol. Phys. 39, 571–574.

Noordijk, E.M., Vecht, C.J., Haaxma-Reiche, H., et al., 1994. The choice of treatment of single brain metastasis should be based on extracranial tumor activity and age. Int. J. Radiat. Oncol. Biol. Phys. 29, 711–717.

Patchell, R.A., Tibbs, P.A., Walsh, J.W., et al., 1990. A randomized trial of surgery in the treatment of single metastases to the brain. N. Engl. J. Med. 322, 494–500.

Phillips, T.L., Scott, C.B., Leibel, S., et al., 1995. Results of a randomized comparison of radiotherapy and bromodeoxyuridine with radiotherapy alone for brain metastasis: a report of RTOG trial 89-05. Int. J. Radiat. Oncol. Biol. Phys. 33, 339–348.

Reggiori, G., Mancosu, P., Castiglioni, S., et al., 2012. Can volumetric modulated arc therapy with flattening filter free beams play a role in stereotactic body radiotherapy for liver lesions? A volume-based analysis. Med. Phys. 39, 1112–1118.

Sause, W.T., Scott, C., Krisch, R., et al., 1993. Phase I/I1 trial of accelerated fractionation in brain metastasis RTOG 85-28. Int. J. Radiat. Oncol. Biol. Phys. 26, 653–657.

Schouten, L.J., Rutten, J., Huveneers, H.A., Twijnstra, A., 2002. Incidence of brain metastases in a cohort of patients with carcinoma of the breast, colon, kidney, lung and melanoma. Cancer 94, 2698–2705.

Scorsetti, M., Alongi, F., Castiglioni, S., et al., 2011. Feasibility and early clinical assessment of flattening filter free (FFF) based stereotactic body radiotherapy (SBRT) treatments. Radiat. Oncol. 12, 113.

Shehata, M.K., Young, B., Reid, B., et al., 2004. Stereotatic radiosurgery of 468 brain metastases $\leq$2 cm: implications for SRS dose and whole brain radiation therapy. Int. J. Radiat. Oncol. Biol. Phys. 59, 87–93.

Sneed, P.K., Larson, D.A., Wara, W.M., 1996. Radiotherapy for cerebral metastases. Neurosurg. Clin. N. Am. 7, 505–515.

Soffietti, R., Ruda, R., Mutani, R., 2002. Management of brain metastases. J. Neurol. 249, 1357–1369.

CHAPTER

14

Brain Metastases from Non-Small Cell Lung Cancer: Clinical Benefits of Erlotinib and Gefitinib

M. Houman Fekrazad, Omid Sanaei, Julie E. Bauman and Dennie V. Jones, Jr.

OUTLINE

Introduction 142

Treatment Options for Brain Metastases 145

Whole Brain Radiotherapy (WBRT) 145

Surgery 145

Stereotactic Radiosurgery (SRS) 145

Systemic Therapy 145

Targeted Therapy 146

Trials of Gefitinib 147

Trials of Erlotinib 148

Obstacles to Drug Activity within the CNS and Ways to Overcome 148

Clinical Implications of EGFR Mutations 150

Prophylactic Role of the Drugs 151

Adverse Reactions of Gefitinib and Erlotinib, Pros and Cons 151

Future Directions/Additional Agents 152

References 153

M.A. Hayat (ed): *Brain Metastases from Primary Tumors, Volume 1*
DOI: http://dx.doi.org/10.1016/B978-0-12-800896-6.00014-0

© 2014 Elsevier Inc. All rights reserved.

INTRODUCTION

A 60-year old never-smoker woman presents with left-sided weakness and ataxia due to innumerable metastatic lesions within the brain originating from an advanced adenocarcinoma of the lung. She receives whole brain radiotherapy (WBRT) and systemic chemotherapy and her symptoms temporarily improve. A few months later her disease recurs both clinically and radiographically within the brain. Institution of erlotinib, a small molecule inhibitor of the epidermal growth factor receptor (EGFR) tyrosine kinase, results in a complete radiographic resolution of brain lesions, improvement in clinical symptoms and performance status, and partial response of the primary lung tumor (Figures 14.1 and 14.2) (Fekrazad et al., 2007).

Metastatic tumors are among the most common mass lesions in the brain. In the USA, up to 200000 people per year, or approximately 40% of patients diagnosed with an invasive malignancy, will develop brain metastases during the course of their illness (Maher et al., 2009; Eichler et al., 2011). Such lesions adversely affect the quality of life as well as the overall survival duration. The incidence of metastatic neoplasms involving the brain is greater than primary central nervous system (CNS) neoplasms. The majority of patients are greater than 60 years old, which is consistent with the median age of most invasive neoplasms. While metastatic disease to the brain may arise from any primary site, the most common sites of origin are the lung, followed by the breast, skin (overwhelmingly, melanomas) and the gut.

Approximately 85% of metastases are supratentorial, while only 1–3% are to the brainstem (Arbit and Wronski, 1995). Approximately 10% of patients will have an unknown primary site and, in 9% with a known source, the brain is the sole site of metastases. Primary lung cancers make up half of all metastatic brain tumors. Of those patients with lung cancer who survive for at least 2 years, 80% will have brain metastases. However, even within lung cancers, there is a differential propensity for the development of brain metastases based upon histology: small cell lung cancers comprise only 15–20% of all lung cancers, but lead to half of all brain metastases from lung cancers. Notably, about 30–40% of patients with non-small cell lung cancer (NSCLC) may develop clinically apparent metastatic disease to the brain; an early autopsy series noted that 55% of patients with NSCLC were found to have brain metastases (Knights, 1954).

A considerable body of work has been dedicated to find effective and safe treatments to improve survival of patients with brain metastases. These include surgery or stereotactic radiosurgery for oligometastatic disease, whole brain radiotherapy, and chemotherapy, either alone or as combined-modality treatments. Most of the larger reports, series or trials of localized treatments of brain metastases include a variety of tumor histologies. More importantly, the natural history of the underlying systemic disease often impacts the overall survival and, in some cases, the clinical benefit of any aggressive treatment specifically directed to the brain metastases. One of the largest retrospective analyses of patients with NSCLC and brain metastases was reported from the Cleveland Clinic (Chidel et al., 1999). The goal was to evaluate the outcome of treatment in patients with newly diagnosed NSCLC who also had an isolated, single, synchronous brain metastasis, with the brain being the sole metastatic site. Over a 14-year period (1982–1996) a total of 219 patients with lung cancer and synchronous brain metastases were identified; of these, only 33 patients had a solitary metastasis, and were further studied. The majority of those patients (64%) were treated with surgical resection followed by whole brain radiotherapy, and the remaining patients were treated with surgery alone or some form of radiotherapy, either as whole brain or

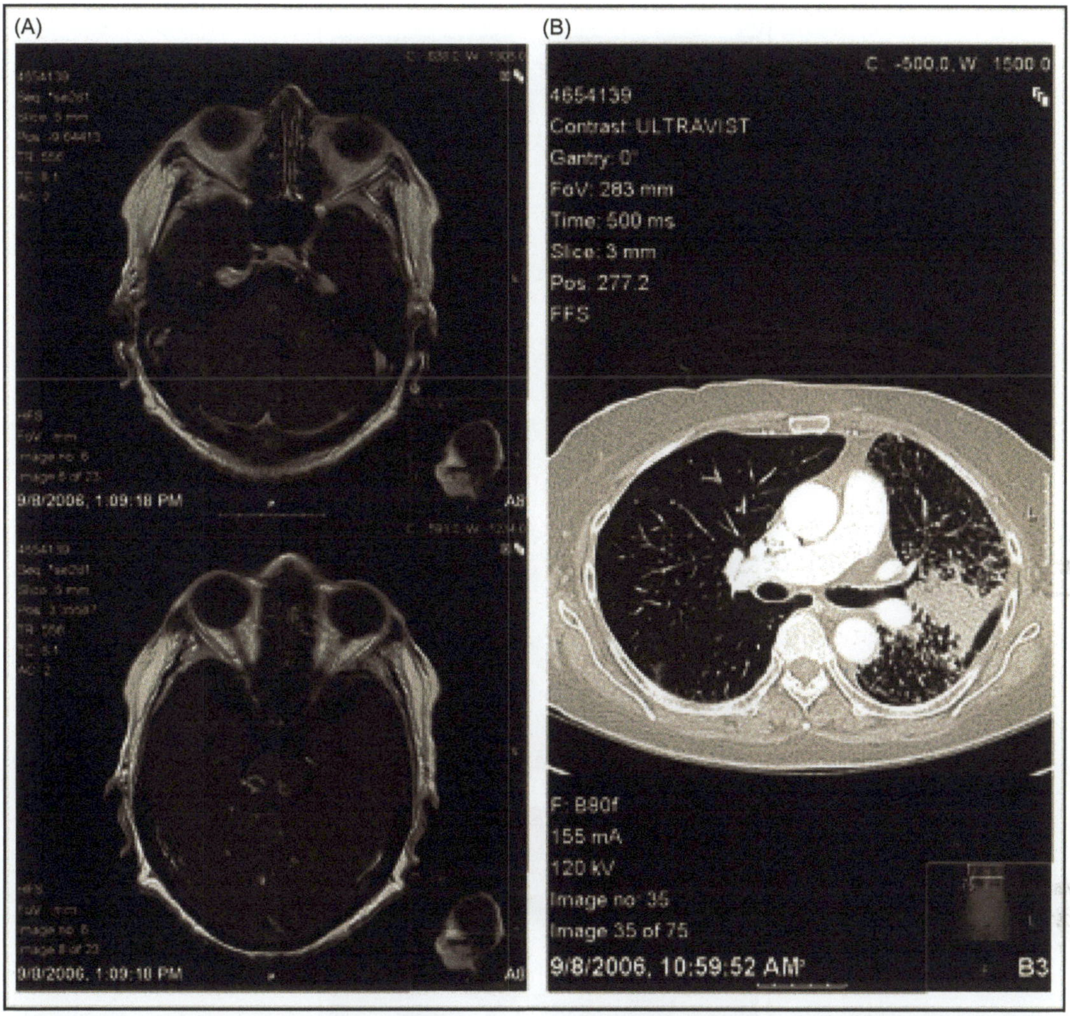

FIGURE 14.1 Magnetic resonance imaging (A) revealed recurrent disease within the brain, and a computed tomography scan of the chest (B) demonstrated progression of her disease (*Fekrazad et al., 2007*).

stereotactic radiotherapy. The disease in the CNS was controlled in 31 patients (94%). The median disease-free survival (DFS) was 3.3 months, with only nine patients suffering brain recurrence. The median overall survival (OS) was 6.9 months, though patients who received whole brain radiotherapy had a markedly prolonged OS compared to those who did not receive WBRT, 9.1 months versus 2.9 months ($p = 0.002$). Most of the patients died from systemic disease progression; control of extracranial disease was associated with a markedly prolonged median OS of 20.1 months. While these results are encouraging, there are several notable factors: this was a very small and highly selected patient population; 85% of the patients in the original cohort had multiple brain metastases, where a surgical resection or stereotactic radiosurgery may not be practical or of benefit. Furthermore, the main cause

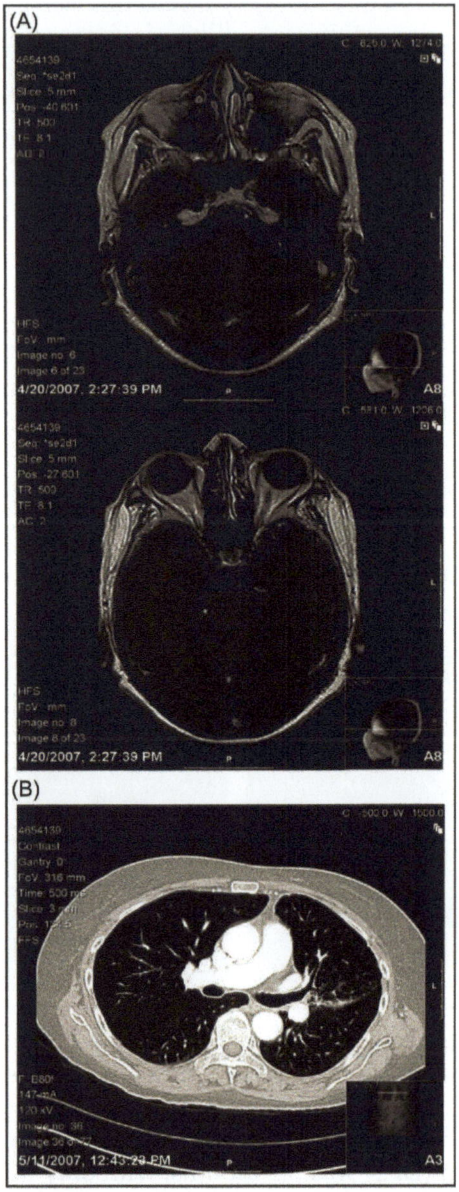

FIGURE 14.2 A follow-up magnetic resonance imaging of the brain obtained after 8 months of erlotinib therapy (A) demonstrated a complete resolution of the brain metastases, and a computed tomography scan of the chest obtained at that time revealed a partial remission of her primary disease (B) (*Fekrazad et al., 2007*).

of death in the studied population was still systemic disease progression, though 27% also had intracranial relapse. The low radiotolerance of normal brain tissue limits the cumulative dose of whole brain radiotherapy. With these factors in mind, it is clear that alternative agents must be developed to treat intracranial metastases from NSCLC.

TREATMENT OPTIONS FOR BRAIN METASTASES

Whole Brain Radiotherapy (WBRT)

Cranial radiotherapy (RT) is most frequently used to control neurologic symptoms caused by brain metastases. An important role for RT, that is a sensitizing effect for epidermal growth factor receptor tyrosine kinase inhibitors (EGFR-TKIs), has also been proposed (Ceresoli et al., 2004; Wu et al., 2007). However, the efficacy of RT is influenced by patient performance status, the number of metastatic lesions in the brain and extracranial tumor histology. Furthermore, RT has acute and chronic side effects which could impact overall quality of life. Overall, WBRT may extend survival by 4–6 months.

Surgery

Surgery is another option to treat brain metastases but is limited to single lesions (oligometastases) with accessible locations. When combined with subsequent RT, surgery improves survival compared to radiotherapy alone in lung cancer patients with oligometastatic disease (Rades et al., 2008). However, as many patients with NSCLC and brain metastases have multiple brain lesions, this option is not widely used.

Stereotactic Radiosurgery (SRS)

SRS treats CNS metastatic lesions by directing high dose radiation precisely to the affected sites with minimal irradiation of the surrounding unaffected tissues. It has been shown that SRS may yield a median survival of 9.4 months with 3-year local control rate of 65% (Alexander et al., 1995). It is possible to target multiple lesions with multiple beams. However, the efficacy of SRS depends on tumor volume and the amount of radiation. Overall, it has been accepted that up to four lesions, each <4 cm in diameter, in properly selected patients may be treated by SRS. When combined with WBRT, SRS improves tumor control, performance status, and decreases post-treatment recurrence of brain metastases compared to WBRT alone but does not usually translate into improvements in overall survival. In a phase III trial, combined use of WBRT plus SRS vs WBRT alone significantly ($p = 0.03$) improved survival, though only in patients with a single lesion; the combination was of no benefit in patients with multiple lesions (Andrews et al., 2004).

Systemic Therapy

Multiple cytotoxic chemotherapeutic drugs have been used to treat intracranial metastases from NSCLC. Several factors have significantly limited the potential efficacy of such agents. Most chemotherapeutic agents do not cross the blood–brain barrier sufficiently to allow for cytocidal levels in the cerebrospinal fluid (CSF) or brain parenchyma. Those agents that provide adequate CSF levels, such as the high doses of methotrexate or cytarabine as utilized in hematologic malignancies, are minimally active against NSCLC, despite being structurally related to pemetrexed and gemcitabine, respectively, which have demonstrated activity in NSCLC. Additionally, adequate CSF levels do not insure adequate parenchymal penetration.

Several agents have been evaluated which do provide CNS responses in other solid tumor malignancies, including temozolomide, topotecan, and capecitabine (Abrey and Christodoulou, 2001; Wong and Berkenblit, 2004; Robins et al., 2006; Kouvaris et al., 2007; Weller, 2007; Addeo et al., 2008; Neuhaus et al., 2009; Paydas et al., 2009; Nagpal et al., 2012). However, the majority of reported clinical experience is in primary CNS tumors (temozolomide) or metastases from other sites, such as small cell lung cancer (topotecan) or breast cancer (capecitabine). With respect to temozolomide, the experience does appear to be modest in most, though not all, of the trials reported of patients with brain metastases from NSCLC. Topotecan does have some activity in NSCLC, but is only approved for SCLC. Capecitabine is approved for treatment of breast cancer and gastrointestinal malignancies, though it is often substituted for 5-fluorouracil in a variety of treatment regimens. However, there are very few data on the activity of capecitabine in NSCLC. Pemetrexed demonstrated benefit in 32 of 39 patients with intracranial metastases in a report by Bearz et al. (2010). This deserves confirmation in a larger trial, though it should be noted that pemetrexed is inactive in the squamous cell type of NSCLC.

TARGETED THERAPY

The discovery of molecular targets within subgroups of neoplasms, some of which are heavily dependent upon a specific aberrantly activated oncogene or pathway, has opened up new opportunities for clinically beneficial treatment. "Targeted therapy", that is, the development of drugs designed to take advantage of specific molecular differences between malignant and normal cells, has existed since the development of agents to interrupt sex steroid signal transduction in subsets of breast and prostate cancer. Recently, a growing number of such targets have been identified in other solid tumors. Data obtained over the past several years have led to a better appreciation of the importance of histology in NSCLC, but even more so, the molecular subtype. For example, specific gene mutations or rearrangements have been identified in over half of all adenocarcinomas, many of which can be targeted with clinically available drugs. More recently, squamous cell carcinomas have likewise been divided into multiple subtypes by activated pathway; in fact, 96% of such NSCLC squamous cell subtypes contained potentially druggable activated tyrosine or serine/threonine kinases (The Cancer Genome Atlas Research Network et al., 2012). Many of these targeted drugs have been evaluated in a variety of neoplasms, and many have demonstrated an ability to provide some clinical benefit in the treatment of intracranial metastases. However, only two such pathways have been investigated in NSCLC to the point where specific agents are now commercially available: (1) the epidermal growth factor receptor (EGFR) pathway and, in particular, EGFR activating mutations in exons 19 and 21, which are potently inhibited by the small molecule tyrosine kinase inhibitors erlotinib (Tarceva) and gefitinib (Iressa); (2) activating anaplastic lymphoma kinase (ALK) gene rearrangements, which are blocked by crizotinib (Xalkori). Erlotinib and gefitinib exert their antitumor activity by binding to the ATP-binding site of the tyrosine kinase domain of the EGFR. This prevents auto/transphosphorylation of the receptors, which is needed for activation of the downstream signal cascade, thereby stopping tumor cell proliferation. In the following sections, we will review trials of the two best studied EGFR-TKIs, gefitinib and erlotinib.

Trials of Gefitinib

The efficacy of gefitinib in patients with NSCLC and brain metastases initially was suggested by several case reports. Thereafter, multiple retrospective or prospective trials evaluated the use of gefitinib in this patient population. In a prospective trial of 41 patients with NSCLC and brain metastases, patients who were treated with gefitinib achieved a median progression-free survival (PFS) and OS of 3 and 5 months, respectively. Four (10%) patients had partial response (PR) and seven (17%) had stable disease (SD) yielding a 27% disease control (DC) rate. Patients who had previously received WBRT attained a significantly higher DC rate than radio-naïve patients ($p = 0.0006$). Finally, adenocarcinoma histology was significantly ($p = 0.04$) associated with longer PFS (Ceresoli et al., 2004).

In another prospective study, 40 patients with brain metastases, all with adenocarcinoma histology and previously treated with chemotherapy, received gefitinib at 250 mg daily. The study showed a 32% objective response rate and 77% DC. The median PFS and OS were 9 and 15 months, respectively. Patients who had been treated previously with WBRT had significantly ($p = 0.041$) improved OS. Similarly, female gender was associated with a significantly improved overall survival, with a male to female hazard ratio of 3.29 (95% CI, 1.36–7.96 $p = 0.008$) (Wu et al., 2007).

Hotta et al. (2004) in a retrospective analysis on 14 NSCLC with brain metastases found 100% DC rate after treatment with gefitinib. The median PFS and median OS for these patients were 8.8 and 9.1 months, respectively. Of these, seven patients simultaneously expressed objective responses to both intra- and extracranial lesions, suggesting the possible correlation between sensitivity of brain metastases to gefitinib and that of extracranial tumors.

None of the patients in these studies were selected for having clinical characteristics associated with increased sensitivity to gefitinib, such as East-Asian ethnicity, female gender and never-smokers, or were molecularly selected for having specific activating EGFR mutations. However, with the striking discovery of the role of EGFR mutations in the responsiveness of patients to EGFR-TKIs, clinical trials conducted thereafter focused on this issue.

In a retrospective study of eight patients with NSCLC and brain metastases harboring EGFR activating mutations in which mutation status was determined by sampling of the primary tumor before the treatment was initiated, patients were treated with gefitinib, five patients experienced objective tumor response in brain lesions. In contrast, in all the remaining three patients in whom no objective tumor response was detected, EGFR mutation was not found (Shimato et al., 2006). Another retrospective analysis identified 14 patients with NSCLC and brain metastases receiving standard dose gefitinib, to assess the importance of EGFR mutation to the CNS response to this drug. Nine out of 14 (65%) with brain metastases and 30 out of 96 (31%) without brain metastases had mutant EGFR genotypes suggesting that development of brain metastases may correlate with EGFR mutation status ($p < 0.05$). Eight out of nine (89%) patients with EGFR mutation and brain metastases objectively responded to gefitinib, highlighting the role of patient selection based on mutation status (Li et al., 2011). As we see in these trials, gefitinib has acceptable efficacy in brain metastases in NSCLC patients who harbor an EGFR mutation.

Trials of Erlotinib

To assess the efficacy of erlotinib in NSCLC patients with brain metastases, several trials have been conducted in East-Asian patients selected either as having a clinical determinant of sensitivity to EGFR-TKIs or having an activating EGFR mutation. In a retrospective study evaluating the efficacy of erlotinib or gefitinib in 23 chemo-naïve, never-smoking Korean patients with lung adenocarcinoma and asymptomatic synchronous brain metastases (EGFR mutation status was undefined), the use of erlotinib was associated with 6.5 and 10.4 months PFS and OS, respectively (Kim et al., 2009).

In another retrospective analysis, 69 patients with NSCLC and brain metastases receiving erlotinib were studied to elucidate the role of EGFR mutation in sensitizing patients to the drug. Seventeen out of 69 patients were found to have an activating EGFR mutation. Most of the patients with EGFR mutations also had clinical determinants of EGFR-TKIs sensitivity [female gender (65%); never-smoker (65%); adenocarcinoma histology (80%)]. The objective response rate in these patients was 82%, of which 47% showed complete resolution of the brain tumors. Interestingly, no objective response was detected in the remaining unselected control group in which EGFR mutational status was either unknown or wild-type, resulting in a significant difference in favor of erlotinib use in patients harboring EGFR mutation ($p < 0.001$). With respect to extracranial disease, all patients with a mutant EGFR achieved an extracranial tumor response or stabilization of disease. The median time to progression in patients with EGFR mutations was significantly ($p < 0.05$) higher (11.7 months) than in those without activating mutations (5.8 months). Similarly, patients harboring EGFR mutations had a significantly higher OS of 12.9 months compared to 3.1 months in patients with a wild-type EGFR ($p < 0.001$) (Porta et al., 2011).

In a phase II study on the efficacy of erlotinib or gefitinib in patients with EGFR mutations, 28 individuals with EGFR mutant NSCLC and measurable brain metastases were enrolled. The rates of objective response and DC in brain metastases were 83% and 93%, respectively. Furthermore, after a median follow-up time of 17.5 months, median PFS and OS were 6.6 and 15.9 months, respectively. There were no statistically significant differences between treatment outcomes with either agent (Park et al., 2012).

Finally, in a more recently phase II study in which erlotinib was used as second-line treatment after failure of first-line chemotherapy in 48 patients with NSCLC and brain metastases, the objective response rate in the brain metastases was 56%, and the median PFS was higher in patients with (23.2 months) than without (8.2 months) EGFR mutations ($p = 0.06$) (Jamal-Hanjani and Spicer, 2012).

OBSTACLES TO DRUG ACTIVITY WITHIN THE CNS AND WAYS TO OVERCOME

The efficacy of EGFR-TKIs in the treatment of CNS metastases is related to their ability to cross an intact blood–brain barrier (BBB). The BBB prevents toxins from entering the brain and spinal cord, with the evolutionary aim of preventing neuronal damage. Unlike capillary beds in the periphery, endothelial cells within brain capillaries bind to each other with tight junctions. Astrocyte foot processes also attach closely to endothelial cells, playing a central role in the BBB function. It has been suggested that the BBB may lose its integrity at sites of metastatic lesions wherein new cellular fenestrations, an increased number of pinocytes, and diminished expression rate of cellular PgP efflux transporters may be found (Deeken and Löscher, 2007). For example, PgP transporters in the capillary beds of brain metastases from lung cancer are expressed at 40% of the level of normal brain capillaries (Deeken and Löscher, 2007). The size of the metastatic lesion is also an important factor for disruption of the BBB; the greater the size of the metastatic lesion, the more likely that BBB integrity will be lost (Deeken and Löscher, 2007). Pharmacologic properties of the drug are also important in its efficacy. For example, OSI-420, the active metabolite of erlotinib, is a PgP substrate which is actively pumped out the brain by this transporter. However, gefitinib is not a PgP substrate and may even inhibit PgP function (Jamal-Hanjani and Spicer, 2012).

Considering the specific obstacles that a drug must circumvent in order to enter the brain, the most important issue is achieving a therapeutic parenchymal concentration with minimal adverse effects. For instance, the usual therapeutic dose of erlotinib, 150 mg daily, is equal to its maximum tolerated dose. However, the maximal tolerated dose for gefitinib is about three times the usual dose of this drug, allowing clinicians to test escalating doses of gefitinib if a patient fails to respond to the usual dose (Togashi et al., 2012). As an example, Jackman et al. (2006) reported a case in which brain metastases from an EGFR-mutated NSCLC responded to escalated doses of gefitinib. In this case, with incremental increasing dose, gefitinib CSF concentration approached the corresponding *in vitro* IC_{50} of the pleural derived malignant cells of the same patient (i.e. 10–50 nmol/L). With each incremental increase in the administered dose, the patient's symptoms improved and radiographic and cytologic examination showed promising results. Ultimately, the patient developed disease progression due to an acquired resistance mutation (T790M in exon 20).

In a retrospective study of seven patients with an EGFR-mutation-positive NSCLC who had developed CNS metastases after a good initial extracranial response to standard dose of gefitinib, the use of erlotinib, instead of escalated-dose gefitinib, was associated with improvement in performance status and clinical symptoms. The median OS after the initiation of erlotinib therapy was 88 days (Katayama et al., 2009). In a separate report, a patient with lung adenocarcinoma and brain metastases harboring an EGFR mutation initially failed to respond to WBRT, gefitinib, chemotherapy and even standard dose erlotinib; however, escalation of the erlotinib dose administered in a pulsatile fashion of 300 mg on alternating days resulted in improvement in the patient's performance status (Hata et al., 2011). Pulsatile high-dose (1500 mg weekly) erlotinib has also been proposed as an option in patients with brain metastases that are initially non-responsive to standard dose erlotinib. In a retrospective study of nine patients with EGFR mutant NSCLC and brain/leptomeningeal metastases, the use of 1500 mg pulsatile weekly erlotinib prolonged survival up to 12 months (Grommes et al., 2011). Although high-dose daily erlotinib has unacceptable adverse events, pulsatile high-dose weekly administration proved to be tolerable with minimal toxicity (Milton et al., 2006; Clarke et al., 2010).

These reports suggest that in patients who are refractory to standard doses of EGFR-TKIs, it is still possible to treat CNS metastatic disease by switching drugs or escalating the dose. This phenomenon may be explained by the impact of the BBB preventing the achievement of therapeutic CSF concentration and permitting CNS metastatic cells to remain sensitive to the drug by not selecting out insensitive mutants, while extracranial tumor cells acquire (or are selected for) resistance mutations.

CLINICAL IMPLICATIONS OF EGFR MUTATIONS

Genetic alterations in the EGFR gene have different clinical phenotypes which confer sensitivity or resistance to EGFR-TKIs. EGFR activating mutations exist in about 77% of NSCLC patients responding to gefitinib or erlotinib. However, the frequency of these mutations in individuals who are refractory to erlotinib or gefitinib is as low as 7%. The activating mutations are most commonly located in exon 19 and 21 of the tyrosine kinase domain of the EGFR gene (Figure 14.3). Despite the prevalence of these mutations in EGFR-TKI responders, about 10–20% of patients who favorably respond to these drugs lack such mutations indicating further unknown mechanisms responsible for drug sensitivity (Sharma et al., 2007).

Besides the striking effects of TKIs in patients with sensitizing mutations, development of resistance during long-term use of these drugs is a problematic issue. Resistance

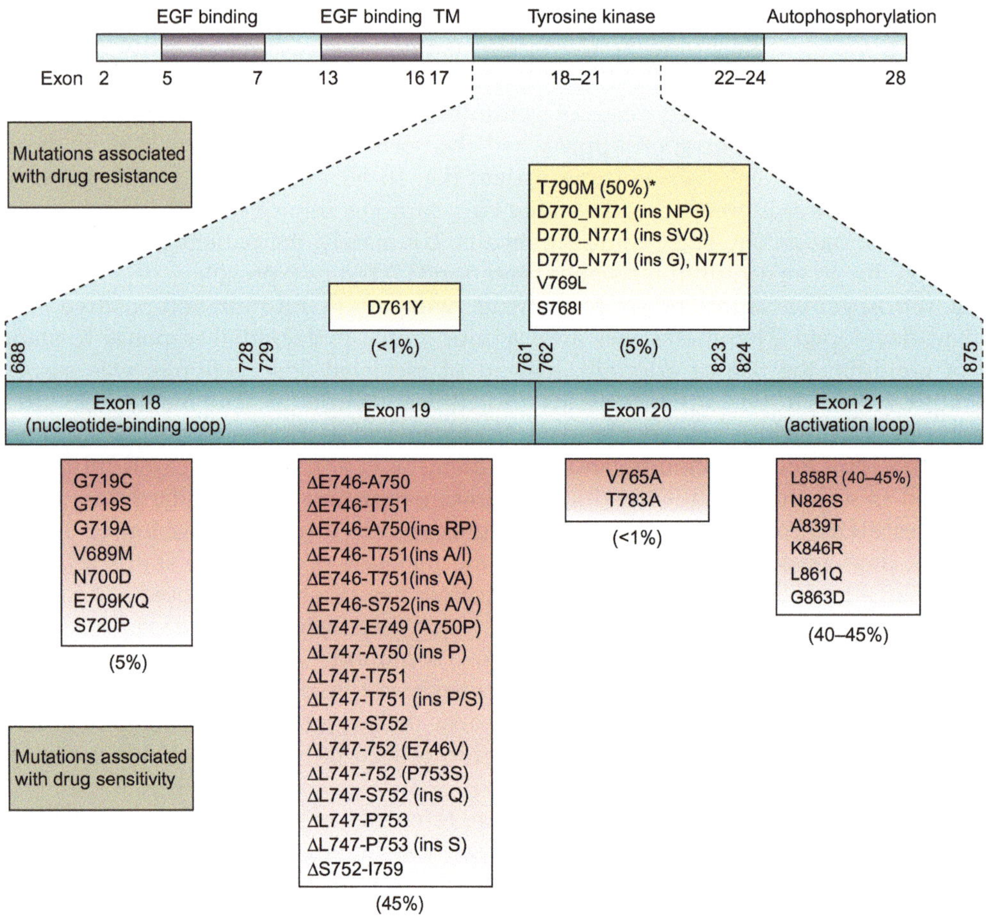

FIGURE 14.3 Activating and resistance mutations most commonly seen in the tyrosine kinase domain of the EGFR gene. *Figure adapted from Sharma et al., 2007.*

mutations may rarely be primary, such as insertion mutations in exon 20. More commonly, resistance mutations are acquired such as T790M in exon 20 which accounts for about half of acquired clinical resistance. D761Y is another less commonly acquired resistance mutation that is located in exon 19 of the EGFR gene and has been suggested to contribute to treatment failure (see Figure 14.3) (Sharma et al., 2007). Other mechanisms include amplification or upregulation of other growth factors such as hepatocyte growth factor or its receptor, c-MET, or other tyrosine kinases such as other HER family members, the insulin-like growth factor 1 receptor, or the AXL kinase (Kosaka et al., 2011; Yano et al., 2011; Zhang et al., 2012). It is unclear at present how prevalent each of these specific mechanisms may be in the clinical setting, but clinical trials targeting some of these mechanisms are already underway.

PROPHYLACTIC ROLE OF THE DRUGS

Recently, in a retrospective series of 36 patients with EGFR-mutant NSCLC and brain metastases at diagnosis, the impact of upfront gefitinib or erlotinib on CNS progression compared to initial chemotherapy was evaluated. This study showed that first-line treatment with EGFR-TKIs instead of chemotherapy in molecularly selected patients with NSCLC and brain metastases may significantly reduce the risk of CNS progression (HR: 0.56 [95% CI, 0.34–0.94]; $p = 0.026$) (Heon et al., 2012). These results are even more compelling when considering a retrospective study of 117 patients where EGFR mutation as compared with wild-type EGFR was a predictive factor for NSCLC recurrence in the CNS (Heon et al., 2012). Thus, upfront EGFR-TKIs therapy may have altered the course of the disease in patients with a mutant EGFR gene. Such a prophylactic role for TKIs should be further studied in larger randomized prospective trials.

ADVERSE REACTIONS OF GEFITINIB AND ERLOTINIB, PROS AND CONS

The most common adverse reactions of gefitinib and erlotinib are skin rash and diarrhea. These side effects are usually mild and controllable, but sometimes grade 3–4 reactions develop and make it necessary to reduce the dose or to discontinue treatment. High-grade adverse reactions may be hematologic or non-hematologic. In a pooled analysis of 15 large clinical trials, gefitinib and erlotinib had more frequent non-hematologic (elevated serum transaminase, interstitial lung disease, skin rash, fatigue, diarrhea, nausea, vomiting) but fewer hematologic (anemia, neutropenia, thrombocytopenia) adverse reactions compared to single-agent chemotherapy with third generation cytotoxic agents (gemcitabine, vinorelbine, taxanes) in patients with advanced NSCLC and poor performance status (Liu et al., 2011).

Among non-hematologic adverse reactions of EGFR-inhibitors, interstitial lung disease (ILD) is an important complication which rarely follows gefitinib or erlotinib administration and may be life threatening. As reported by United States Food and Drug Administration (FDA), the overall incidence of ILD following gefitinib and erlotinib is 1% and 1.1%, respectively. ILD in these situations may be seen as diverse entities such as alveolitis, pneumonitis or interstitial pneumonia. With gefitinib, the incidence of ILD has been reported to be higher (2%) among patients with Japanese ethnicity (Barber and Ganti, 2011). This may also translate to increase mortality in the Asian population following EGFR-TKIs (ter Heine et al., 2012). As reported by the FDA, approximately one-third of patients who develop ILD after gefitinib administration may have a fatal outcome. Similarly, a recent literature review showed that 11 out of 19 reported cases with erlotinib-induced ILD did not survive this complication (ter Heine et al., 2012).

Interestingly, skin toxicity is not only an adverse reaction to gefitinib and erlotinib, but may be a good prognostic factor. Correlation of skin toxicity with better outcome in NSCLC patients with brain metastases has been studied in a prospective trial using the approved 250 mg daily dosing of gefitinib. In this study, the occurrence of skin toxicity was associated with higher overall response rate ($p = 0.041$) and the results were consistent with respect to increasing grades of skin toxicity ($p = 0.007$). The rate of disease control was also increased significantly ($p < 0.001$) as higher grades of skin toxicity developed (Chiu et al., 2005). In a recent meta-analysis of gefitinib or erlotinib use in NSCLC, development of skin rash was associated with reduced risk of death with similar results between patients treated with gefitinib and those treated with erlotinib ($p < 0.0001$). Skin rash development was also significantly ($p < 0.0001$) associated with a reduced risk of disease progression; the results were similar in trials of both drugs. Patients with higher grades of skin rash also had higher rates of treatment response; this was also true for patients with any grade of skin involvement compared to those with intact skin (Petrelli et al., 2012).

FUTURE DIRECTIONS/ADDITIONAL AGENTS

Apart from gefitinib and erlotinib, new molecularly-targeted drugs are emerging as new pathophysiologic mechanisms are identified for NSCLC. In this regard, afatinib, a new ErbB-family blocker which binds to EGFR, HER2 and HER4, has entered clinical trials in recent years. This drug also has the advantage of blocking EGF receptors harboring T790M – the dominant EGFR-TKI resistance mutation. To date there are few data with mixed results about the impact of afatinib on brain metastases in patients with NSCLC.

In a phase I trial evaluating afatinib in 59 patients with advanced solid tumors, one individual developed brain metastases while on the 10 mg daily dose of afatinib. However, escalation of afatinib to 40 mg daily subsequently caused regression of the brain metastases (Yap et al., 2010). In a phase II trial (LUX-lung2), afatinib efficacy was assessed in 129 TKI-naïve patients with lung adenocarcinoma and an activating EGFR mutation (Yang et al., 2010). These patients had a good performance status (0–2), and had received no more than one prior chemotherapeutic regimen. Among them, 31 individuals had brain metastases. The objective response rate (primary study endpoint) was not different between the two subgroups with or without brain metastases (20 out of 31 [65%] vs 59 out of 98 [60%]; odds ratio 1.20, 95% CI 0.52–2.78). Unfortunately, clinical evidence evaluating afatinib efficacy specifically in patients with EGFR-TKI resistant brain metastases is lacking.

Another novel antitumor agent is icotinib, which also targets EGFR-TKI. In a recently finished phase III head-to-head double blind trial, icotinib had non-inferior efficacy with a superior safety profile to gefitinib (Tan et al., 2012). Similarly, in a prospective trial evaluating patients with NSCLC and brain metastases, icotinib was used simultaneously with, or subsequent to, gefitinib or erlotinib through selected arterial infusion to involved organs including the brain. In this study, systemically administered EGFR targeted therapy was combined with selected arterial icotinib and the results were promising. The reported overall response rate was 38.7% and the rate of disease control was 74.2% (Li and Guo, 2012).

Another newly developed targeted therapy in NSCLC inhibits ALK. ALK gene activation occurs following translocation, usually with the Echinoderm Microtubule-associated protein Like 4, forming a novel fusion protein, EML4–ALK; this is found in approximately 4% of patients with NSCLC (Preusser et al., 2012). Crizotinib, an ALK inhibitor, has been promising in early phase clinical trials in patients with NSCLC but the evidence regarding its efficacy on brain metastases in such patients is limited and conflicting. In a recently published case series, three EML4–ALK positive patients with NSCLC, developed isolated brain metastases while on crizotinib, in spite of good response in extracranial sites. This report suggests that the CNS may be a sanctuary site for EML4–ALK positive NSCLC cells (Chun et al., 2012). This phenomenon may be explained by very low CSF-to-plasma (0.0026) concentration of the drug (Costa et al., 2011). By contrast, the use of crizotinib in a 37-year-old man with NSCLC and miliary brain metastases was associated with an objective improvement in miliary disease (Falk et al., 2012). Overall, complementary trials are needed to explore mechanisms responsible for response or resistance to this drug. Notably, crizotinib also inhibits c-MET and ROS, both of which play a role in the development or maintenance of the malignant state of subsets of NSCLC; as noted previously, c-MET is involved in the development of clinical resistance to EGFR-TKIs in a portion of patients.

The efficacy of several other novel drugs with different mechanisms of action, such as GRN1005, enzastaurin, veliparib, patupilone and vorinostat, is currently under investigation in NSCLC patients with brain metastases.

References

Abrey, L.E., Christodoulou, C., 2001. Temozolomide for treating brain metastases. Semin. Oncol. 28, 34–42.

Addeo, R., De Rosa, C., Faiola, V., et al., 2008. Phase 2 trial of temozolomide using protracted low-dose and whole-brain radiotherapy for nonsmall cell lung cancer and breast cancer patients with brain metastases. Cancer 113, 2524–2531.

Alexander, E., 3rd, Moriarty, T.M., Davis, R.B., et al., 1995. Stereotactic radiosurgery for the definitive, noninvasive treatment of brain metastases. J. Natl. Cancer Inst. 87, 34–40.

Andrews, D.W., Scott, C.B., Sperduto, P.W., et al., 2004. Whole brain radiation therapy with or without stereotactic radiosurgery boost for patients with one to three brain metastases: phase III results of the RTOG 9508 randomised trial. Lancet 363, 1665–1672.

Arbit, E., Wronski, M., 1995. The treatment of brain metastases. Neurosurg. Q. 5, 1–17.

Barber, N.A., Ganti, A.K., 2011. Pulmonary toxicities from targeted therapies: a review. Target Oncol. 6, 235–243.

Bearz, A., Garassino, I., Tiseo, M., et al., 2010. Activity of pemetrexed on brain metastases from non-small cell lung cancer. Lung Cancer 68, 264–268.

Cancer Genome Atlas Research Network, 2012. Comprehensive genomic characterization of squamous cell lung cancers. Nature 489, 519–525.

Ceresoli, G.L., Cappuzzo, F., Gregorc, V., Bartolini, S., Crino, L., Villa, E., 2004. Gefitinib in patients with brain metastases from non-small-cell lung cancer: a prospective trial. Ann. Oncol. 15, 1042–1047.

Chidel, M.A., Suh, J.H., Greskovich, J.F., Kupelian, P.A., Barnett, G.H., 1999. Treatment outcome for patients with primary nonsmall-cell lungcancer and synchronous brain metastasis. Radiat. Oncol. Investig. 7, 313–319.

Chiu, C.H., Tsai, C.M., Chen, Y.M., Chiang, S.C., Liou, J.L., Perng, R.P., 2005. Gefitinib is active in patients with brain metastases from non-small cell lung cancer and response is related to skin toxicity. Lung Cancer 47, 129–138.

Chun, S.G., Choe, K.S., Iyengar, P., Yordy, J.S., Timmerman, R.D., 2012. Isolated central nervous system progression on Crizotinib: an Achilles heel of non-small cell lung cancer with EML4-ALK translocation? Cancer Biol. Ther. 13.

Clarke, J.L., Pao, W., Wu, N., Miller, V.A., Lassman, A.B., 2010. High dose weekly erlotinib achieves therapeutic concentrations in CSF and is effective in leptomeningeal metastases from epidermal growth factor receptor mutant lung cancer. J. Neurooncol. 99, 283–286.

Costa, D.B., Kobayashi, S., Pandya, S.S., et al., 2011. CSF concentration of the anaplastic lymphoma kinase inhibitor crizotinib. J. Clin. Oncol. 29, e443–e445.

Deeken, J.F., Löscher, W., 2007. The blood-brain barrier and cancer: transporters, treatment, and Trojan horses. Clin. Cancer Res. 13, 1663–1674.

Eichler, A.F., Chung, E., Kodack, D.P., Loeffler, J.S., Fukumura, D., Jain, R.K., 2011. The biology of brain metastases – translation to new therapies. Nat. Rev. Clin. Oncol. 8, 344–356.

Falk, A.T., Poudenx, M., Otto, J., Ghalloussi, H., Barrière, J., 2012. Adenocarcinoma of the lung with miliary brain and pulmonary metastases with echinoderm microtubule-associated protein like 4-anaplastic lymphoma kinase translocation treated with crizotinib: A case report. Lung Cancer 78, 282–284.

Fekrazad, M.H., Ravindranathan, M., Jones Jr., D.V., 2007. Response of intracranial metastases to erlotinib therapy. A case report. J. Clin. Oncol. 25, 5024–5026.

Grommes, C., Oxnard, G.R., Kris, M.G., et al., 2011. "Pulsatile" high-dose weekly erlotinib for CNS metastases from EGFR mutant non-small cell lung cancer. Neuro. Oncol. 13, 1364–1369.

Hata, A., Kaji, R., Fujita, S., Katakami, N., 2011. High-dose erlotinib for refractory brain metastases in a patient with relapsed non-small cell lung cancer. J. Thorac. Oncol. 6, 653–654.

Heon, S., Yeap, B.Y., Lindeman, N.I., et al., 2012. The impact of initial gefitinib or erlotinib versus chemotherapy on central nervous system progression in advanced non-small cell lung cancer with EGFR mutations. Clin. Cancer Res. 18, 4406–4414.

Hotta, K., Kiura, K., Ueoka, H., et al., 2004. Effect of gefitinib ('Iressa', ZD1839) on brain metastases in patients with advanced non small-cell lung cancer. Lung Cancer 46, 255–261.

Jackman, D.M., Holmes, A.J., Lindeman, N., et al., 2006. Response and resistance in a non-small-cell lung cancer patient with an epidermal growth factor receptor mutation and leptomeningeal metastases treated with high-dose gefitinib. J. Clin. Oncol. 24, 4517–4520.

Jamal-Hanjani, M., Spicer, J., 2012. Epidermal growth factor receptor tyrosine kinase inhibitors in the treatment of epidermal growth factor receptor-mutant non-small cell lung cancer metastatic to the brain. Clin. Cancer Res. 18, 938–944.

Katayama, T., Shimizu, J., Suda, K., et al., 2009. Efficacy of erlotinib for brain and leptomeningeal metastases in patients with lung adenocarcinoma who showed initial good response to gefitinib. J. Thorac. Oncol. 4, 1415–1419.

Kim, J.E., Lee, D.H., Choi, Y., et al., 2009. Epidermal growth factor receptor tyrosine kinase inhibitors as a first-line therapy for never smokers with adenocarcinoma of the lung having asymptomatic synchronous brain metastasis. Lung Cancer 65, 351–354.

Kosaka, T., Yamaki, E., Mogi, A., Kuwano, H., 2011. Mechanisms of resistance to EGFR TKIs and development of a new generation of drugs in non-small-cell lung cancer. J. Biomed. Biotechnol. 165214, Epub 2011.

Kouvaris, J.R., Miliadou, A., Kouloulias, V.E., et al., 2007. Phase II study of temozolomide and concomitant whole-brain radiotherapy in patients with brain metastases from solid tumors. Onkologie 30, 361–366.

Knights Jr., E.M., 1954. Metastatic tumors of the brain and their relation to primary and secondary pulmonary cancer. Cancer 7, 259–265.

Li, J., Guo, Z., 2012. Selected arterial infusion chemotherapy combined with target drugs for non-small cell lung cancer with multiple brain metastase. Zhongguo Fei Ai Za Zhi 15, 305–308.

Li, Z.L.J., Zhao, Y., Guo, H., 2011. The retrospective analysis of the frequency of EGFR mutations and efficacy of gefitinib in NSCLC patients with brain metastases. J. Clin. Oncol. 29 (Suppl; abstr, e18065).

Liu, S., Wang, D., Chen, B., Wang, Y., Zhao, W., Wu, J., 2011. The safety and efficacy of EGFRTKIs monotherapy versus single-agent chemotherapy using third-generation cytotoxics as the first-line treatment for patients with advanced non-small cell lung cancer and poor performance status. Lung Cancer 73, 203–210.

Maher, E.A., Mietz, J., Arteaga, C.L., DePinho, R., Mohla, S., 2009. Brain metastasis: opportunities in basic and translational research. Cancer Res. 69, 6015–6020.

Milton, D.T., Azzoli, C.G., Heelan, R.T., et al., 2006. A phase I/II study of weekly high-dose erlotinib in previously treated patients with nonsmall cell lung cancer. Cancer 107, 1034–1041.

Nagpal, S., Riess, J., Wakelee, H., 2012. Treatment of leptomeningeal spread of NSCLC: a continuing challenge. Curr. Treat. Options Oncol. 13, 491–504.

Neuhaus, T., Ko, Y., Muller, R.P., et al., 2009. A phase III trial of topotecan and whole brain radiation therapy for patients with CNS-metastases due to lung cancer. Br. J. Cancer 100, 291–297.

Park, S.J., Kim, H.T., Lee, D.H., et al., 2012. Efficacy of epidermal growth factor receptor tyrosine kinase inhibitors for brain metastasis in non-small cell lung cancer patients harboring either exon 19 or 21 mutation. Lung Cancer 77, 556–560.

Paydas, S., Bicakci, K., Yavuz, S., 2009. Dramatic response with capecitabine after cranial radiation to the brain parenchymal and leptomeningeal metastases from lung cancer. Eur. J. Intern. Med. 20, 96–99.

Petrelli, F., Borgonovo, K., Cabiddu, M., Lonati, V., Barni, S., 2012. Relationship between skinrash and outcome in non-small-cell lung cancer patients treated with anti-EGFR tyrosine kinase inhibitors: a literature-based meta-analysis of 24trials. Lung Cancer 78, 8–15.

Porta, R., Sanchez-Torres, J.M., Paz-Ares, L., et al., 2011. Brain metastases from lung cancer responding to erlotinib: the importance of EGFR mutation. Eur. Respir. J. 37, 624–631.

Preusser, M., Capper, D., Ilhan-Mutlu, A., et al., 2012. Brain metastases: pathobiology and emerging targeted therapies. Acta Neuropathol. 123, 205–222.

Rades, D., Kieckebusch, S., Haatanen, T., Lohynska, R., Dunst, J., Schild, S.E., 2008. Surgical resection followed by whole brain radiotherapy versus whole brain radiotherapy alone for single brain metastatsis. Int. J. Radiat. Oncol. Biol. Phys. 70, 1319–1324.

Robins, H.I., Traynor, A.M., Mehta, M., 2006. Temozolomide as prophylaxis for brain metastasis in non-small cell lung cancer. J. Thorac. Oncol. 1, 732–733.

Sharma, S.V., Bell, D.W., Settleman, J., Haber, D.A., 2007. Epidermal growth factor receptor mutations in lung cancer. Nat. Rev. Cancer 7, 169–181.

Shimato, S., Mitsudomi, T., Kosaka, T., et al., 2006. EGFR mutations in patients with brain metastases from lung cancer: association with the efficacy of gefitinib. Neuro. Oncol. 8, 137–144.

Tan, F., Shen, X., Wang, D., et al., 2012. Icotinib (BPI-2009H), a novel EGFR tyrosine kinase inhibitor, displays potent efficacy in preclinical studies. Lung Cancer 76, 177–182.

ter Heine, R., van den Bosch, R.T., Schaefer-Prokop, C.M., et al., 2012. Fatal interstitial lung disease associated with high erlotinib and metabolite levels. A case report and a review of the literature. Lung Cancer 75, 391–397.

Togashi, Y., Masago, K., Masuda, S., et al., 2012. Cerebrospinal fluid concentration of gefitinib and erlotinib in patients with non-small cell lungcancer. Cancer Chemother. Pharmacol. 70, 399–405.

Weller, M., 2007. Radiochemotherapy for brain metastasis: how to define a role for temozolomide. Onkologie 30, 350–351.

Wong, E.T., Berkenblit, A., 2004. The role of topotecan in the treatment of brain metastases. Oncologist 9, 68–79.

Wu, C., Li, Y.L., Wang, Z.M., Li, Z., Zhang, T.X., Wei, Z., 2007. Gefitinib as palliative therapy for lung adenocarcinoma metastatic to the brain. Lung Cancer 57, 359–364.

Yang, J.C., Shih, J.Y., Su, W.C., et al., 2010. Afatinib for patients with lung adenocarcinoma and epidermal growth factor receptor mutations (LUX-Lung 2): a phase 2 trial. Lancet Oncol. 13, 539–548.

Yano, S., Yamada, T., Takeuchi, S., et al., 2011. Hepatocyte growth factor expression in EGFR mutant lung cancer with intrinsic and acquired resistance to tyrosine kinase inhibitors in a Japanese cohort. J. Thorac. Oncol. 6, 2011–2017.

Yap, T.A., Vidal, L., Adam, J., et al., 2010. Phase I trial of the irreversible EGFR and HER2 kinase inhibitor BIBW 2992 in patients with advanced solid tumors. J. Clin. Oncol. 28, 3965–3972.

Zhang, Z., Lee, J.,C., Lin, L., et al., 2012. Activation of the AXL kinase causes resistance to EGFR-targeted therapy in lung cancer. Nat. Genet. 44, 852–860.

CHAPTER

15

Bispecific Targeted Toxin DTATEGF Against Metastatic NSCLC Brain Tumors

Walter A. Hall, Jun Huang, Yan Michael Li and Daniel A. Vallera

OUTLINE

Introduction 157

Diphtheria Toxin (DT) 159

DTATEGF 160
DTATEGF Construction 160
NSCLC Cell Preparation 161
In vitro DTATEGF Efficacy 161
Intracranial NSCLC Tumor Model 161
Pump Implantation and DTATEGF Delivery 162
Bioluminescent Imaging (BLI) 162
Body Weights, Histology, and Statistical Analysis 162

DTATEGF *in vitro* and *in vivo* Results 163

Discussion 164
Targeted Toxin Limitations 166

References 166

INTRODUCTION

Brain metastases affect 25% of patients with systemic cancer and are at least four times more common than primary brain tumors (Kaal et al., 2005). Nearly half of brain metastases arise from the lung and involve the cerebral hemispheres 80% of the time (Delattre et al., 1988). Non-small cell lung cancer (NSCLC) constitutes 80% of lung cancer in patients that

M.A. Hayat (ed): *Brain Metastases from Primary Tumors, Volume 1*
DOI: http://dx.doi.org/10.1016/B978-0-12-800896-6.00015-2

© 2014 Elsevier Inc. All rights reserved.

usually have advanced systemic disease or metastatic spread (Jemal et al., 2008). Despite treatment with corticosteroids and whole brain radiation therapy, the median survival for patients with NSCLC brain metastases is only 6 months leading clinicians to seek new innovative treatments (Olson et al., 2010). Targeting intracellular pathways that are responsible for tumor growth and progression is one direction being pursued by some investigators. The epidermal growth factor receptor (EGFR) and the vascular endothelial growth factor receptor (VEGF) pathways can be blocked in patients with NSCLC metastases (Socinski et al., 2009). A high therapeutic response rate and poor prognosis have been associated with EGFR expression (Wu et al., 2007). The EGFR tyrosine kinase inhibitors erlotinib and gefitinib have been used clinically (Wu et al., 2007). High levels of urokinase plasminogen activator receptor (uPAR) expression in NSCLC and other human cancers are associated with poor prognosis. Because uPAR is expressed on tumor cells and the endothelial cells of tumor blood vessels, it is suitable for targeting when attempting to interfere with pathogenic plasminogen activation (Duriseti et al., 2010).

Radiotherapy and chemotherapy represent the primary treatment modalities for metastatic NSCLC, although both therapies are of limited benefit because they are not selective for cancer cells and they cause serious side effects due to toxicity to normal cells. Surgical resection and stereotactic radiosurgery represent focal therapies that do not address the micrometastatic disease that is present outside the treatment field. In order to address this problem, one option is to combine a targeting ligand that will recognize tumor cells with a toxin that kills the tumor cells. Targeted toxins or immunotoxins are extremely potent compounds that bind to antigens on the surface of tumor cells that block protein synthesis after cellular entry (Hall, 1996). Targeted toxins are effective *in vitro* against numerous cell lines and *in vivo* in flank tumor models in athymic mice where complete tumor regression was seen (Tsai et al., 2011). The systemic delivery of these compounds is impractical because of the large size of these compounds and their inability to cross the blood–brain barrier (BBB) into the central nervous system (CNS) and the innate toxicity of these agents to some normal cells. Another factor that has diminished the efficacy of targeted toxins includes the immunogenicity of the toxin component of the molecule. In order to gain entry to the CNS by bypassing the BBB, a delivery technique that was introduced in the 1990s was convection enhanced delivery (CED) whereby the drug was infused into the brain parenchyma at a slow continuous rate. By inducing a fluid wave through positive pressure, the drug is administered into the brain. The potential application of this technique was recognized and confirmed in preclinical studies and in early phase clinical trials (Hall et al., 2003, 2006, 2009).

A bispecific immunotoxin DTATEGF was constructed with two different carrier ligands, epidermal growth factor (EGF) and the amino-terminal fragment (ATF) of urokinase plasminogen activator (uPA) that targeted the EGF receptor (EGFR) and uPA receptor (uPAR), respectively, linked to a truncated diphtheria toxin (DT). Compared to the monospecific targeted toxins, DTATEGF was more potent against some cell lines (Oh et al., 2011). DTATEGF was tested against a human metastatic NSCLC PC9-BrM3 cell line *in vitro* and *in vivo* (Huang et al., 2012). In the human NSCLC mouse xenograft brain tumor model, the cells were genetically labeled with the firefly luciferase reporter gene to allow for real-time bioluminescent imaging (BLI). DTATEGF was administered directly into the intracerebral PC9-BrM3 NSCLC tumor cell via CED over 7 days using an implanted osmotic minipump.

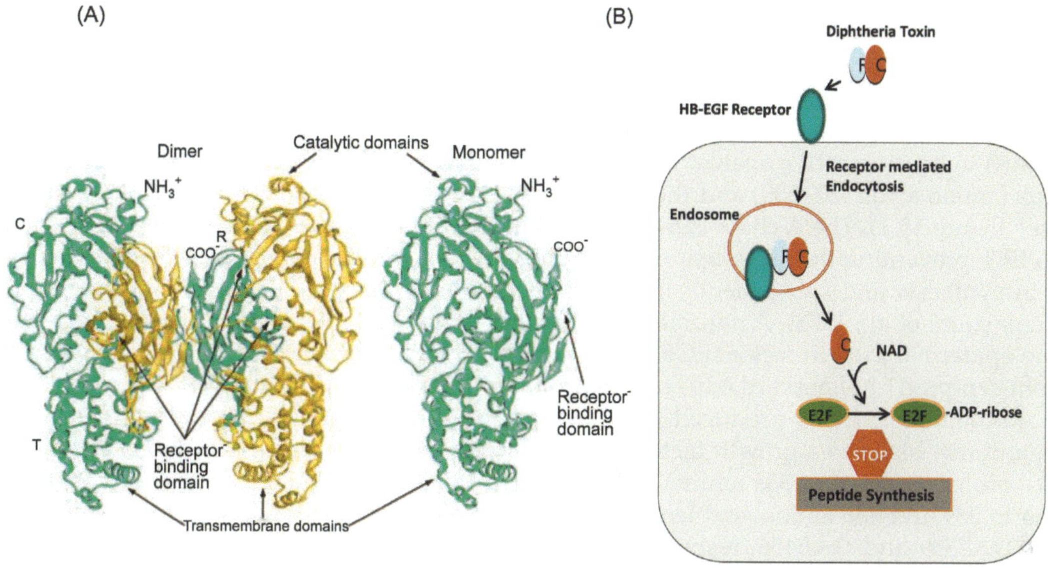

FIGURE 15.1 Diphtheria Toxin Protein. (A) View of diphtheria toxin (DT) showing swapped domains of a dimer of the toxin and a monomer of the toxin (PDB code: 1SGK). The amino terminus has a catalytic domain (C-domain) consisting of 8 β strands and 7 α helices. The carboxy terminal end has two domains, a transmembrane domain (T-domain) consisting of nine α helices and a receptor binding domain (R domain) consisting of 10 β strands. It has four cysteine residues, which form two internal disulfide bonds linking C186–C201 and C461–C471. (B) This image demonstrates the mechanism in which the diphtheria bacterial toxin invades the host's cell membrane. The binding of the HB-EGF receptor on the host's plasma membrane with R domain results in the activation of receptor-mediated endocytosis. When the toxin enters the endosome it is separated into R domain and C domain. The C domain is discharged into the cell cytoplasm and prevents protein synthesis by catalyzing ADP-ribosylation of elongation factor-2 (EF-2).

DIPHTHERIA TOXIN (DT)

Diphtheria toxin (DT) functions like other toxins by inhibiting protein synthesis either by modifying elongation factor-2 (EF2) or by acting directly on the ribosome (Siegall, 1994). Most toxins are polypeptide chains with several domains that include a cell recognition chain that attaches to cell surface receptors on the target tumor; a translocation domain that enables the toxin to cross the cell membrane and enter the cell; and an inactivation chain that blocks an important intracellular function leading to cell death (Rustamzadeh et al., 2003; Pastan et al., 2006). After the toxin binds to the overexpressed antigens or receptors on cancer cells, it is endocytosed into the cell and transferred by an endosome to a lysosome or to the Golgi apparatus. The toxin is then separated from the carrier ligand allowing it to inhibit protein synthesis. Toxins can inactivate over 200 EF2s per minute (Figure 15.1). Compared to conventional chemotherapy where 10^5 molecules are needed to kill one cell, a single toxin molecule can kill a cancer cell (Siegall, 1994).

Corynebacterium diphtheriae is a non-encapsulated, non-motile, Gram-positive bacillus that produces the 62-kDa protein DT (Sandvig and Olsnes, 1981; Zovickian et al., 1987).

The gene for DT is carried beside the promoter and operator sequences, however, the bacterium carries a repressor sequence that regulates gene expression. Gene regulation is dependent on iron concentration. After the repressor binds iron, the resulting complex attaches to the operator to prevent gene transcription (De Zoysa et al., 2005). The single polypeptide chain must be enzymatically nicked at an arginine-rich site for the A and B chains to become active against human cells. DT has a cell-binding domain at the C terminus (amino acids 482–539) and the A chain has ADP-ribosylation activity at the N terminus (see Figure 15.1). The A chain catalyzes the transfer of adenosine-diphosphate (ADP)-ribose to EF2, preventing the translocation of peptidyl-t-RNA on ribosomes, thereby blocking protein synthesis and subsequently killing the cell (Boquet et al., 1977; Pappenheimer, 1977; Yamaizumi et al., 1978). A natural ligand for DT on the cell membrane is the heparin-binding epidermal growth factor (EGF)-like precursor (Naglich et al., 1992) http://www.nature.com.ezp-prod1.hul.harvard.edu/nrc/journal/v6/n7/full/nrc1891.html - B6#B6.

Recombinant DT is produced by replacing the C terminal cell-binding domain with a ligand that binds to a growth factor receptor or the Fv fragment of an antibody. The native DT protein consists of 535 amino acids. Variable truncation of the binding segments resulting in 389 and 486 amino acid length toxin conjugates has resulted in the formation of toxins DAB389 and DAB486, respectively (Siegall, 1994). These modified DTs cannot enter a cell without selective binding of their carrier ligand to a receptor. Another modification of DT involves the substitution of two amino acids in the B chain resulting in a new molecule cross-reacting material-107 (CRM-107) (Greenfield et al., 1987; Johnson and Youle, 1989; Johnson et al., 1989). This modification reduced the non-specific binding of DT to human cells by 8000-fold and increased the toxin's tumor-specificity 10000-fold.

DTATEGF

DTATEGF Construction

DNA shuffling and DNA cloning techniques were used to synthesize and assemble the hybrid genes encoding the single-chain DTATEGF (Figure 15.2) (Vallera et al., 2002; Oh et al., 2009). From the 5′ to 3′ end, the assembled fusion gene contained an *Nco*1 restriction site, an ATG initiation codon, the first 389 amino acids of the DT molecule (DT390), the seven-amino-acid EASGGPE linker, the genes for human EGF and 135-ATF from uPA linked by 20-amino-acid segment of human muscle aldolase, and a *Xho*I restriction site (Huang et al., 2012). The resulting *Nco*I/*Xho*I fragment gene was spliced into the pET21d expression vector under the control of an isopropyl-*h*-D-thiogalactopyranoside-inducible T7 promoter. Verification that the gene was correct in sequence and had been cloned in frame was confirmed using DNA sequencing analysis. The monospecific targeted toxins DTAT and DTEGF were created using the same techniques (Vallera et al., 2002; Oh et al., 2009). A Novagen pET expression system was used for protein expression and purification from inclusion bodies. Fast protein liquid chromatography-ion exchange chromatography (Q Sepharose Fast Flow, Sigma) was used to purify refolded proteins. Sodium dodecyl sulfate polyacrylamide gel electrophoresis followed by Coomassie brilliant blue staining was performed to determine protein purity.

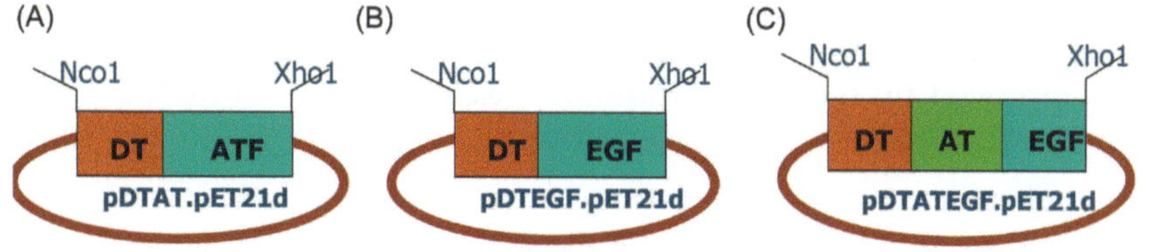

FIGURE 15.2 Construction of bispecific and monospecific ligand directed DT cytotoxins. The diagram illustrating the construction of (A) DTAT that consists of truncated DT and the ATF of uPA targeting uPAR; (B) DTEGF that consists of truncated DT and EGF ligand; (C) DTATEGF that consists of truncated DT and two different ligands, EGF and the ATF of uPA.

NSCLC Cell Preparation

Memorial Sloan-Kettering Cancer Center provided the human brain metastasis NSCLC cell line PC9-BrM3 which was then transfected with the luciferase reporter gene. The PC9-BrM3 cells were cultured in Dulbecco's modified Eagle medium with 10% fetal bovine serum and 5% streptomycin (Mediatech Inc., Manassas, VA) and maintained at 37°C in a humidified atmosphere of 5% CO_2. Cells with >95% viability were used for experiments as determined by Trypan blue exclusion.

In vitro DTATEGF Efficacy

An MTT assay was performed to test the *in vitro* cytotoxicity of DTATEGF against PC9-BrM3 NSCLC tumor cells. Cells were incubated overnight at 37°C with 5% CO_2 in a 96-well flat-bottomed plate containing 10^4 cells/well. The following day control DT, DTATEGF, DTAT, or DTEGF were added in varying concentrations to the wells. After 72 hours of incubation, MTT was added to each well for the last 4 hours. The cells were then washed, dried and counted using standard scintillation techniques. The data from the proliferation assays was reported as a percentage of the control counts. All assays were performed in triplicate and the results were obtained in three independent experiments.

Intracranial NSCLC Tumor Model

The mice used for intracranial tumor experiments were 6-week-old female athymic mice weighing 17–19 grams (Taconic, Hudson, NY). Intraperitoneal ketamine (80 mg/kg) was used to anesthetize the mice for the tumor implantation using a David Kopf stereotactic frame (David Kopf Instruments, Tujunga, CA) for immobilization. Using a midline incision the skull was accessed in order to place a burr hole 0.5 mm anterior to bregma and 2.5 mm lateral to the midline using a drill (Foredom Electric Co., Bethel, CT). A 25-gauge needle was attached to a 10-μL Hamilton syringe in order to deliver the tumor cells stereotactically. The needle was inserted into the brain to a depth of 3.2 mm from the skull surface and kept in place for 2 minutes before injecting tumor cells. Over a period of 5 minutes 4×10^5 PC9-BrM3 cells in 1.4 μL were injected into the brain. After completion of the injection the needle was left in place for 5 minutes before it was withdrawn slowly and the burr hole was covered with sterile bone wax. The skin incision was closed with surgical glue. All surgical procedures were approved by the animal care and use committee of SUNY Upstate Medical University and performed under sterile conditions.

Pump Implantation and DTATEGF Delivery

An implantable osmotic minipump system (ALZET model 1007D, Durect Corporation, Cupertino, CA) was chosen because of its infusion characteristics and size. The system contains a disposable filling tube, flow moderator and an osmotic pump. The PC9-BrM3 cells were implanted intracranially as described above. Four days after the cells were implanted, the first bioluminescent imaging (BLI) was performed to confirm the presence of tumor. The mice were divided into two groups each with six mice; the DTATEGF treatment group and the DT control group. The osmotic minipump system was assembled according to the manufacturer's instructions and contained 1.5 cm of infusion tubing attached to a 25-gauge 3-mm needle. After the mice were anesthetized and immobilized in the stereotactic frame, the drug-loaded pumps were implanted subcutaneously on the back. The treatment pumps were filled with 1 μg of DTATEGF in 100 μL and the control group pumps received 1 μg DT in 100 μL. The infusion rate was 0.5 μL/hour continuously for 7 days. The animals were again anesthetized on day 8 and all components of the pump system were removed to prevent interference with the BLI or the future potential for hardware exposure over time.

Bioluminescent Imaging (BLI)

Prior to BLI, the animals were anesthetized using isoflurane gas inhalation. BLI was performed with the IVIS 50 imaging system (Xenogen Corporation, Alameda, CA) and the results were analyzed with Living Image 2.5 software (Figure 15.3). An intraperitoneal injection of 150 mg/kg aqueous D-luciferin solution was administered to the mice 10 minutes before BLI. The BLI obtained represents 2 minutes of exposure time and the total number of photons per second per steradian per square centimeter was recorded. BLI was performed on days 4, 14, 30, 60, and 90 after PC9-BrM3 cell implantation.

Body Weights, Histology, and Statistical Analysis

Animals were weighed every 3 days for the first month and then once a week to monitor for toxicity. Animals were monitored for neurologic symptoms suggesting toxicity such as serious ataxic movements. In the presence of neurologic worsening or after weight loss of more than 20% body weight, animals were euthanized with an overdose of inhaled CO_2. The brains were then harvested en bloc and fixed overnight in 4% formalin before being placed in a 20% sucrose solution at 4°C. Once the brains sank to the bottom of the sucrose they were then embedded in ice and 7 μm sections were cut with a microtome (Leica Biosystems Richmond, Inc., Richmond, IL). The slides were stained with hematoxylin and eosin.

Kaplan–Meier survival curves were generated for the treatment and control groups and the differences between both groups was compared using GraphPad software version 4

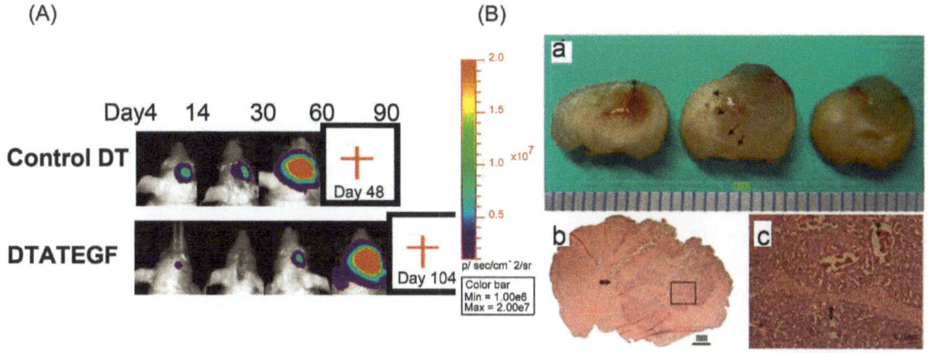

FIGURE 15.3 Bioluminescence and histopathological photomicrographs show the mouse xenograft brain tumor of human metastatic NSCLC. (A) Bioluminescence is shown on each picture as a function of photons/s/cm^2/sr. The intensity of the signal is illustrated by the color bar, with red representing the highest signal intensity. Red crosses indicate death of the animal. (B). Histopathologic photomicrographs show the mouse xenograft brain tumor of human metastatic NSCLC. a: a representative figure is shown in 1-mm coronal section of the mouse brain. b: Photomicrographs of H & E-stained coronal sections show metastatic brain tumor invading the brain tissue with a relatively clear boundary. c: Photomicrographs demonstrate tumor cellular patterns and multiple areas of necrosis, hemorrhage, and neovasculature.

(Graph-Pad Software, Inc., La Jolla, CA). Body weights and the proliferation indices were analyzed with the student t test. Statistical significance was considered present at $p \leq 0.05$.

DTATEGF *IN VITRO* AND *IN VIVO* RESULTS

Cell proliferation assays were performed to determine whether the bispecific DTATEGF could selectively kill PC9-BrM3 cells in tissue culture. Monospecific DTAT demonstrated an IC_{50} of 1 nM against PC9-BrM3 cells. Monospecific DTEGF was more effective against PC9-BrM3 cells than DTAT with an IC_{50} of 0.1 nM. DTATEGF was significantly more effective than either monospecific conjugate with an IC_{50} of less than 0.001 nM which represents a more than 100–1000-fold increase in cytotoxic activity. DT was used as an irrelevant control and demonstrated no activity against the cells. Antibody blocking experiments to EGFR and uPAR inhibited the antiproliferation effect of DTATEGF toward PC9-BrM3 cells confirming the expression of EGFR and uPAR on the surface of these cells.

There was no morbidity or mortality related to any surgical procedure in the 12 experimental animals. No neurologic deficits were seen in the early stages of the experiments in any animal after tumor cell inoculation, pump implantation, or drug delivery. In the late stages of the study, mild contralateral forelimb weakness developed and progressed rapidly within 1–2 weeks due to tumor proliferation. Seizures often occurred in the late stages. Even though body weight loss is often used as an indicator of systemic toxicity in catalytic toxin studies, our mice did not demonstrate this finding because they were still in the process of development in the 2 weeks following tumor cell inoculation. Even after DTATEGF administration there was no demonstrable weight loss in the animals indicating that the treatment dose was well tolerated. Body weight sharply declined in the last week of life as the tumor growth progressed.

Based on the results of animal survival studies for the intracerebral implantation of PC9-BrM3 cells in athymic mice, 4×10^5 cells were chosen to study the efficacy of DTATEGF *in vivo*. Previous studies of brain toxicity in non-tumor bearing mice supported the use of 1 μg DTATEGF for intracerebral administration. Either 1 μg of DTATEGF or DT was delivered into an intracerebral PC9-BrM3 tumor over 7 days at a rate of 0.5 μL/h by CED using the ALZET 1007D osmotic minipump system. BLI was used to confirm viable tumor cell implantation and to measure the response to treatment of metastatic intracranial PC9-BrM3 tumor xenografts to DTATEGF. There was a progressive increase in luminescence as determined from the normalized luminescence plot in the DT control group until symptoms developed in the animals necessitating their sacrifice once moribund. Luminescence was reduced in the treatment group at day 14 when the treatment was completed and remained low until 30 days after PC9-BrM3 cell implantation. Survival curve analysis revealed that the DTATEGF treatment group had a statistically significant prolongation in their median survival compared to the control group (87 days vs 63 days, $p = 0.006$). No mouse survived more than 120 days with their relapse due to tumor recurrence.

All mice implanted with 4×10^5 PC9-BrM3 cells developed tumors. There was no histopathological difference between the tumors in the treatment and the control groups. These tumors compressed the lateral ventricle and displaced the midline. Histopathological examination of the tumors showed highly cellular neoplasms infiltrating into the adjacent white matter with fine fibrillary backgrounds (see Figure 15.3). There was abundant necrosis present within the tumors surrounded by pseudopalisading cells. The cells were pleomorphic with bizarre nuclear patterns. Occasionally, multinucleated cells were seen and mitotic figures were present. Endothelial proliferation and alternate areas of angiogenesis were present.

DISCUSSION

NSCLC brain metastases are associated with a median survival of 6 months despite treatment with whole brain radiation therapy (Gaspar et al., 1997). New strategies are being developed that target growth factor receptor tyrosine kinase signaling pathways that are responsible for tumor growth, survival, and angiogenesis. Erlotinib is a tyrosine kinase inhibitor of the EGFR that was active against NSCLC brain metastases in clinical trials (Porta et al., 2011). The EGFR is expressed on 14–91% of NSCLC cells with overexpression associated with a poor prognosis (Koo and Kim, 2011). Agents that target the EGFR on tumor cells can exert direct and indirect anti-angiogenic effects. High levels of uPAR are associated with a poor prognosis in a number of human cancers that include NSCLC (Jacobsen and Ploug, 2008; Almasi et al., 2011). Targeting uPAR can result in disrupting angiogenesis because uPAR are expressed on endothelial cells. In animal models, targeting uPAR interferes with pathogenic plasminogen activation (Jacobsen and Ploug, 2008).

DTEGF13 is a bispecific targeted toxin that targets the EGFR and the interleukin 13 receptor. This compound was effective against human glioblastoma multiforme (GBM) *in vivo* and had greater activity than did either of the monospecific agents or a mixture of both (Oh et al., 2009). DTATEGF is a more recently developed targeted toxin than DTEGF13. DTATEGF was highly effective *in vivo* in a mouse xenograft model of intracerebral metastatic NSCLC created using PC3-BrM3 cells. Toxicity was not seen *in vivo* due to the absence of animal weight loss. The *in vitro* activity of DTATEGF also confirms that EGF and uPA are effective carrier ligands for the protein toxin DT. DTATEGF offers the additional benefit that both carrier ligands target both the tumor cells and the tumor vasculature.

Approaches to enhancing drug penetration into the CNS have been a major focus of investigators for the past two decades. The presence of the BBB prevents the passage of molecules larger that 180 kilodaltons into the brain (Kroll and Neuwelt, 1998). Based on their size, most targeted toxins will not cross the BBB. In the face of systemic delivery failure of most drugs to brain tumors, new more direct routes of administration are being pursued. Local delivery of a drug directly into a brain tumor will result in high local concentrations that may provide high antitumor activity. CED represents a promising technique that allows for the direct delivery of agents into brain tumors (Vogelbaum, 2007; Vogelbaum et al., 2007; Hall, 2009). This technique maintains a constant infusion of a drug into the brain which distinguishes this methodology from simple diffusion. Positive infusion pressures of up to 70 mmHg have been well tolerated in the brain (Hall, 2009).

Another factor that can significantly influence the distribution of a drug being given by CED in the brain is the design of the infusion catheter. When a targeted toxin is delivered directly into the brain there can be backflow along the catheter as a result of being administered under pressure (Sampson et al., 2007). More effective catheter designs will allow for the increased delivery of the drug being administered to the tumor with less delivery to the surrounding non-target brain parenchyma hopefully resulting in a reduced potential for toxicity. A hollow fiber catheter that reduces back flow is highly effective for drug delivery (Oh et al., 2007).

Prior studies of CED have utilized either a shunt catheter or a syringe to deliver a large drug volume over a short time interval. These higher flow rates have been shown to create a deforming force on tissue that results in tearing the tissue or causing reflux back along the infusion catheter away from the target tissue (Morrison et al., 1999; Vogelbaum, 2005). The osmotic minipump system used to perform CED in a mouse model demonstrated several distinct advantages: (1) the continuous infusion pressure allowed for the delivery of the drug at a constant rate; (2) the drug is delivered continuously over several days without an external connection; (3) there is less stress on the animals since they do not need to be handled; and (4) the drug is administered directly to the immunologically privileged CNS avoiding systemic exposure which could cause an immune reaction since most humans are immunized to DT. Another unique feature of these studies is the use of the luciferase reporter gene which is an efficient, accurate, and cost-effective means of monitoring tumor growth and response to treatment. After intracranial implantation of PC3-BrM3 NSCLC cells in the nude mouse xenograft brain tumor model, the bioluminescent signal was detectable on day 4 and was then followed at periodic intervals in real-time with BLI. The antitumor effect of DTATEGF was readily apparent on BLI and correlated with the extended survival seen in the treatment group. BLI does possess one limitation which is that luciferin metabolism and photon emission can occur in non-dividing cells indicating that signal loss does not always correspond with cell killing (Dinca et al., 2007).

Targeted Toxin Limitations

Targeted toxins are proteins that could stimulate immunogenicity and systemic antibody production. Targeted toxins with mutated toxin portions retain their functional activity with an 80–90% reduction in the generation of antitoxin antibodies in mice (Stish et al., 2009; Oh et al., 2011; Tsai et al., 2011). There is also the potential result that DTATEGF could have adverse vascular effects leading to intracranial hemorrhage or stroke.

In conclusion, DTATEGF was highly efficacious when delivered by CED intracranially into a metastatic NSCLC brain tumor. The osmotic minipump system performed well and delivered DTATEGF by CED with a therapeutic effect that was confirmed by BLI. The drug was also effective *in vitro* against the PC9-BrM3 metastatic NSCLC cell line. The drug represents a potential alternative therapy in patients who have failed whole brain radiation therapy and developed recurrent intracerebral tumors from NSCLC. DTATEGF should be further developed for future clinical use.

References

Almasi, C.E., Christensen, I.J., Hoyer-Hansen, G., et al., 2011. Urokinase receptor forms in serum from non-small cell lung cancer patients: relation to prognosis. Lung Cancer 74, 510–515.

Boquet, P., Silverman, M.S., Pappenheimer Jr., A.M., 1977. Interaction of diphtheria toxin with mammalian cell membranes. Prog. Clin. Biol. Res. 17, 501–509.

De Zoysa, A., Efstratiou, A., Hawkey, P.M., 2005. Molecular characterization of diphtheria toxin repressor (dtxR) genes present in nontoxigenic Corynebacterium diphtheriae strains isolated in the United Kingdom. J. Clin. Microbiol. 43, 223–228.

Delattre, J.Y., Krol, G., Thaler, H.L., Posner, J.B., 1988. Distribution of brain metastases. Arch. Neurol. 45, 741–744.

Dinca, E.B., Sarkaria, J.N., Schroeder, M.A., et al., 2007. Bioluminescence monitoring of intracranial glioblastoma xenograft: response to primary and salvage temozolomide therapy. J. Neurosurg. 107, 610–616.

Duriseti, S., Goetz, D.H., Hostetter, D.R., LeBeau, A.M., Wei, Y., Craik, C.S., 2010. Antagonistic anti-urokinase plasminogen activator receptor (uPAR) antibodies significantly inhibit uPAR-mediated cellular signaling and migration. J. Biol. Chem. 285, 26878–26888.

Gaspar, L., Scott, C., Rotman, M., et al., 1997. Recursive partitioning analysis (RPA) of prognostic factors in three Radiation Therapy Oncology Group (RTOG) brain metastases trials. Int. J. Radiat. Oncol. Biol. Phys. 37, 745–751.

Greenfield, L., Johnson, V.G., Youle, R.J., 1987. Mutations in diphtheria toxin separate binding from entry and amplify immunotoxin selectivity. Science 238, 536–539.

Hall, W.A., 1996. Immunotoxin therapy. Neurosurg. Clin. N. Am. 7, 537–546.

Hall, W.A., 2009. Convection-enhanced delivery: neurosurgical issues. Curr. Drug Targets 10, 126–130.

Hall, W.A., Vallera, D.A., 2006. Efficacy of antiangiogenic targeted toxins against glioblastoma multiforme. Neurosurg. Focus 20, E23.

Hall, W.A., Rustamzadeh, E., Asher, A.L., 2003. Convection-enhanced delivery in clinical trials. Neurosurg. Focus 14, E2.

Huang, J., Li, Y.M., Massague, J., Sicheneder, A., Vallera, D.A., Hall, W.A., 2012. Intracerebral infusion of the bispecific targeted toxin DTATEGF in a mouse xenograft model of a human metastatic non-small cell lung cancer. J. Neurooncol. 109, 229–238.

Jacobsen, B., Ploug, M., 2008. The urokinase receptor and its structural homologue C4.4A in human cancer: expression, prognosis and pharmacological inhibition. Curr. Med. Chem. 15, 2559–2573.

Jemal, A., Siegel, R., Ward, E., et al., 2008. Cancer statistics 2008. CA Cancer J. Clin. 58, 71–96.

Johnson, V.G., Youle, R.J., 1989. A point mutation of proline 308 in diphtheria toxin B chain inhibits membrane translocation of toxin conjugates. J. Biol. 264, 17739–17744.

Johnson, V.G., Wrobel, C., Wilson, D., et al., 1989. Improved tumor-specific immunotoxins in the treatment of CNS and leptomeningeal neoplasis. J. Neurosurg. 70, 240–248.

Kaal, E.C., Niel, C.G., Vecht, C.J., 2005. Therapeutic management of brain metastasis. Lancet Neurol. 4, 289–298.

Koo, J.S., Kim, S.H., 2011. EGFR and HER-2 status of non-small cell lung cancer brain metastasis and corresponding primary tumor. Neoplasma 58, 27–34.

Kroll, R.A., Neuwelt, E.A., 1998. Outwitting the blood-brain barrier for therapeutic purposes: osmotic opening and other means. Neurosurgery 42, 1083–1099.

Morrison, P.F., Chen, M.Y., Chadwick, R.S., Lonser, R.R., Oldfield, E.H., 1999. Focal delivery during direct infusion to the brain: role of flow rate, catheter diameter, and tissue mechanics. Am. J. Physiol. 277, R1218–R1229.

Naglich, J.G., Metherall, J.E., Russell, D.W., Eidels, L., 1992. Expression cloning of a diphtheria toxin receptor: identity with a heparin-binding EGF-like growth factor precursor. Cell 69, 1051–1061.

Oh, S., Odland, R., Wilson, S.R., et al., 2007. Improved distribution of small molecules and viral vectors in the murine brain using a hollow fiber catheter. J. Neurosurg. 107, 568–577.

Oh, S., Ohlfest, J.R., Todhunter, D.A., et al., 2009. Intracranial elimination of human glioblastoma brain tumors in nude rats using the bispecific ligand-directed toxin, DTEGF13 and convection enhanced delivery. J. Neurooncol. 95, 331–342.

Oh, S., Tsai, A.K., Ohlfest, J.R., Panoskaltsis-Mortari, A., Vallera, D.A., 2011. Evaluation of a bispecific biological drug designed to simultaneously target glioblastoma and its neovasculature in the brain. J. Neurosurg. 114, 1662–1671.

Olson, J.J., Paleologos, N.A., Gaspar, L.E., et al., 2010. The role of emerging and investigational therapies for metastatic brain tumors: a systematic review and evidence-based clinical practice guideline of selected topics. J. Neurooncol. 96, 115–142.

Pappenheimer Jr., A.M., 1977. Diphtheria toxin. Annu. Rev. Biochem. 46, 69–94.

Pastan, I., Hassan, R., Fitzgerald, D.J., Kreitman, R.J., 2006. Immunotoxin therapy of cancer. Nat. Rev. Cancer 6, 559–565.

Porta, R., Sanchez-Torres, J.M., Paz-Ares, L., et al., 2011. Brain metastases from lung cancer responding to erloyinib: the importance of EGFR mutation. Eur. Respir. J. 37, 624–631.

Rustamzadeh, E., Low, W.C., Vallera, D.A., Hall, W.A., 2003. Immunotoxin therapy for CNS tumor. J. Neurooncol. 64, 101–116.

Sampson, J.H., Brady, M.L., Petry, N.A., et al., 2007. Intracerebral infusate distribution by convection-enhanced delivery in humans with malignant gliomas: descriptive effects of target anatomy and catheter positioning. Neurosurgery 60, ONS89–ONS98.

Sandvig, K., Olsnes, S., 1981. Rapid entry of nicked diphtheria toxin into cells at low pH. Characterization of the entry process and effects of low pH on the toxin molecule. J. Biol. Chem. 256, 9068–9076.

Siegall, C.B., 1994. Targeted toxins as anticancer agents. Cancer 74, 1006–1012.

Socinski, M.A., Langer, C.J., Huang, J.E., et al., 2009. Safety of bevacizumab in patients with non-small-cell lung cancer and brain metastases. J. Clin. Oncol. 27, 5255–5261.

Stish, B.J., Oh, S., Chen, H., Dudek, A.Z., Kratzke, R.A., Vallera, D.A., 2009. Design and modification of EGF4KDEL 7Mut, a novel bispecific ligand-directed toxin, with decreased immunogenicity and potent anti-mesothelioma activity. Br. J. Cancer 101, 1114–1123.

Tsai, A.K., Oh, S., Chen, H., Shu, Y., Ohlfest, J.R., Vallera, D.A., 2011. A novel bispecific ligand-directed toxin designed to simultaneously target EGFR on human glioblastoma cells and uPAR on tumor neovasculature. J. Neurooncol. 103, 255–266.

Vallera, D.A., Li, C., Jin, N., Panoskaltsis-Mortari, A., Hall, W.A., 2002. Targeting urokinase-type plasminogen activator receptor on human glioblastoma tumors with diphtheria toxin fusion protein DTAT. J. Natl. Cancer Inst. 94, 597–606.

Vogelbaum, M.A., 2005. Convection enhanced delivery for the treatment of malignant gliomas: symposium review. J. Neurooncol. 73, 57–69.

Vogelbaum, M.A., 2007. Convection enhanced delivery for treating brain tumors and selected neurological disorders: symposium review. J. Neurooncol. 83, 97–109.

Vogelbaum, M.A., Sampson, J.H., Kunwar, S., et al., 2007. Convection-enhanced delivery of cintredekin besudotox (interleukin-13-PE38QQR) followed by radiation therapy with and without temozolomide in newly diagnosed malignant gliomas: phase 1 study of final safety results. Neurosurgery 61, 1031–1037.

Wu, W., Onn, A., Isobe, T., et al., 2007. Targeted therapy of orthotopic human lung cancer by combined vascular endothelial growth factor and epidermal growth factor and epidermal growth factor receptor signaling blockade. Mol. Cancer Ther. 6, 471–483.

Yamaizumi, M., Mekada, E., Uchida, T., Okada, Y., 1978. One molecule of diphtheria toxin fragment A introduced into a cell can kill the cell. Cell 15, 245–250.

Zovickian, J., Johnson, V.G., Youle, R.J., 1987. Potent and specific killing of human malignant brain tumor cells by an anti-transferrin receptor antibody-ricin immunotoxin. J. Neurosurg. 66, 850–861.

CHAPTER

16

Intracranial Disease in Patients with Non-Small Cell Lung Cancer: Treatment with Erlotinib

Mazhar Ajaz, Fiona McDonald, Jaishree Bhosle, Paola Bordi and Mary O'Brien

OUTLINE

Introduction 170

First-Line Treatment for Advanced NSCLC 170

Development and Management of NSCLC Brain Metastases 171

Do EGFR Mutated NSCLC Patients have a Higher Risk of Developing Brain Metastases? 172

Are Brain Metastases in EGFR-Mutated Patients Radiosensitive? 172

Erlotinib 172

Do EGFR TKIs have Efficacy in Treatment and Prevention of Intracranial Disease from NSCLC? 174

What is the Efficacy and Safety of Combining Erlotinib with Radiotherapy for Brain Metastases? 175

Is there a Role for Rechallenge and Pulsed dose Escalation of Erlotinib? 176

Summary 176

References 177

M.A. Hayat (ed): *Brain Metastases from Primary Tumors, Volume 1*
DOI: http://dx.doi.org/10.1016/B978-0-12-800896-6.00016-4

© 2014 Elsevier Inc. All rights reserved.

INTRODUCTION

Lung cancer affects approximately 1.6 million persons a year globally. In the West, it accounts for approximately 10–15% of new cancer cases and 20–30% of cancer deaths (Ferlay et al., 2007). Metastasis to the brain is responsible for death in up to half of cancer patients. Lung cancer is the most frequent primary site of origin, making up 40–50% of cases (Barnholtz-Sloan et al., 2004). Metastasis involving the central nervous system (CNS) affects approximately 20–40% of patients with non-small cell lung cancer (NSCLC) at some stage in their illness, and is present in about 10% at diagnosis (Mujoomdar et al., 2007). It is highly likely that brain metastasis from NSCLC will present an increasing clinical challenge, due to improvements in initial radiological staging and longer survival following successful treatment of primary and systemic disease.

Patients developing brain metastases are not a homogeneous population. Developments in both neuro-oncology and thoracic oncology have brought about a change in perspective in recent years. First, improved clinical data have resulted in meaningful stratification of patients with brain metastasis, allowing treatment to be adapted according to therapy context and anticipated outcome. In particular, the use of magnetic resonance imaging (MRI) means the extent of intracranial lesions can be more accurately defined. Classic prognostic classification systems (Gaspar et al., 1997) have been refined to take into account these data as well as primary site of origin. Second, the technical capabilities of both surgery and radiotherapy have improved including highly focused stereotactic irradiation techniques. Third, within medical thoracic oncology, a new generation of drugs has expanded the treatment options for molecularly-defined NSCLC subsets. We now have the first and second generation of epidermal growth factor receptor (EGFR) tyrosine kinase inhibitors (TKIs), erlotinib, gefitinib, and now afatinib, which have proven activity against brain metastases in case reports, retrospective case series and prospective clinical trials.

This chapter discusses the characteristics and standard clinical management of intracranial disease in patients with NSCLC. We focus on the pharmacologic aspects of erlotinib and pre-clinical evidence for intracerebral activity. We review the evidence for the activity of erlotinib in patients with brain metastases in various treatment settings. Lastly, we discuss opportunities for further research in improving the efficacy of erlotinib as a treatment for intracranial disease in NSCLC patients.

FIRST-LINE TREATMENT FOR ADVANCED NSCLC

Primary chemotherapy for advanced NSCLC has for a long time been centered on platinum agents, with adjunctive roles for the taxanes, gemcitabine, vinorelbine and pemetrexed. However, in the last decade, NSCLC has joined a short list of malignancies that display major vulnerability to targeted inhibition of single aberrant kinases, derived from so-called "driver" mutations. One such target is a receptor tyrosine kinase, EGFR, which activates major survival and proliferation signaling pathways. In an initial large phase III trial, the EGFR-TKI erlotinib improved survival overall in previously treated unselected NSCLC patients (Shepherd et al., 2005). However, it became apparent that a subset of these patients demonstrated significant and prolonged treatment responses. These patients displayed common clinical characteristics: often female, light or never smokers, with adenocarcinoma and a greater frequency in East-Asians. *Post-hoc* analysis revealed that their tumors contained mutations in the tyrosine kinase domain of the *EGFR* gene, specifically an exon 19 deletion and a point mutation in exon 21 (L858R). Preclinical evidence confirmed that these are driver mutations, defining a specific subtype of adenocarcinoma, distinct from the more highly mutated cancers that are associated with long-term cigarette smoking (Lynch et al., 2004).

While erlotinib remains licensed for unselected patients with NSCLC in the second- and third-line setting, its major clinical benefit is in those with sensitizing *EGFR* mutations. Subsequent trials have addressed the role of tyrosine kinase inhibition as primary therapy in this patient subpopulation and confirmed that erlotinib is effective in the first-line treatment of *EGFR*-mutated NSCLC with better progression-free survival and quality of life when compared to chemotherapy (Mok et al., 2009).

DEVELOPMENT AND MANAGEMENT OF NSCLC BRAIN METASTASES

Development of intracranial metastasis from NSCLC requires multiple pathophysiologic steps. After dissemination from the primary tumor, cancer cells must enter and survive in the bloodstream, arrest in the brain capillary bed, extravasate and proliferate. Stromal cells associated with the primary tumor, as well as co-opted brain microglia and astrocytes, have been shown to assist this process and are likely to be an increasing focus of therapeutic attention (Fidler, 2011). Establishment and propagation of a blood vessel supply has been shown to occur by a variety of mechanisms, probably varying by tumor type and disease progression; growth of brain metastasis from NSCLC is at least partly dependent on neoangiogenesis via vascular endothelial growth factor.

Intracranial metastasis is not only a distinct clinical problem in disseminated NSCLC (Ortuzar et al., 2012), but is also a frequent site of initial failure in patients with localized disease who have received treatment with curative intent. A review of 112 NSCLC patients found that brain metastasis was observed in 29% of all recurrences, with a median time to brain recurrence of 9 months (Robnett et al., 2001). Young age, primary tumor size and lymph node metastasis were associated with a higher risk of intracranial involvement. In one retrospective study, the predicted probabilities of developing brain metastasis from node-negative, primary adenocarcinomas measuring 2 or 6 cm were 0.14 and 0.72, respectively (Robnett et al., 2001; Ceresoli et al., 2002). However, tumor size does not fully explain the development of brain metastasis with cases of small or even occult NSCLC metastasizing early to the brain, while other patients with large tumors, or locoregionally or systemically advanced disease may never establish overt intracranial growth. Prophylactic cranial irradiation (PCI) has been shown to reduce the risk of brain metastasis in high-risk NSCLC, but without disease-free or overall survival benefits (Pöttgen et al., 2007; Gore et al., 2011).

NSCLC patients with brain metastases may present with severe debility and the least-harm, symptom-based approach to maintain quality of life may be the most appropriate management. However, more commonly some permutation of surgery, whole brain radiotherapy (WBRT) and/or stereotactic radiosurgery is usual. In the presence of multiple brain metastases, the basis of treatment is WBRT, combined with short-course corticosteroid therapy to control peritumoral edema. This is historically associated with a median survival of 3–5 months with 10% of patients alive at 1 year. In the presence of three or fewer brain metastases, addition of a second treatment to WBRT (surgery or stereotactic radiotherapy) confers improved prognosis (Patchell et al., 1990). Furthermore, radiosurgery has been widely adopted as primary sole treatment for patients with oligometastatic disease to the brain. Subsequent systemic cytotoxic chemotherapy is feasible and may confer benefits in a subset of patients with good functional status and a limited number of brain metastases.

DO EGFR MUTATED NSCLC PATIENTS HAVE A HIGHER RISK OF DEVELOPING BRAIN METASTASES?

There does appear to be a higher incidence of brain metastasis in patients with *EGFR*-mutated NSCLC. In a retrospective review of 93 patients who developed brain metastasis, 44% demonstrated an *EGFR* mutation (Eichler et al., 2010). Median survival in the presence of brain metastasis was higher in the *EGFR* mutation group, 14.5 vs 7.6 months, although this did not reach independent statistical significance.

ARE BRAIN METASTASES IN EGFR-MUTATED PATIENTS RADIOSENSITIVE?

EGFR overactivation was initially viewed as a cause of radioresistance (Lammering, 2005), yet NSCLC with *de novo* EGFR activation as a driver mutation displays marked radiosensitivity. *In vitro*, *EGFR*-mutant lung cancer cell lines show up to 3-log greater sensitivity to ionizing radiation than wild-type cells (Das et al., 2006). A retrospective clinical study of 63 patients with lung adenocarinoma suggested a higher response rate to WBRT in the presence of *EGFR*-mutated primaries (54% vs 24% wild-type), although interpretation was confounded by concurrent administration of EGFR-targeted drug therapy (Gow et al., 2008). Trials with PCI have demonstrated some benefit in patients with NSCLC but it has not been studied in the subset of patient with EGFR mutations. This may be a population in which the benefits of PCI with regard to risk reduction in development of brain metastases, disease-free and overall survival should be studied in a randomized trial.

ERLOTINIB

Erlotinib (OSI-774) is a quinazoline derivative [6,7-bis(2-methoxy-ethoxy)-quinazolin-4-yl-(3-ethynylphenyl)amine] which inhibits EGFR kinase activity. It is structurally similar to gefitinib (Figure 16.1). It binds reversibly to the intracellular kinase domain, competing with adenosine triphosphate, and thereby impairing autophosphorylation and the downstream signal cascade. Fifty percent growth inhibition of cell lines with the L858R *EGFR* mutation is achieved at 100 nanomolar (nM) (Hidalgo et al., 2001).

Clinical pharmacology studies have established a standardized oral dose of erlotinib at a 150 milligrams (mg) daily. Adverse effects are principally diarrhea and skin rash, although

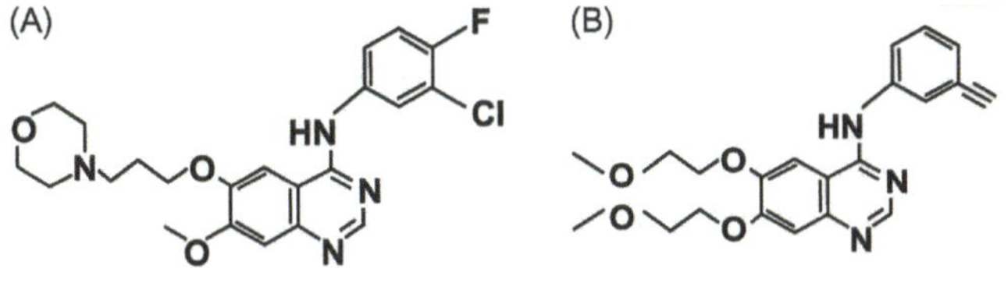

FIGURE 16.1 Chemical structures of (A) gefitinib and (B) erlotinib.

interstitial lung disease is a rare and potentially life-threatening association. Metabolism is hepatic, mainly via CYP3A4, to the active metabolite desmethyl-erlotinib (OSI-420). The time after administration when the maximum plasma concentration is reached is 3–4 hours with a half-life of 24–36 hours. Concomitant smoking decreases erlotinib exposure. The drug is 93% bound to albumin and alpha-1 acid glycoprotein (Hidalgo et al., 2001), disfavoring CNS uptake. It has a molecular weight of 393.4 Dalton (Da) which approaches the limit of blood–brain barrier diffusibility versus active transport. Notably gefitinib has a molecular weight of 446 Da. Erlotinib has moderately high lipophilicity, underlying both relatively good oral absorption and potential for penetration.

Preclinical studies have shown that erlotinib is liable to efflux by components of the blood–brain barrier, P-glycoprotein (P-gp) and breast cancer resistance protein (BCRP). Transgenic mice with double deletions of the genes for P-gp and BCRP demonstrate significantly higher brain accumulation of erlotinib than wild-type animals. P-gp function appears to be the dominant barrier to erlotinib uptake into brain tissue (de Vries et al., 2012). Empiric evidence for brain penetration by erlotinib derives in part from studies in primary brain tumors. In an early pharmacokinetic study, erlotinib was administered in a pulsed schedule of 450 mg or 900 mg every 72 h, the dose chosen according to concurrent usage of enzyme-inducing antiepileptic drugs (EIAEDs). The use of EIAEDs was associated with increased hepatic metabolism to OSI-420 and increased clearance. Cerebrospinal fluid (CSF) concentrations ranged from 1 to 3% of peak plasma concentrations and the schedule was tolerable (Buie et al., 2007). In a pharmacokinetic study in patients undergoing resection for glioblastoma, tumor concentrations of erlotinib and OSI-420 were measured after a week of erlotinib 150 mg daily, 24 h after the last dose. Target site concentrations of erlotinib and OSI-420 were 6–8% and 5–11%, respectively, of concomitant plasma concentrations in evaluable patients (Lassman et al., 2005).

Gefitinib has demonstrated similar characteristics of low CSF concentrations. The CSF concentrations of gefitinib and erlotinib were directly compared in a series of 15 Japanese patients, the majority receiving either drug and two receiving both drugs sequentially (Togashi et al., 2012). The mean steady state CSF concentration and penetration rate of gefitinib 250 mg daily were 8.2 nM and 1.13%, respectively. For erlotinib 150 mg daily these figures were 66.9 nM and 2.77%, respectively. Erlotinib therefore had higher CSF penetration than gefitinib in this report.

Radiolabeling of drugs with carbon-11, which decays by positron emission, allows *in vivo* human biodistribution analyses without tissue sampling. In a case report, [11C]-erlotinib (Memon et al., 2009) was administered to a 32-year-old patient with exon 19-mutant NSCLC accompanied by multiple brain metastases and meningeal carcinomatosis (Weber et al., 2011). Positron emission tomography (PET)/computed tomography (CT) of the brain was performed during treatment and coregistered with magnetic resonance imaging (MRI).

[11C]-erlotinib progressively accumulated in two cerebellar metastases over a 60-minute period, with minimal uptake in the cerebral cortex, giving tumor-to-cortex ratios up to 10:1.

DO EGFR TKIS HAVE EFFICACY IN TREATMENT AND PREVENTION OF INTRACRANIAL DISEASE FROM NSCLC?

Early observations with gefitinib showed the potential for treating NSCLC brain metastases with EGFR-TKI. A first report in 2003 of four heavily pretreated patients, three of whom had intracranial progression after WBRT, described three partial responses and one complete response (Cappuzzo et al., 2003). Several groups have also now reported response in leptomeningeal disease (Kim et al., 2005).

Similar cases reports have appeared for erlotinib since 2006 (Jackman et al., 2006). A recently reported phase II trial in 48 patients from a Chinese population has assessed the efficacy of erlotinib as second-line therapy for NSCLC brain metastases (Wu et al., 2013). Inclusion criteria included adenocarcinoma or confirmed activating *EGFR* mutation and asymptomatic brain metastases without extracranial progressive disease after first-line platinum-based chemotherapy. Erlotinib 150 mg daily was associated with 10.1 month median intracranial progression-free survival, extending to 15.2 months for those with *EGFR*-mutant disease vs 4.4 months for those without *EGFR* mutation.

In a case-control study of NSCLC patients with brain metastases treated with erlotinib ± WBRT, an *EGFR*-mutant population was compared to a population with unknown or wild-type EGFR. The objective response rate of the brain metastases was 82% in the mutant population compared to 0% in the control group despite all control group patients additionally receiving WBRT (Porta et al., 2011). Interestingly, eight of the patients with mutations did not receive WBRT and erlotinib was their sole treatment. The objective response rate of the brain metastases in these patients was striking at 75%. Interestingly, across all patients receiving erlotinib in this series, more complete responses were attained in brain than at primary lung sites, suggesting at minimum that CNS drug delivery considerations are not an obstacle to efficacy, at least initially in the context of macroscopic intracranial disease. This analysis did not however provide comparative time-to-progression data for those patients receiving erlotinib alone vs WBRT plus erlotinib. In retrospective series, with mixed wild-type and mutated patients, conclusions have not been definitive and have not changed practice, but highlight the need for studies in subgroups with the same biological profile.

There is increasing interest in maintenance drug therapy in the management of advanced NSCLC, with evidence for progression and/or overall survival advantages from docetaxel (Fidias et al., 2009), pemetrexed (Paz-Ares et al., 2012) and erlotinib (Cappuzzo et al., 2010). In unselected treatment populations, erlotinib does not prevent the development of brain metastasis. In the BR21 trial of maintenance erlotinib, some patients were observed to develop brain metastases despite ongoing erlotinib (Shepherd et al., 2005). This was recorded as disease progression but patients continued on-study if there was evidence of extracranial control of disease. Data are unavailable from this study regarding the influence of *EGFR*-mutation status and the development of brain metastases while taking erlotinib. The most convincing evidence derives from a comparison of upfront EGFR-TKI versus chemotherapy in *EGFR*-mutant lung cancer in 155 patients. At a median follow up of 25 months, 33% of patients in the

EGFR-TKI group and 48% in the chemotherapy group had developed CNS progression, with a hazard ratio of 0.56 (Heon et al., 2012).

WHAT IS THE EFFICACY AND SAFETY OF COMBINING ERLOTINIB WITH RADIOTHERAPY FOR BRAIN METASTASES?

As brain metastases from *EGFR*-mutated NSCLC could exhibit higher radiosensitivity than brain metastases from *EGFR*-wild type tumors (Das et al., 2006), it is possible that little or no extra benefit accrues from upfront combination of radiotherapy with EGFR-targeting agents. However, erlotinib will frequently need to be commenced due to the synchronous development or presentation of extracranial disease, and the question that arises then is whether erlotinib alone would be enough to control brain metastases for the life time of a lung cancer patient with an EGFR mutation. In practice, we see patients who have control for long periods of time in the brain but, in general, relapse occurs at some point. A trial of erlotinib with or without WBRT would answer this question but may be difficult to recruit to in the absence of phase I data on the long-term toxicities. A trial has been terminated early in unselected patients of erlotinib plus WBRT versus WBRT alone but some data will become available (Tactic trial NCT 00554775). Before this, we would need to be convinced that erlotinib and radiotherapy can be combined without prejudicing the efficacy or safety of either treatment option in sequence. Notably, while antibody-mediated EGFR inhibition is an efficacious combination partner for radiotherapy for head and neck cancer (Bonner et al., 2010), toxicity needs to be managed. Likewise, the combination of erlotinib with radical thoracic irradiation has been associated with high toxicity (Socinski et al., 2012). Treatment-related damage in the brain parenchyma is of special consideration due to the acute risk of progressive radiation necrosis and the chronic risk of radiation-induced dementia (DeAngelis et al., 1989).

A prospective trial of gefitinib in 41 NSCLC patients with brain metastases from a European population was reported in 2004 (Ceresoli et al., 2004). It predated knowledge and application of *EGFR*-mutation testing and only four patients demonstrated a partial response. Adenocarcinoma histology was associated with response and, importantly, prior WBRT was also associated with a higher disease control rate. A phase II trial in a Chinese population combined gefitinib 250mg daily with WBRT (40Gy in 20 fractions) and found a 19% complete and 62% partial response rate (Ma et al., 2009). There was no apparent synergistic damage of the normal brain. Similarly, a pediatric study found erlotinib to be a tolerable partner to cranial irradiation, including brainstem treatments (Geoerger et al., 2011). In contrast, unexpectedly severe toxicities occurred with the combination of erlotinib and WBRT in a series of seven patients (Olmez et al., 2010), one of whom suffered neurologic deterioration without clear signs of disease progression. However, all seven patients showed durable intracranial disease control.

A two-stage dose-escalation phase I trial evaluated the safety of WBRT with concurrent and maintenance erlotinib in patients with previously untreated brain metastases from NSCLC and a phase II trial assessing concurrent WBRT and erlotinib in patients with brain metastases from NSCLC, both found the combination was feasible (Lind et al., 2009; Welsh et al., 2013). The numbers of patients with EGFR mutations in these studies were either small or unknown and therefore the combination still needs to be studied more extensively in the *EGFR*-mutant population. Interesting, survival was related to the severity of dermatitis: 3.7 months with grade zero, 10 months with grade one and 17 months with grade two or higher skin toxicity. Six patients had grade three skin toxicity requiring dose reduction. The prevalence of skin toxicity with combined EGFR inhibition and radiotherapy has been well documented in head and neck cancer (Bonner et al., 2010), and there is an association of higher grade skin toxicity and sensitivity to lower doses of TKIs in patients with EGFR mutations (Myerson et al., 2010).

IS THERE A ROLE FOR RECHALLENGE AND PULSED DOSE ESCALATION OF ERLOTINIB?

In a case report published from the Royal Marsden Hospital in 2007, a recurrent response of brain metastases to erlotinib was demonstrated. The patient was a 42-year-old female never-smoker who presented with widely disseminated extracranial NSCLC and brain metastases. Following WBRT and initial cytotoxic systemic chemotherapy she received erlotinib 150mg/day. The intracranial disease showed a partial response but the intrathoracic disease progressed. Three cycles of docetaxel were administered but she then developed symptoms of intracranial progression, confirmed by demonstration of a new cerebral lesion on CT. She was rechallenged with erlotinib and achieved a partial response in the brain (Popat et al., 2007).

Anecdotal active strategies in patients who have developed brain metastases on TKI include increasing the dose of TKI within the recommended therapeutic window if has been reduced because of toxicity, rechallenge with the original TKI and a crossover to an alternate TKI (Togashi et al., 2011). A Japanese patient developed brain metastases after a 12-month progression-free interval taking erlotinib 75mg, reduced from 150mg due to grade 3 fatigue. She received WBRT without early radiological response. Her erlotinib dose was increased to 150mg and a partial response was shown in the brain (Togashi et al., 2011).

An alternative approach to intracranial progression during EGFR-TKI treatment is to develop a dose escalation strategy to allow CNS penetration of gefitinib or erlotinib to increase and achieve therapeutic concentrations (Jackman et al., 2006). Even within a low range this may have some effect. A 56-year-old never-smoker showed a major response to erlotinib rechallenge at 600mg orally every 4 days. This resulted in clinical, radiologic and cytologic improvements in her leptomeningeal disease that were maintained for 10 months (Hata et al., 2011). There are an increasing number of such reports in the literature including doses of erlotinib up to 2000mg once weekly being tolerated (Milton et al., 2006) and a schedule of erlotinib at a dose of 1500mg weekly showing activity. A series of nine patients with *EGFR*-mutant lung cancer and brain or leptomeningeal metastasis were treated at a median weekly dose of 1500mg after progression on conventional daily erlotinib or gefitinib (Grommes et al., 2011). This is clearly an area for further study.

SUMMARY

The reliance on and heterogeneity of case reports in this field illustrates the complexity of the clinical landscape of patients with brain metastases from NSCLC. It is thus difficult to gain direct evidence for every scenario. Instead, erlotinib should be viewed as an active treatment option added to the armamentarium of surgery, radiotherapy and chemotherapy for intracranial disease. However, a few clinical scenarios can be identified based on an evolution from current standard practice. The evidence suggests that the brain as a site of disease should not be an exclusion factor for patients entering trials of TKIs. These patients should be included and either stratified at entry or a pre-planned analysis carried out in the subgroup with brain metastases. Equally for patients with progressing disease, it is a missed opportunity not to try dose escalation at the point of progression in the brain.

For patients with multiple brain metastases who are in poor functional condition and unlikely to draw net benefit from WBRT, primary erlotinib is a very reasonable option and may be sufficient as sole therapy for control of intracranial disease. Erlotinib is also a clear option for those who have failed standard neuro-oncological therapies and have *EGFR*-mutant tumors. Erlotinib can be safely combined in non-selected patients with cranial irradiation, but more data are needed in the group with mutated disease. In general, erlotinib can be given as first-line definitive therapy, with a deferred radiotherapy/surgery strategy if there is other uncontrolled extracranial disease. Importantly, *EGFR*-mutant NSCLC may display high radiosensitivity and, where feasible, a first-line radiotherapy/surgery strategy remains standard. The pulsed high-dose erlotinib concept clearly requires further large-scale validation. Overall, erlotinib is an effective option for intracranial disease from *EGFR*-mutant NSCLC and its use is likely to increase with growing practitioner confidence in its efficacy and tolerability.

References

Barnholtz-Sloan, J.S., Sloan, A.E., Davis, F.G., Vigneau, F.D., Lai, P., Sawaya, R.E., 2004. Incidence proportions of brain metastases in patients diagnosed (1973 to 2001) in the Metropolitan Detroit Cancer Surveillance System. J. Clin. Oncol. 22, 2865–2872.

Bonner, J.A., Harari, P.M., Giralt, J., et al., 2010. Radiotherapy plus cetuximab for locoregionally advanced head and neck cancer: 5-year survival data from a phase 3 randomised trial, and relation between cetuximab-induced rash andsurvival. Lancet Oncol. 11, 21–28.

Buie, L.W., et al., 2007. Plasma pharmacokinetics and cerebrospinal fluid concentrations of erlotinib in high-grade gliomas: a novel, phase I, dose escalation study. J. Clin. Oncol. 25, 2054.

Cappuzzo, F., Ardizzoni, A., Soto-Parra, H., et al., 2003. Epidermal growth factor receptor targeted therapy by ZD 1839 (Iressa) in patients with brain metastases from non-small cell lung cancer (NSCLC). Lung Cancer 41, 227–231.

Cappuzzo, F., et al., 2010. Erlotinib as maintenance treatment in advanced non-small-cell lung cancer: a multicentre, randomised, placebo-controlled phase 3 study. Lancet Oncol. 11, 521–529.

Ceresoli, G.L., Cappuzzo, F., Gregorc, V., Bartolini, S., Crinò, L., Villa, E., 2004. Gefitinib in patients with brain metastases from non-small-cell lung cancer: a prospective trial. Ann. Oncol. 15, 1042–1047.

Ceresoli, G.L., Reni, M., Chiesa, G., et al., 2002. Brain metastases in locally advanced nonsmall cell lung carcinoma after multimodality treatment: risk factors analysis. Cancer 95, 605–612.

Das, A.K., Sato, M., Story, M.D., et al., 2006. Non-small-cell lung cancers with kinase domain mutations in the epidermal growth factor receptor are sensitive to ionizing radiation. Cancer Res. 66, 9601–9608.

DeAngelis, L.M., Delattre, J.Y., Posner, J.B., 1989. Radiation-induced dementia in patients cured of brain metastases. Neurology 39, 789–796.

de Vries, N.A., Buckle, T., Zhao, J., Beijnen, J.H., Schellens, J.H., van Tellingen, O., 2012. Restricted brain penetration of the tyrosine kinase inhibitor erlotinib due to the drug transporters P-gp and BCRP. Invest. New Drugs 30, 443–449.

Eichler, A.F., Kahle, K.T., Wang, D.L., et al., 2010. EGFR mutation status and survival after diagnosis of brain metastasis in nonsmallcell lung cancer. Neuro-oncology 12, 1193–1199.

Ferlay, J., Autier, P., Boniol, M., Heanue, M., Colombet, M., Boyle, P., 2007. Estimates of the cancer incidence and mortality in Europe in 2006. Ann. Oncol. 18, 581–592.

Fidias, P.M., et al., 2009. Phase III study of immediate compared with delayed docetaxel after front-line therapy with gemcitabine plus carboplatin in advanced non-small-cell lung cancer. J. Clin. Oncol. 27, 591–598.

Fidler, I.J., 2011. The role of the organ microenvironment in brain metastasis. Semin. Cancer Biol. 21, 107–112.

Gaspar, L., et al., 1997. Recursive partitioning analysis (RPA) of prognostic factors in three Radiation Therapy Oncology Group (RTOG) brain metastases trials. Int. J. Radiat. Oncol. Biol. Phys. 37, 745–751.

Geoerger, B., et al., 2011. Innovative Therapies for Children with Cancer pediatric phase I study of erlotinib in brainstem glioma and relapsing/refractory brain tumors. Neuro-oncol. 13, 109–118.

Gore, E.M., Bae, K., Wong, S.J., et al., 2011. Phase III comparison of prophylactic cranial irradiation versus observation in patients with locally advanced non-small-cell lung cancer: primary analysis of radiation therapy oncology group study RTOG 0214. J. Clin. Oncol. 29, 272–278.

Gow, C.H., Chien, C.R., Chang, Y.L., et al., 2008. Radiotherapy in lung adenocarcinoma with brain metastases: effects of activating epidermal growth factor receptor mutations on clinical response. Clin. Cancer Res. 14, 162–168.

Grommes, C., et al., 2011. "Pulsatile" high-dose weekly erlotinib for CNS metastases from EGFR mutant non-small cell lung cancer. Neuro-oncol. 13, 1364–1369.

Hata, A., Kaji, R., Fujita, S., Katakami, N., 2011. High-dose erlotinib for refractory brain metastases in a patient with relapsed non-small cell lung cancer. J. Thorac. Oncol. 6, 653–654.

Heon, S., Yeap, B.Y., Lindeman, N.I., et al., 2012. The impact of initial gefitinib or erlotinib versus chemotherapy on central nervous system progression in advanced non-small cell lung cancer with EGFR mutations. Clin. Cancer Res. 18, 4406–4414.

Hidalgo, M., Siu, L.L., Nemunaitis, J., et al., 2001. Phase I and pharmacologic study of OSI-774, an epidermal growth factor receptor tyrosine kinase inhibitor, in patients with advanced solid malignancies. J. Clin. Oncol. 19, 3267–3279.

Jackman, D.M., Holmes, A.J., Lindeman, N., et al., 2006. Response and resistance in a non-small-cell lung cancer patient with an epidermal growth factor receptor mutation and leptomeningeal metastases treated with high-dose gefitinib. J. Clin. Oncol. 24, 4517–4520.

Kim, M.K., Lee, K.H., Lee, J.K., Choi, J.H., Hyun, M.S., 2005. Gefitinib is also active for carcinomatous meningitis in NSCLC. Lung Cancer 50, 265–269.

Lammering, G., 2005. Molecular predictor and promising target: will EGFR now become a star in radiotherapy? Radiother. Oncol. 74, 89–91.

Lassman, A.B., Rossi, M.R., Raizer, J.J., et al., 2005. Molecular study of malignant gliomas treated with epidermal growth factor receptor inhibitors: tissue analysis from North American Brain Tumor Consortium Trials 01-03 and 00-01. Clin. Cancer Res. 11, 7841–7850.

Lind, J.S., Lagerwaard, F.J., Smit, E.F., Senan, S., 2009. Phase I study of concurrent whole brain radiotherapy and erlotinib for multiple brain metastases from non-small-cell lung cancer. Int. J. Radiat. Oncol. Biol. Phys. 74, 1391–1396.

Lynch, T.J., Bell, D.W., Sordella, R., et al., 2004. Activating mutations in the epidermal growth factor receptor underlying responsiveness of non-small-cell lung cancer to gefitinib. N. Engl. J. Med. 350, 2129–2139.

Ma, S., Xu, Y., Deng, Q., Yu, X., 2009. Treatment of brain metastasis from non-small cell lung cancer with whole brain radiotherapy and Gefitinib in a Chinese population. Lung Cancer 65, 198–203.

Memon, A.A., Jakobsen, S., Dagnaes-Hansen, F., Sorensen, B.S., Keiding, S., Nexo, E., 2009. Positron emission tomography (PET) imaging with [11C]-labeled erlotinib: a micro-PET study on mice with lung tumor xenografts. Cancer Res. 69, 873–878.

Milton, D.T., et al., 2006. A phase I/II study of weekly high-dose erlotinib in previously treated patients with non-small cell lung cancer. Cancer 107, 1034–1041.

Mok, T.S., Wu, Y.L., Thongprasert, S., et al., 2009. Gefitinib or carboplatin-paclitaxel in pulmonary adenocarcinoma. N. Engl. J. Med. 361, 947–957.

Mujoomdar, A., Austin, J.H., Malhotra, R., et al., 2007. Clinical predictors of metastatic disease to the brain from non-small cell lung carcinoma: primary tumor size, cell type, and lymph node metastases. Radiology 242, 882–888.

Myerson, J.S., Iqbal, S.A., O'Brien, M.E., Popat, S., 2010. Supersensitive mutation: two case reports of non-small-cell lung cancer treated with epidermal growth factor receptor tyrosine kinase inhibitors. Clin. Lung Cancer 11, E5–E8.

Olmez, I., Donahue, B.R., Butler, J.S., Huang, Y., Rubin, P., Xu, Y., 2010. Clinical outcomes in extracranial tumor sites and unusual toxicities with concurrent whole brain radiation (WBRT) and Erlotinib treatment in patients with non-small cell lung cancer (NSCLC) with brain metastasis. Lung Cancer 70, 174–179.

Ortuzar, W., Hanna, N., Pennella, E., et al., 2012. Brain metastases as the primary site of relapse in two randomized phase III pemetrexed trials in advanced non-small-cell lung cancer. Clin. Lung Cancer 13, 24–30.

Patchell, R.A., Tibbs, P.A., Walsh, J.W., et al., 1990. A randomized trial of surgery in the treatment of single metastases to the brain. N. Engl. J. Med. 322, 494–500.

Paz-Ares, L., et al., 2012. Maintenance therapy with pemetrexed plus best supportive care versus placebo plus best supportive care after induction therapy with pemetrexed plus cisplatin for advanced non-squamous non-small-cell lung cancer (PARAMOUNT): a double-blind, phase 3, randomised controlled trial. Lancet Oncol. 13, 247–255.

Popat, S., Hughes, S., Papadopoulos, P., et al., 2007. Recurrent response to non small cell lung cancer brain metastases with erlotinib. Lung Cancer 56, 135–137.

Porta, R., Sánchez-Torres, J.M., Paz-Ares, L., et al., 2011. Brain metastases from lung cancer responding to erlotinib: the importance of EGFR mutation. Eur. Respir. J. 37, 624–631.

Pöttgen, C., Eberhardt, W., Grannass, A., et al., 2007. Prophylactic cranial irradiation in operable stage IIIA non small-cell lung cancer treated with neoadjuvant chemoradiotherapy: results from a German multicenter randomized trial. J. Clin. Oncol. 25, 4987–4992.

Robnett, T.J., Machtay, M., Stevenson, J.P., Algazy, K.M., Hahn, S.M., 2001. Factors affecting the risk of brain metastases after definitive chemoradiation for locally advanced non-small-cell lung carcinoma. J. Clin. Oncol. 19, 1344–1349.

Shepherd, F.A., Pereira, J., Ciuleanu, T., National Cancer Institute of Canada Clinical Trials Group, 2005. Erlotinib in previously treated non-small-cell lung cancer. N. Engl. J. Med. 353, 123–132.

Socinski, M.A., Stinchcombe, T.E., Moore, D.T., et al., 2012. Incorporating bevacizumab and erlotinib in the combined-modality treatment of stage III non-small-cell lung cancer: results of a phase I/II trial. J. Clin. Oncol. 30, 3953–3959.

Togashi, Y., Masago, K., Fukudo, M., et al., 2011. Efficacy of increased-dose erlotinib for central nervous system metastases in non-small cell lung cancer patients with epidermal growth factor receptor mutation. Cancer Chemother. Pharmacol. 68, 1089–1092.

Togashi, Y., Masago, K., Masuda, S., et al., 2012. Cerebrospinal fluid concentration of gefitinib and erlotinib in patients with non-small cell lung cancer. Cancer Chemother. Pharmacol. 70, 399–405.

Weber, B., Winterdahl, M., Memon, A., et al., 2011. Erlotinib accumulation in brain metastases from non-small cell lung cancer: visualization by positron emission tomography in a patient harboring a mutation in the epidermal growth factor receptor. J. Thorac. Oncol. 6, 1287–1289.

Welsh, J.W., Komaki, R., Amini, A., et al., 2013. Phase II trial of erlotinib plus concurrent whole-brain radiation therapy for patientswith brain metastases from non-small-cell lung cancer. J. Clin. Oncol. 31, 895–902.

Wu, Y.L., Zhou, C., Cheng, Y., et al., 2013. Erlotinib as second-line treatment in patients with advanced non-small-cell lung cancer and asymptomatic brain metastases: a phase II study (CTONG-0803). Ann. Oncol. 24, 993–999.

CHAPTER

17

Radiation Management of Synchronous Brain Metastases from Non-Small Cell Lung Cancer

Allison Ashworth, David Palma and George Rodrigues

OUTLINE

Introduction 182

Management of Brain Metastases in Patients with NSCLC 182

General Considerations for the Management of Brain Metastases 182

Management of Patients with Single Brain Metastases 183

Surgery vs SRS for Single Brain Metastases 184

Management of Patients with Multiple Brain Metastases 184

Emerging Techniques in the Radiation Management of Brain Metastases 185

Surgery for Multiple Brain Metastases 185

Is Whole Brain Radiotherapy Necessary after Surgical Resection or SRS? 185

Which Patients Benefit from Aggressive Management of Brain Metastases? 186

Prognostic Factors Specific to NSCLC Patients with Brain Metastases 187

Management of NSCLC Patients with Synchronous Brain Metastases 187

Rationale for Aggressive Treatment of Oligometastatic Disease 188

Management of Oligometastatic NSCLC 188

Prognostic Factors Affecting Survival in NSCLC Patients with Synchronous Brain Metastases 189

Factors of Undetermined or No Prognostic Significance 189

Other Prognostic Factors for NSCLC 191

M.A. Hayat (ed): *Brain Metastases from Primary Tumors, Volume 1*
DOI: http://dx.doi.org/10.1016/B978-0-12-800896-6.00017-6

© 2014 Elsevier Inc. All rights reserved.

Radiation Management of Thoracic Disease in NSCLC Patients with Synchronous Brain Metastases 191
Surgical Management of Thoracic Disease in NSCLC Patients with Synchronous Brain Metastases 193
Staging Workup of NSCLC Patients with Synchronous Brain Metastases 193
Management Algorithm for NSCLC Patients with Synchronous Brain Metastases 194
Future Directions in the Management of Oligometastatic NSCLC 194
Conclusion 194
References 195

INTRODUCTION

Lung cancer is the leading cause of cancer-related mortality worldwide (Jemal et al., 2011). The majority of patients with NSCLC present with locally advanced or metastatic disease. The development of brain metastases is a common site of recurrence and spread (Law et al., 2001). The synchronous development of a lung cancer with metastatic disease to the brain without other metastatic foci can frequently occur in routine clinical practice. The management of this patient population can be complex due to the integration of separately acquired medical evidence relating to the management of both sites into a coherent treatment plan that can be feasibly executed. The purpose of this chapter will review the current evidence for the management of brain metastases in patients with non-small cell lung cancer (NSCLC), with a specific focus on the recent literature surrounding the radiation management of NSCLC patients with synchronous brain metastases. The execution of evidence-based management of both intracranial metastases and the primary thoracic disease will be a major focus of this review.

MANAGEMENT OF BRAIN METASTASES IN PATIENTS WITH NSCLC

General Considerations for the Management of Brain Metastases

Brain metastases cause significant morbidity and mortality. Approximately one-quarter of NSCLC patients will develop clinically detectable brain metastases (Sørensen et al., 1988). The outcomes for this population are generally poor; median survival in the absence of treatment is about 1 month and may be extended to 2 months by the use of steroids (Zimm et al., 1981). Symptoms that are associated with brain metastases may be a result of increased intracranial pressure from cerebral edema, resulting in headaches, nausea, and vomiting. Focal neurological symptoms due to brain metastases include seizures, focal motor and sensory deficits, ataxia, speech problems and cognitive deficits.

Standard treatment options for patients with brain metastases include comfort measures, steroids, anticonvulsants, whole brain radiotherapy (WBRT), stereotactic radiosurgery (SRS), surgical resection, or a combination of these modalities. The optimal treatment for brain metastases is highly dependent on individual patient characteristics, tumor factors, and treatment considerations. The clinician must take these factors into consideration to determine if the goal of treatment is palliation of symptoms or whether long-term disease control with more aggressive treatment modalities might be achievable.

For most patients with multiple brain metastases, WBRT is considered the standard of care. WBRT alone is most commonly used in patients with multiple brain metastases with a limited life expectancy due to poorly controlled extracranial disease or poor performance status. The use of WBRT in NSCLC patients with brain metastases improves quality of life (Order et al., 1968), neurologic function, and results in an improvement in median survival to approximately 3–6 months (Zabel and Debus, 2004). Various dose and fractionation schedules for WBRT have been investigated and no altered dose-fractionation schedule has proven to be superior to the commonly prescribed schedules of 20 Gy in five fractions or 30 Gy in 10 fractions with respect to survival or symptom control (neurologic functional status, symptom relief, palliative index or performance status) (Tsao et al., 2012). Other commonly used fractionation schedules routinely employed in clinical practice are 40 Gy in 20 fractions or 37.5 Gy in 15 fractions.

Management of Patients with Single Brain Metastases

For selected patients with a good performance status and a single brain metastasis, higher rates of local control and survival have been achieved with the use of SRS or surgical resection with WBRT compared to WBRT alone. The first trial to demonstrate a benefit to surgical resection randomized 48 patients with a single brain metastasis and a Karnofsky performance status (KPS) of ≥70 to WBRT alone versus surgical resection followed by WBRT (Patchell et al., 1990). Those patients who received surgery had fewer recurrences at the site of the original metastasis (20 vs 52%, $p < 0.02$), a higher overall median survival (40 vs 15 weeks, $p < 0.01$) and remained functionally independent for longer (38 weeks vs 8 weeks, $p < 0.005$) than those who had WBRT alone.

Stereotactic radiosurgery, a highly precise, typically single-fraction treatment of high dose radiation, has also been shown to improve local control and overall survival when combined with WBRT in patients with a single brain metastasis, as demonstrated by Andrews et al. (2004). Three-hundred and thirty-three patients with a KPS of at least 70 and one to three brain metastases from a variety of primary malignancies were randomized to WBRT or WBRT followed by SRS boost to the metastases. Metastases had to be less than 4 cm in diameter for the largest lesion and additional lesions could not exceed 3 cm. The addition of SRS resulted in a local control benefit at 1 year for all patients compared to WBRT alone (82% vs 71%, $p = 0.01$). No survival benefit was observed for patients in the SRS group (6.5 vs 5.7 months) but, on subset analysis, patients with single metastases who received an SRS boost had a significantly better survival (median survival time 6.5 vs 4.9 months, $p = 0.0393$). On multivariate analysis, RTOG RPA Class 1 patients had a survival advantage whether they had a single or multiple tumors. The use of SRS was not associated with any significant additional toxicity.

To summarize, the evidence suggests that the standard of care for patients with a KPS ≥70 and a single brain metastasis should be SRS or surgical excision, integrated with adjuvant WBRT. Though these options have never been directly compared to each other in a randomized controlled trial, non-randomized data suggest that both options are considered equally effective. Unfortunately, the only randomized controlled trial designed to address the question failed to accrue enough patients to permit any firm conclusions (Roos et al., 2011).

Surgery vs SRS for Single Brain Metastases

The choice of surgery vs SRS depends on several factors including: whether the patient is a surgical candidate; the presence of severe neurologic symptoms; the location, size and resectability of the lesion; and the need for histopathological confirmation. The ASTRO evidence-based guideline on the radiotherapeutic and surgical management of newly diagnosed brain metastases recommends that good prognosis patients with a single brain metastasis less than 3 or 4 cm in maximum dimension and amenable to surgical excision can be considered for either surgery or radiosurgery (Tsao et al., 2012). In general, surgical resection should be considered in patients who have a surgically accessible lesion, patients with severe neurologic deficits due to mass effect or in patients for whom histopathological confirmation is required (Patchell, 2003). Radiosurgery should be considered in good prognosis patients with single brain metastasis less than 3–4 cm in maximal dimension, in eloquent areas not amenable to safe total resection, or in patients who are unfit for surgery (Tsao et al., 2012).

Management of Patients with Multiple Brain Metastases

For patients with two to four brain metastases, the randomized data (RCT) have not demonstrated a survival advantage with the addition of SRS to WBRT. This fact is often used as the rationale for treating patients with multiple brain metastases with WBRT alone. Guidelines published by the American Association of Neurosurgeons suggest that the lack of survival benefit observed in the studies examining patients with more than two brain metastases may be due to crossover of study participants and insufficient power in the available RCTs (Linskey et al., 2010). Furthermore, some non-randomized data have demonstrated a survival advantage for patients with multiple brain metastases treated with SRS. A retrospective study by Bhatnagar et al. (2006) of 205 patients with four or more intracranial metastases from various primary cancers treated with SRS found a survival benefit compared to historical controls treated with WBRT alone. Total intracranial treatment volume was found to be an important predictor of survival and the authors suggest that this factor be of primary consideration, rather than the total number of metastases.

Though it is unclear whether a survival benefit exists for patients with multiple brain metastases, there is level I evidence that SRS boost results in improved local tumor control, reduced steroid dependence, and improved performance status. Kondziolka et al. (1999) randomized 27 patients with two to four brain metastases measuring <2.5 cm and with a KPS $\geq$ 70 to WBRT alone vs WBRT + SRS. The study was stopped early after an interim analysis revealed substantial improvements in the rate of local failure at 1 year (100% vs 8%) and median time to local failure (6 vs 36 months). No survival benefit was found with the use of SRS boost and WBRT compared to WBRT alone. The RTOG 9508 study (Andrews et al., 2004), discussed previously, found a statistically significant improvement in KPS and a reduction in steroid use with the addition of SRS to WBRT in patients with one to three brain metastases. This study did not find statistically significant differences in mental status, overall time to intracranial tumor progression, neurologic death rates, or toxicity between the two treatment arms.

Emerging Techniques in the Radiation Management of Brain Metastases

Various radiation therapy approaches (e.g. helical tomotherapy (HT), volumetric arc therapy, and intensity modulated radiation therapy) using image-guided fractionated radiotherapy regimens are being investigated as a non-invasive alternative to SRS in the management of patients with brain metastases. This technique combines intensity modulated fan-beam radiotherapy delivery with megavoltage computed tomography imaging, providing the capability of on-line image-guided conformal radiation delivery. The addition of SRS to WBRT requires separate localization and treatment procedures that add some cost and inconvenience to patients, caregivers and providers. Some SRS systems require invasive immobilization devices, which can add to patient discomfort and patients with multiple lesions can experience long treatment times.

For example, a phase II multi-institutional study (Rodrigues et al., 2012b) assessing a simultaneous in-field boost HT technique for brain metastases (TOMO-BII) is now open for accrual. Patients with one to three brain metastases are treated with a simultaneous in-field boost technique yielding a total intralesional dose of 60 Gy with a surrounding whole brain dose of 30 Gy. Outcomes will be compared with historical controls treated with SRS and WBRT. The purpose of the trial is to provide patients with a shorter course, dose intense and non-invasive radiotherapy treatment with equivalent or improved CNS control, survival, quality of life and toxicity. Other clinical trials using alternative radiotherapy platforms are also accruing patients (www.clinicaltrials.gov).

Surgery for Multiple Brain Metastases

The role of neurosurgical resection for patients with multiple brain metastases remains undefined. The current ASTRO guidelines do not address the utility of surgical resection in patients with more than one brain metastasis. In practice, palliative surgery is considered in patients with multiple brain metastases who have one life-threatening brain lesion that is surgically accessible (i.e. impending herniation, large lesions in critical areas, hemorrhage) to provide rapid decompression or for patients in whom a tissue diagnosis is required. This approach is consistent with the NCCN guidelines on the use of surgery for multiple brain metastases (http://www.nccn.org/professionals/physician_gls/pdf/cns.pdf.).

Is Whole Brain Radiotherapy Necessary after Surgical Resection or SRS?

Another point of controversy in the brain metastases literature is the need for adjuvant WBRT following surgical resection or SRS. The rationale for the use of adjuvant WBRT is to prevent recurrence in the tumor bed and to control microscopic disease that may be present elsewhere in the brain. The randomized trial by Patchell et al. (1998) found that the omission of radiotherapy after surgical resection of a single brain metastasis significantly increased the risk of recurrence at the tumor bed and at other sites in the brain. These patients were more likely to die of neurologic causes. Aoyama et al. (2006) randomized 132 patients with one to four brain metastases to SRS and WBRT versus SRS alone. Those patients who did not receive WBRT were more likely to experience intracranial relapse, however, there were no statistically significant differences in the rates of neurologic death.

Thus far, no randomized trial has demonstrated a clear survival benefit to adjuvant WBRT. Given the apparent lack of survival benefit and the concern for the potential long-term neurotoxicity, some investigators advocate withholding WBRT, reserving it for salvage therapy. A recent randomized trial, using a single measure for neurocognitive decline at a single time-point, found that patients with one to three brain metastases treated with SRS and WBRT were found to have a significantly higher risk of deterioration in memory and learning at 4 months, compared to patients who had only SRS (Chang et al., 2009). The EORTC 22952-26001 trial compared observation versus WBRT after surgical resection or SRS in 359 patients with one to three brain metastases (Kocher et al., 2011). The primary endpoint was duration of functional independence. Adjuvant WBRT reduced the intracranial relapse rate and decreased the rate of neurologic death. No significant difference in the duration of functional independence was observed, however, the rate of neurologic death due to intracranial failure was significantly lower in patients who received WBRT. In summary, both of these studies suggest that WBRT may be withheld in patients with one to three brain metastases treated with SRS if frequent serial brain imaging is performed to detect early failures requiring salvage treatment.

In contrast, it is well established that patients who do not receive WBRT are at higher risk for recurrence in the tumor bed and elsewhere in the brain. Whether the morbidity of recurrence is more severe than the morbidity related to WBRT remains unclear, since data on quality of life outcomes and neurocognitive function in patients who do not receive WBRT are limited. In a retrospective study of 36 patients treated with SRS and observation, Regine et al. (2002) found that 47% had a recurrence of brain metastases and 71% of these patients were symptomatic. Of those patients with recurrent tumors, 59% had neurologic deficits that did not improve after salvage radiotherapy. These findings suggest that uncontrolled brain tumors can cause a substantial decrease in mental performance that far outweighs any decrement seen with cranial irradiation (Patchell, 2003) and that recurrent brain metastases may be less amenable to successful treatment. Therefore, ASTRO guidelines recommend that treatment options for patients with one to three brain metastases and stable systemic disease include any of the following: SRS or surgical resection alone with serial imaging for follow up; SRS with WBRT; or WBRT alone. For patients with a single brain metastasis treated with surgical resection, it is strongly recommended that adjuvant WBRT be considered, as WBRT reduces the risk of tumor bed recurrence (Tsao et al., 2012).

Which Patients Benefit from Aggressive Management of Brain Metastases?

Predicting which patients with brain metastases may benefit from aggressive treatment can be very challenging for the clinician. Several major factors have been identified in the literature that influence prognosis and predict for therapeutic benefit. The RTOG developed a recursive partitioning model based on 1960 patients with brain metastases treated with WBRT alone, WBRT and radiosensitizers or WBRT and radiosurgery and divided these patients into three prognostic groups based on pre-treatment prognostic variables: age, performance status, primary tumor status, presence/absence of extracranial systemic metastases (Gaspar et al., 1997). Patients with the highest median survival (7.1 months) were <65 years old, had a KPS ≥70, with a controlled primary and no extracranial disease. The poorest median survival of 2.3 months was observed in Class III patients (KPS <70). Class II (all others patient combinations) had a median survival of 4.2 months.

The number of brain metastases is another important prognostic factor. The prognostic significance of the number of brain metastases was demonstrated in the RTOG 9508 randomized controlled trial that compared WBRT and SRS versus WBRT alone in patients with one to three brain metastases (Andrews et al., 2004). They found a survival benefit in only those patients with a single brain metastasis. No survival benefit was observed in those patients who had two or three brain metastases.

A recent systematic review of brain metastases prognostic indices for a variety of primary cancers found that nine prognostic systems have been published in the medical literature (Rodrigues et al., 2012a). Four of the nine prognostic systems include control of the primary malignancy as an important prognostic factor. Other factors commonly used in these prognostic indices are performance status, age, number of brain metastases, control of the primary malignancy and presence of extracranial metastases.

Prognostic Factors Specific to NSCLC Patients with Brain Metastases

The RTOG recursive partitioning analysis was refined by Sperduto et al. (2010) to include the primary disease site as a parameter in 4259 patients treated with surgery, WBRT, SRS or various treatment combinations to define a disease-specific graded prognostic assessment (DS-GPA) score. For patients with brain metastases from NSCLC, age, KPS, presence of extracranial metastases, and number of brain metastases were identified as prognostic factors. The median overall survival for all NSCLC patients with brain metastases was 7 months. A median survival of 14.78 months was achieved in patients with the highest DS-GPA score (≤50 years old, KPS 90–100, absence of extracranial metastases and a single brain metastasis). In contrast, those with the lowest DS-GPA score (>60 years, KPS <70, presence of ECM, more than three brain metastases) had a median survival of only 3.02 months.

MANAGEMENT OF NSCLC PATIENTS WITH SYNCHRONOUS BRAIN METASTASES

Patients with NSCLC can present with brain metastases at the time of diagnosis (synchronous metastases) or may develop brain metastases subsequent to diagnosis of the primary lung malignancy (metachronous metastases). Synchronous brain metastases are identified in approximately 10% of patients with NSCLC at the time of diagnosis (Schuette, 2004) and the proportion of patients who develop metachronous metastases is higher, in the range of 30–50% (Knights, 1954). Synchronous brain metastases are thought to confer a poorer prognosis than metachronous brain metastases, since they are felt to be the result of inherently more aggressive disease, yet in the literature, there is no conclusive evidence that patients with metachronous brain metastases survive longer. In the case of a synchronous presentation, typically, the intracranial disease is treated first, to avoid the potentially life-threatening consequences of neurologic progression.

With recent advances in the management of brain metastases, patients with single brain metastases and favorable prognostic features can achieve long-term survival with aggressive neurosurgical or stereotactic radiosurgical treatments. However, the optimal treatment of the primary intrathoracic disease in patients with NSCLC who present with synchronous brain metastasis is less well defined.

Rationale for Aggressive Treatment of Oligometastatic Disease

In 1995, Hellman and Weichselbaum proposed the existence of an "oligometastatic state": an intermediate disease state between locoregionally confined and widely metastatic cancer, where tumors early in the evolution of metastatic progression produce metastases limited in number and location (Hellman and Weichselbaum, 1995). The extension of this hypothesis is that selected patients with oligometastatic cancer may benefit from local aggressive treatment to eradicate all measurable disease, with the goal of higher rates of local control or even cure. Ablation of metastatic deposits can be achieved surgically (metastatectomy), or through stereotactic ablative radiotherapy (SABR, also known as stereotactic body radiotherapy/SBRT), a new radiotherapy technology that delivers very large, highly conformal, hypofractionated doses of radiotherapy to small tumor targets, usually in five fractions or less, with observed high rates of local control.

Management of Oligometastatic NSCLC

Evidence to support the oligometastatic hypothesis is supported by the long-term survival of some patients who have had surgical resection of pulmonary, hepatic and brain metastases (Macdermed et al., 2008) and patients who have received SABR for lung oligometastases (Siva et al., 2010). Studies examining the patterns of failure of advanced or metastatic NSCLC after first-line systemic therapy have demonstrated that the predominant sites of failure are local, rather than systemic, providing further rationale for using SABR in patients with oligometastases (Rusthoven et al., 2009). Furthermore, it is interesting to note that in the seventh edition of the TNM classification of lung tumors, the survival of patients with pathologic stage IV disease is higher than patients with stage IIIB disease (Detterbeck et al., 2009) possibly due to specific subgroups of stage IV patients who had aggressive surgical management of metastatic disease.

Patients with oligometastatic NSCLC are increasingly being treated aggressively, with encouraging results. Several single institution series have reported long-term survival in NSCLC patients with solitary brain metastases who received aggressive treatment of both the brain metastasis and the primary lung disease, as summarized in a recent review of the literature (Villarreal-Garza et al., 2012). Papers cited within this review generally managed patients by surgical resection or SRS $\pm$ WBRT for brain metastases and either surgical resection or primary radiotherapy $\pm$ systemic chemotherapy for the primary lung tumor. The majority of patients had a solitary brain metastasis, however, several series included patients with multiple (two to six) brain metastases. Patients who received surgical resection of the primary had pneumonectomy, lobectomy, or wedge resection, in some cases followed

TABLE 17.1 Outcomes of Selected Series Utilizing Radical Cranial and Thoracic Treatments for NSCLC Patients with Synchronous Brain Metastases

Series	No. Patients Who Received Cranial and Thoracic Rx	Cranial Rx	Thoracic Rx	Median Survival with Thoracic Rx (months)	Median Survival without Thoracic Rx (months)	1 yr OS* (%)	2 yr OS* (%)	5 yr OS* (%)
Billing (Billing et al., 2001)	28	Surgery	Surgery	24	NA	64.3	54	2%
Lind (Lind et al., 2011)	24	Surgery and WBRT or SRS and salvage WBRT	Surgery ($n = 10$) or Chemoradiation ($n = 6$) or SABR ($n = 8$)	28.4	12.1 (Chemotherapy) 5.6 (supportive therapy)	≈70	≈50	NR
Hu (Hu et al., 2006)	44	Surgery ± WBRT SRS ± WBRT	RT ± chemotherapy	15.5	5.9	70	18.5	NR

*WBRT: whole brain radiotherapy; SRS: stereotactic radiosurgery; SABR: stereotactic ablative body radiotherapy; NA: not applicable; NR: not reported; * patients who received thoracic Rx.*

by thoracic radiotherapy and/or systemic chemotherapy. Radical chest radiotherapy was delivered using 3D conformal or IMRT techniques.

In the review by Garza-Villarreal et al., the median survival of those patients who received surgical resection of the lung primary ranged from 19 to 27 months, with 1-, 2- and 5-year overall survivals (OS) of 56–69%, 28–54% and 11–24% respectively. Those patients who received primary thoracic radiotherapy had similar survival rates, with median survival ranging from 15.5 to 31.8 months, 1- and 2-year OS of 50–71% and 16–60% respectively, with a small proportion of patients surviving beyond 5–10 years (Villarreal-Garza et al., 2012). These outcomes are quite favorable in comparison to the 7-month median survival of stage IV NSCLC patients treated for brain metastases (Sperduto et al., 2010) and the 1-year overall survival of 10–20% in NSCLC patients treated with WBRT alone (Zabel and Debus, 2004). The outcomes of selected series are summarized in Table 17.1.

Prognostic Factors Affecting Survival in NSCLC Patients with Synchronous Brain Metastases

Several prognostic factors influencing survival have been reported in the medical literature and are summarized in Table 17.2 (Villarreal-Garza et al., 2012).

Factors of Undetermined or No Prognostic Significance

It is controversial whether the burden of thoracic disease is an important prognostic factor in NSCLC patients with synchronous brain metastases. As shown in Table 17.1, several

TABLE 17.2 Prognostic Factors Influencing Survival in NSCLC Patients with Synchronous Brain Metastases

Control of the primary thoracic malignancy: use of definitive thoracic therapy (surgical resection, chemoradiotherapy, or SABR)
N-stage (N0 better outcomes than N1/N2/N3)
Age (younger patients had better outcomes)
Sex: females had better survival
Performance status
Histology (adenocarcinoma better prognosis than other types)
Absence of extracranial metastases
Location of brain metastases (supratentorial better than infratentorial)
Response to induction chemotherapy prior to focal thoracic treatment (Girard et al., 2006)
Thoracic stage: stage I or II better (Hu et al., 2006; Lind et al., 2011; Louie et al., 2009)
Time to thoracic intervention: better survival if thoracic treatment <8 weeks from initial brain treatment (Louie et al., 2009)
Radiotherapy dose (>63 Gy better than <63 Gy) (Lopez Guerra et al., 2012)

series have found longer overall survival with stage I or II thoracic disease, compared to stage III, whereas other studies have found no impact of locoregional stage on survival (Villarreal-Garza et al., 2012). Though patients with thoracic stage III disease may have relatively poor outcomes, it is important to note that patients with stage III thoracic disease who receive aggressive management of both thoracic disease and brain metastases can achieve better survival than stage III patients who receive aggressive treatment of brain metastases only or those who receive only WBRT (Lind et al., 2011).

Similarly, there is variable evidence regarding the prognostic value of the burden of nodal disease (N-stage), where some series have found better survival in lymph node negative patients (NO) compared with lymph node positive patients, whereas others have found no survival difference (Villarreal-Garza et al., 2012). The prognostic significance of synchronous versus metachronous brain metastases is also uncertain, with conflicting reports in the literature. The number of brain metastases appears to be a significant prognostic factor in patients with brain metastases from a variety of primary cancers, however, it has not been found to be a prognostic factor in NSCLC patients with brain metastases who receive aggressive treatments to both the primary and intracranial metastases.

Standard treatment for stage IV NSCLC includes the consideration for systemic chemotherapy. Platinum-based regimens are most commonly used, which have been found to prolong survival and improve symptom control and quality of life compared to best supportive care, however, failure at the original sites of disease is common after chemotherapy. The role of chemotherapy in NSCLC patients with synchronous brain metastases is poorly defined. The response rates of brain metastases to systemic chemotherapy are poor and there is no high quality evidence to support the use of chemotherapy in the management of brain metastases (Tsao et al., 2012). However, several series have used systemic chemotherapy as part of the aggressive management approach for the primary thoracic disease in patients with synchronous brain metastases, delivered concurrently, or sequentially with thoracic radiotherapy. The response to induction chemotherapy prior to local thoracic treatment has been found to be prognostic in one study (Girard et al., 2006).

Other Prognostic Factors for NSCLC

Prognostic factors have been identified in the NSCLC populations that are associated with better survival outcomes: female sex, Asian ethnicity, non-smoker history, adenocarcinoma histology and presence of EGFR-activating mutations.

Radiation Management of Thoracic Disease in NSCLC Patients with Synchronous Brain Metastases

The optimal radiotherapeutic management of the primary thoracic disease in patients with synchronous brain metastases remains unclear, owing to the small number of patients in the published series and to incomplete reporting on the dose and fractionation schedules used. The aggressive management of thoracic disease in these series is similar to management of thoracic disease in non-metastatic NSCLC (Figure 17.1). Small thoracic tumors (T1–T2) with limited nodal disease (N0–1) or T3N0 tumors can be considered for surgical resection or primary radiotherapy. Tumors ≤5 cm, in the absence of nodal disease, can be considered for SABR in patients deemed unfit for surgery. Unresectable primary tumors, advanced nodal disease (N2, N3) found on mediastinoscopy, or non-surgical candidates should be considered for radical radiotherapy with or without chemotherapy.

Most published reports utilized conventional 3D-conformal or IMRT radiation-planning techniques to deliver radical radiation dose and fractionation schedules similar to those used in non-metastatic NSCLC. A variety of radical radiation dose and fractionation schedules have been reported with doses in the range of 60 Gy in 30 fractions, or a biologically equivalent dose, most commonly being used (Villarreal-Garza et al., 2012). These doses are consistent with doses prescribed in non-metastatic NSCLC, where there are emerging data from the RTOG 0617 phase III trial that suggest there is no survival benefit to dose escalation beyond 60 Gy when given concurrently with chemotherapy in patients with stage III NSCLC (www.rtog.org). Furthermore, one study that examined prognostic factors associated with survival in patients with NSCLC and oligometastatic disease in intracranial and extracranial sites reported that patients with a KPS >80 who received at least 63 Gy to the primary tumor had a significantly lower incidence of mortality than those receiving <63 Gy (Lopez Guerra et al., 2012). Data on the use of SABR for aggressive management of the lung primary in this setting are scant and to our knowledge there is only one published report in the literature describing its use, where doses of 60 Gy in three fractions of 20 Gy, or 60 Gy in five fractions of 12 Gy were used (Lind et al., 2011). The standard dose fractionation schedules for early-stage NSCLC SABR in our institution are risk-adapted, with 54 Gy in three fractions as the standard dose, 55 Gy in five fractions for any tumor with broad chest wall

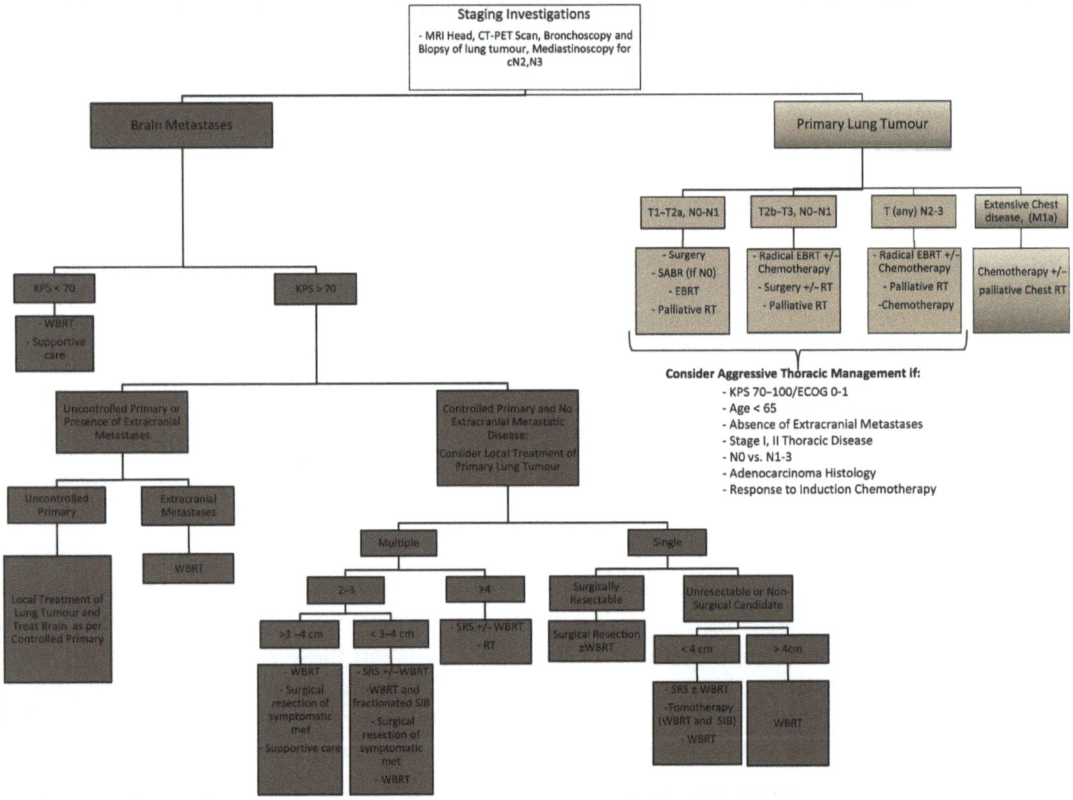

FIGURE 17.1 Management algorithm for NSCLC patients with synchronous brain metastases.

involvement, and 60 Gy in eight fractions for central tumors near the brachial plexus or within 2 cm of the mediastinum. Doses are prescribed to the 80% isodose line and have a biologically effective dose (BED10) of >100 Gy, based upon a study that found better local control and survival rates for BED ≥100 Gy in stage I NSCLC patients treated with SABR (Onishi et al., 2004).

Patients with synchronous brain metastases with a poor performance status or extensive thoracic disease not amenable to aggressive radiotherapy or surgery can be treated with palliative radiotherapy. A dose of 30 Gy in 10 fractions or a biologically effective dose-equivalent (BED 35 Gy_{10}) or greater are associated with improvements in total symptom scores and survival, at the cost of an increased risk of radiation esophagitis, primarily in patients with a high performance status when compared to schedules of lower BED. More abbreviated courses of palliative radiotherapy (e.g. 17 Gy in two fractions, 2000 cGy in five fractions and 8–10 Gy in a single fraction) can provide good symptomatic relief and can be considered for patients with a poor performance status or patients who request shorter treatment schedules (Rodrigues et al., 2011).

Surgical Management of Thoracic Disease in NSCLC Patients with Synchronous Brain Metastases

A variety of surgical approaches have been used in studies that have evaluated surgical treatment of primary thoracic disease in patients with brain metastases (pneumonectomy, lobectomy, wedge resection) (Villarreal-Garza et al., 2012). Some series report the addition of postoperative radiotherapy ± chemotherapy. No particular surgical approach has been shown to be associated with superior outcomes. The timing of thoracic intervention was found to be of prognostic importance in one study, where patients who received thoracic treatment within 8 weeks after the initial brain treatment had better overall survival.

Staging Workup of NSCLC Patients with Synchronous Brain Metastases

Identification of patients who might benefit from aggressive treatment to the brain and chest requires a thorough panel of staging investigations. Patients should be selected for curative intent treatments only after staging investigations have excluded the presence of metastatic disease elsewhere in the body.

1. Pathological confirmation of the lung tumor with bronchoscopy and biopsy, or CT-guided core biopsy.
2. Positron emission tomography–computed tomography (PET-CT) of the whole body should be performed to rule out extracranial metastases.
3. As noted previously, the presence of N2 or N3 lymphadenopathy has been found to be an adverse prognostic factor and thus pathological confirmation of mediastinal disease (N2 or N3 lymph nodes) with mediastinoscopy or endobronchial ultrasound (EBUS)-guided biopsy is important.
4. Imaging of the brain:
   a. Common practice is first to obtain a contrast-enhanced CT of the head. If a single brain metastasis is found on contrast-enhanced CT, or the diagnosis of brain metastases is in question, an MRI should be ordered to determine if other brain metastases are present and to rule out the presence of infarcts, abscesses, or other non-metastatic CNS lesions. Gadolinium-enhanced MRI of the brain, including T1- and T2-weighted and FLAIR sequences are recommended.
   b. Brain metastases tend to be found at the junction of the gray and white matter, with associated surrounding edema that appears as hypodense areas on non-contrast enhanced CT. Metastases commonly show a ring-enhancement pattern on contrast-enhanced CT.
5. In those patients who are deemed to have surgically inaccessible brain metastases, a stereotactic biopsy is recommended if the diagnosis on cranial imaging is in doubt.
6. Pulmonary function tests for those patients in whom radical chest radiotherapy or thoracic surgery is being considered, including FEV1, FEV1/FVC and DLCO measurements.
7. Multidisciplinary tumor board discussion regarding management with input from specialists from radiation oncology, medical oncology, thoracic surgery, radiology and pathology.

Management Algorithm for NSCLC Patients with Synchronous Brain Metastases

Prognostic factors may help to identify those NSCLC patients with brain metastases who are most likely to benefit from curative intent treatment. An important caveat is that each patient must be considered on an individual basis and the absence of particular prognostic factors should not be used as justification to exclude patients who might otherwise benefit from aggressive management. A proposed algorithm of management for NSCLC patients with synchronous brain metastases is shown in Figure 17.1.

Future Directions in the Management of Oligometastatic NSCLC

It is apparent that NSCLC patients with synchronous oligometastatic brain metastases may benefit from aggressive management of both the primary lung tumor and brain metastases. Though the available evidence is limited, most authors would agree that aggressive management should be considered a therapeutic option in a select group of patients. Randomized controlled trials are underway to answer definitively the question as to whether there is a survival benefit associated with such treatments.

The randomized, phase II SWOG/NCCTG N0724 study, recently closed to accrual, aims to evaluate whether consolidative radiation to areas of gross disease after systemic chemotherapy will enhance the survival of oligometastatic NSCLC patients. NSCLC patients with one to three successfully treated, non-progressive brain metastases or one to three extracranial metastases were randomized to further radiotherapy (45 Gy in 15 fractions or 60 Gy in 30 fractions) to residual disease post-chemotherapy versus no further treatment. All patients had previously received systemic chemotherapy. The primary endpoint is overall survival and secondary endpoints include progression-free survival, time-to-disease progression, time-to-treatment failure, confirmed response rate, duration of response and adverse events.

To elucidate further the role of SABR in oligometastatic patients, a multi-institutional clinical trial, Stereotactic Ablative Radiotherapy for Comprehensive Treatment of Oligometastatic Tumors (SABR-COMET) is now open for accrual (registered at www.clinicaltrials.gov). In this randomized phase II clinical trial, patients with a variety of primary tumor types with up to five metastases (no more than three in any single organ system) are randomized to either the standard of care (palliative radiotherapy with further chemotherapy at the discretion of the medical oncologist) versus SABR to all known sites of metastatic disease. The primary endpoint of this study is overall survival, with secondary endpoints evaluating toxicity, quality of life and progression-free survival.

CONCLUSION

In summary, patients with brain metastases have an overall poor survival. However, there is evidence from prospective randomized controlled trials to support consideration of aggressive, curative-intent treatment options in select patients with favorable prognostic factors. For patients with a solitary brain metastasis, whether synchronous or metachronous, treatment options include surgical resection or stereotactic radiosurgery, followed by whole brain radiotherapy. Prognostic factors for improved overall survival in this population include KPS >70, age <65, controlled primary disease, absence of extracranial disease, and presence of a single brain metastasis. Patients with one to four brain metastases and favorable prognostic features may be considered for SRS followed by WBRT. Patients with multiple brain metastases and poor prognostic factors should be considered for WBRT. Techniques under investigation in the management of brain metastases include helical tomotherapy WBRT with simultaneous in-field boost. The optimal treatment for patients presenting with synchronous brain metastases from NSCLC remains to be defined. There is increasing evidence that survival is improved in oligometastastic NSCLC patients who receive radical intracranial and thoracic treatments. Chemotherapy is not routinely used in the management of brain metastases. Clinical trials are underway better to define the role of aggressive treatment options in patients with synchronous brain metastases.

References

Andrews, D.W., Scott, C.B., Sperduto, P.W., et al., 2004. Whole brain radiation therapy with or without stereotactic radiosurgery boost for patients with one to three brain metastases: phase iii results of the rtog 9508 randomised trial. Lancet 363, 1665.

Aoyama, H., Shirato, H., Tago, M., et al., 2006. Stereotactic radiosurgery plus whole-brain radiation therapy vs stereotactic radiosurgery alone for treatment of brain metastases: a randomized controlled trial. J. Am. Med. Assoc. 295, 2483–2491.

Bhatnagar, A.K., Flickinger, J.C., Kondziolka, D., Lunsford, L.D., 2006. Stereotactic radiosurgery for four or more intracranial metastases. Int. J. Radiat. Oncol. Biol. Phys. 64, 898–903.

Billing, P.S., Miller, D.L., Allen, M.S., Deschamps, C., Trastek, V.F., Pairolero, P.C., 2001. Surgical treatment of primary lung cancer with synchronous brain metastases. J. Thorac. Cardiovasc. Surg. 122, 548–553.

Chang, E.L., Wefel, J.S., Hess, K.R., et al., 2009. Neurocognition in patients with brain metastases treated with radiosurgery or radiosurgery plus whole-brain irradiation: a randomised controlled trial. Lancet Oncol. 10, 1037–1044.

Detterbeck, F.C., Boffa, D.J., Tanoue, L.T., 2009. The new lung cancer staging system. Chest 136, 260–271.

Gaspar, L., Scott, C., Rotman, M., et al., 1997. Recursive partitioning analysis (RPA) of prognostic factors in three radiation therapy oncology group (RTOG) brain metastases trials. Int. J. Radiat. Oncol. Biol. Phys. 37, 745–751.

Girard, N., Cottin, V., Tronc, F., et al., 2006. Chemotherapy is the cornerstone of the combined surgical treatment of lung cancer with synchronous brain metastases. Lung Cancer 53, 51–58.

Hellman, S., Weichselbaum, R.R., 1995. Oligometastases. J. Clin. Oncol. 13, 8–10.

Hu, C., Chang, E.L., Hassenbusch 3rd, S.J., et al., 2006. Nonsmall cell lung cancer presenting with synchronous solitary brain metastasis. Cancer 106, 1998–2004.

Jemal, A., Bray, F., Center, M.M., Ferlay, J., Ward, E., Forman, D., 2011. Global cancer statistics. CA Cancer J. Clin. 61, 69–90.

Knights, E.M., 1954. Metastatic tumors of the brain and their relation to primary and secondary pulmonary cancer. Cancer 7, 259–265.

Kocher, M., Soffietti, R., Abacioglu, U., et al., 2011. Adjuvant whole-brain radiotherapy versus observation after radiosurgery or surgical resection of one to three cerebral metastases: results of the EORTC 22952-26001 study. J. Clin. Oncol. 29, 134–141.

Kondziolka, D., Patel, A., Lunsford, L.D., Kassam, A., Flickinger, J.C., 1999. Stereotactic radiosurgery plus whole brain radiotherapy versus radiotherapy alone for patients with multiple brain metastases. Int. J. Radiat. Oncol. Biol. Phys. 45, 427–434.

Law, A., Karp, D.D., Dipetrillo, T., Daly, B.T., 2001. Emergence of increased cerebral metastasis after high-dose preoperative radiotherapy with chemotherapy in patients with locally advanced nonsmall cell lung carcinoma. Cancer 92, 160–164.

Lind, J.S.W., Lagerwaard, F.J., Smit, E.F., Postmus, P.E., Slotman, B.J., Senan, S., 2011. Time for reappraisal of extracranial treatment options? Cancer 117, 597–605.

Linskey, M., Andrews, D., Asher, A., et al., 2010. The role of stereotactic radiosurgery in the management of patients with newly diagnosed brain metastases: A systematic review and evidence-based clinical practice guideline. J. Neurooncol. 96, 45–68.

Lopez Guerra, J.L., Gomez, D., Zhuang, Y., et al., 2012. Prognostic impact of radiation therapy to the primary tumor in patients with non-small cell lung cancer and oligometastasis at diagnosis. Int. J. Radiat. Oncol. Biol. Phys. 84, e61–e67.

Louie, A.V., Rodrigues, G., Yaremko, B., Yu, E., Dar, A.R., Dingle, B., et al., 2009. Management and prognosis in synchronous solitary resected brain metastasis from non–small-cell lung cancer. Clin. Lung Cancer 10 (3), 174–179.

Macdermed, D.M., Weichselbaum, R.R., Salama, J.K., 2008. A rationale for the targeted treatment of oligometastases with radiotherapy. J. Surg. Oncol. 98, 202–206.

Onishi, H., Araki, T., Shirato, H., et al., 2004. Stereotactic hypofractionated high-dose irradiation for stage I non-small cell lung carcinoma: clinical outcomes in 245 subjects in a Japanese multiinstitutional study. Cancer 101, 1623–1631.

Order, S.E., Hellman, S., Von Essen, C.F., Kligerman, M.M., 1968. Improvement in quality of survival following whole-brain irradiation for brain metastasis. Radiology 91, 149–153.

Patchell, R.A., 2003. The management of brain metastases. Cancer Treat. Rev. 29, 533–540.

Patchell, R.A., Tibbs, P.A., Regine, W.F., et al., 1998. Postoperative radiotherapy in the treatment of single metastases to the brain: a randomized trial. J. Am. Med. Assoc. 280, 1485–1489.

Patchell, R.A., Tibbs, P.A., Walsh, J.W., et al., 1990. A randomized trial of surgery in the treatment of single metastases to the brain. N. Engl. J. Med. 322, 494–500.

Regine, W.F., Huhn, J.L., Patchell, R.A., et al., 2002. Risk of symptomatic brain tumor recurrence and neurologic deficit after radiosurgery alone in patients with newly diagonised brain metastases: results and implications. Int. J. Radiat. Oncol. Biol. Phys. 52, 333–338.

Rodrigues, G., Bauman, G., Palma, D., et al., 2012a. Systematic review of brain metastases prognostic indices. Pract. Radiat. Oncol. in press.

Rodrigues, G., Videtic, G.M.M., Sur, R., et al., 2011. Palliative thoracic radiotherapy in lung cancer: an American Society for Radiation Oncology evidence-based clinical practice guideline. Pract. Radiat. Oncol. 1, 60–71.

Rodrigues, G., Yartsev, S., Tay, K.Y., Pond, G.R., Lagerwaard, F., Bauman, G., 2012b. A phase II multi-institutional study assessing simultaneous in-field boost helical tomotherapy for 1-3 brain metastases. Radiat. Oncol. 7, 42.

Roos, D.E., Smith, J.G., Stephens, S.W., 2011. Radiosurgery versus surgery, both with adjuvant whole brain radiotherapy, for solitary brain metastases: a randomised controlled trial. Clin. Oncol. 23, 646–651.

Rusthoven, K.E., Hammerman, S.F., Kavanagh, B.D., Birtwhistle, M.J., Stares, M., Camidge, D.R., 2009. Is there a role for consolidative stereotactic body radiation therapy following first-line systemic therapy for metastatic lung cancer? A patterns-of-failure analysis. Acta. Oncol. 48, 578–583.

Schuette, W., 2004. Treatment of brain metastases from lung cancer: chemotherapy. Lung Cancer 45 (Suppl. 2), S253–S257.

Siva, S., MacManus, M., Ball, D., 2010. Stereotactic radiotherapy for pulmonary oligometastases: a systematic review. J. Thorac. Oncol. 5, 1091–1099.

Sørensen, J.B., Hansen, H.H., Hansen, M., Dombernowsky, P., 1988. Brain metastases in adenocarcinoma of the lung: frequency, risk groups, and prognosis. J. Clin. Oncol. 6, 1474–1480.

Sperduto, P.W., Chao, S.T., Sneed, P.K., et al., 2010. Diagnosis-specific prognostic factors, indexes, and treatment outcomes for patients with newly diagnosed brain metastases: a multi-institutional analysis of 4,259 patients. Int. J. Radiat. Oncol. Biol. Phys. 77, 655–661.

Tsao, M.N., Rades, D., Wirth, A., et al., 2012. Radiotherapeutic and surgical management for newly diagnosed brain metastasis(es): an American Society for Radiation Oncology Evidence-based Guideline. Pract. Radiat. Oncol. 2, 210–225.

Villarreal-Garza, C., de la Mata, D., Zavala, D.G., Macedo-Perez, E.O., Arrieta, O., 2012. Aggressive treatment of primary tumor in patients with non-small-cell lung cancer and exclusively brain metastases. Clin. Lung Cancer in press.

Zabel, A., Debus, J., 2004. Treatment of brain metastases from non-small-cell lung cancer (NSCLC): radiotherapy. Lung Cancer 45 (Suppl. 2), S247–S252.

Zimm, S., Wampler, G.L., Stablein, D., Hazra, T., Young, H.F., 1981. Intracerebral metastases in solid-tumor patients: natural history and results of treatment. Cancer 48, 384–394.

PART III

BRAIN METASTASES FROM SMALL CELL LUNG CARCINOMA

18 *Brain Metastasis after Prophylactic Cranial Irradiation in Patients with Small Cell Lung Cancer* 199

19 *Brain Metastasis from Small-Cell Lung Cancer with High Levels of Placental Growth Factor* 213

20 *Brain Metastases from Lung Cancer* 227

21 *Lambert–Eaton Myesthenic Syndrome and Brain Metastasis from Occult Small Cell Lung Carcinoma: A Clinician's Perspective* 243

CHAPTER

18

Brain Metastasis after Prophylactic Cranial Irradiation in Patients with Small Cell Lung Cancer

Patricia Tai, Avi Assouline, Kurian Joseph, Joseph Siu-kie Au and Edward Yu

OUTLINE

Introduction 200

Brain Metastasis after Prophylactic Cranial Irradiation 201

How Often does Brain Relapse Occur after PCI? 201

Does the Timing of PCI Affect the Rate of Brain Relapse? 201

Does the Timing of Chest RT Affect the Rate of Brain Relapse after PCI? 204

Is the Rate of Brain Relapse Affected by the Dose of PCI? 205

When do they Occur after PCI? 205

How to Detect them? 206

Treatment Options 206

Stereotactic Radiotherapy 206

Whole Brain Re-Irradiation 207

Chemotherapy 208

Outcome and Conclusion 209

References 209

M.A. Hayat (ed): *Brain Metastases from Primary Tumors, Volume 1*
DOI: http://dx.doi.org/10.1016/B978-0-12-800896-6.00018-8

© 2014 Elsevier Inc. All rights reserved.

INTRODUCTION

Small cell lung cancer (SCLC) accounts for about 15–20% of all lung cancers. It is both chemo- and radiosensitive. The brain is a common site of metastases. Unfortunately, because of the blood–brain barrier, chemotherapy may not be able to achieve a sufficient tumoricidal dose. Some patients achieve a complete response (CR) to treatment in the chest, only to develop brain metastases (BM) later. In 1974, Newman and Hansen reported that central nervous system (CNS) metastases were more common in SCLC than in other types of lung cancer, and postulated that CNS prophylaxis might decrease the frequency of CNS relapse (Hansen et al., 1973; Newman and Hansen, 1974). Attempts to diminish the frequency of CNS relapse with chemotherapeutic agents, including those that cross the blood–brain barrier, have been unsuccessful even with modern chemotherapy. Prophylactic cranial irradiation (PCI), initially employed in leukemic patients, has been extended to SCLC. In the literature, researchers have tested the efficacy of PCI in patients with limited stage SCLC who achieved CR after combined chemotherapy and thoracic radiation. In a well-known study from Institut Gustave-Roussy in France, the 5-year cumulative rate of BM as an isolated first site of relapse was 37% in the control group and 20% in the PCI group ($p < 0.001$) (Arriagada et al., 2002). The overall 5-year rates of BM were 59% and 43%, respectively [relative risk (RR) 0.50; $p < 0.001$]. The 5-year overall survival rates were 15% in the control group and 18% in the PCI group (RR 0.84; $p = 0.06$).

Slotman et al. (2007) recently challenged the traditional idea that only patients with limited stage SCLC with CR benefit from PCI. In their report, PCI is also beneficial in extensive stage SCLC with any chemotherapy response. Irradiated patients had a lower risk of symptomatic BM (hazard ratio, 0.27; 95% confidence interval [CI], 0.16–0.44; $p < 0.001$). The cumulative risk of BM within 1 year was 14.6% in the irradiation group (95% CI, 8.3–20.9) and 40.4% in the control group (95% CI, 32.1–48.6).

PCI is better than therapeutic cranial irradiation (Arriagada et al., 1995), since the mean duration of survival is brief (approximately 4.5 months) after BM are detected. In a clinical trial with 370 patients, 50 relapsed initially in the brain and 20 in the liver (Felletti et al., 1985). Those who relapsed in the brain suffered a greater deterioration in performance status, and spent a greater proportion of their remaining life in hospital than did patients whose initial relapse was in the liver. This difference was most marked in patients who died soon after relapse. Radiotherapy (20 Gy in five fractions over one week or 30 Gy in 10 fractions over 2 weeks) and dexamethasone were not very effective treatments for brain relapse though subjective responses were common.

Another study also demonstrated that the palliative treatment of overt BM is relatively unsuccessful. Thirty-nine of 225 patients with SCLC developed BM after the initiation of chemotherapy (Lucas et al., 1986). Treatment with high-dose dexamethasone in all 39 patients and cranial irradiation in 32 patients resulted in a complete neurologic recovery in only eight of 39 patients (20%). Twenty-one of 39 patients (53%) failed to derive lasting benefit from their palliative treatment. Thirteen of 24 patients with limited disease with cranial relapse had no clinical evidence of other distant metastases prior to death and, in these patients, the CNS disease was an important cause of morbidity.

The outcome of BM after PCI will be even worse as the general condition of patients and responsiveness to further therapy would be worse after previous treatment. Factors affecting the relapse rate, detection and management of BM after PCI will be the focus of this chapter.

BRAIN METASTASIS AFTER PROPHYLACTIC CRANIAL IRRADIATION

How Often does Brain Relapse Occur after PCI?

The incidence varies from 6% to 33.3%, as seen in the following studies. An overview in 1988 that included nine earlier trials found fewer patients who received PCI had clinically detected BM (6% irradiated versus 22% non-irradiated patients) (Pedersen et al., 1988). In a meta-analysis of seven randomized trials, 33.3% versus 58.6% of patients in the PCI group and control group had BM respectively (Auperin et al., 1999). Tai et al. found the brain relapse rate after PCI was 19% (24/128) patients with CR and 28% (11/40) patients with response less than CR (Tai et al., 2013; Table 18.1). The authors pointed out that, in the past, most randomized studies were on complete responders after chemoradiation. Some studies did not give PCI to partial responders, while others did. Partial responders represent a heterogeneous group of patients with responses ranging from minimal to almost complete response. Partial responders do benefit from PCI with longer progression-free intervals and decreased rates of BM.

Another retrospective study included 133 unselected patients with histologically proven SCLC from 1985 to 1990 (Stiess et al., 1995). The primary therapy consisted of combined radiochemotherapy or only chemotherapy. Sixteen patients were treated only by irradiation. The overall incidence of CNS metastases for all 133 patients was 33.1%. The incidence of new BM in the group of CR patients given PCI was 21.7%, with an average time to development of BM after primary diagnosis of 15.4 months.

Apart from radiotherapy or chemotherapy, there is a small subgroup of SCLC patients who are treated with surgery as the sole definitive local treatment modality. The controversy is whether all such patients or only those with more advanced stages need PCI. Lewinski et al. (1990) reported 13/29 patients without PCI developed BM at 19 months (13/29), while 0/17 patients who received PCI had BM at 4 years.

The incidence of BM would be slightly higher if the hippocampal sparing technique was used for PCI, as only 2.3% BM involves the hippocampus (Marsh et al., 2010). The authors identified 697 intracranial metastases in 107 patients after reviewing contrast-enhanced computerized tomography (CT) and/or magnetic resonance (MR) image sets for each patient. Patients had different histology (e.g. non-SCLC, SCLC, breast cancer, and others). There were 36 limbic metastases (5.2% of all metastases) identified in 22 patients who had a median of 16.5 metastases/patient. Sixteen metastases (2.29%) involved the hippocampus, and 20 (2.86%) involved the rest of the limbic circuit. Another contemporary study is from Denmark (Ramlov et al., 2012). From 2007 to 2010 a total of 118 consecutive patients underwent PCI (25Gy in 10 fractions). Five of the 21 patients had brain relapses after PCI within the limbic system. There is a Radiation Therapy Oncology Group (RTOG)-0933 study on the hippocampal sparing technique which has just completed accrual. Results are pending.

Does the Timing of PCI Affect the Rate of Brain Relapse?

The rate of BM relapse reported in the literature appears to depend on the timing of PCI. Proponents of early PCI state: (1) Suwinski et al. (1998) performed radiobiological estimation and felt that PCI started within 60 days of chemotherapy is more effective since we are

TABLE 18.1 Summary of Studies of Prophylactic Cranial Irradiation (PCI) in Small Cell Lung Cancer

Study	Treatment Sequence			Overall Survival	Other Results	
Rosen, prospective 1983	136 LD, 196 ED patients:			PCI+		
	76 group 1: PCI 20 Gy/10f on day 1 of induction chemoRT			18–20%		
	80 group 2: PCI 24 Gy/8f at week 12 or 24 for both CR and PR			PCI–		
	176 group 3: no PCI, with less intensive chemo			5% (2 y), $p < 0.005$		
Murray, NCIC 1993	308 LD patients:			Initial ChRT 40%,	High rate of BM at 2 y – initial ChRT 15.8%,	
	155 initial ChRT, 153 late ChRT (40 Gy/15f). PCI 25 Gy/10f to patients without progressive disease after chemo and ChRT			late ChRT 34% (2 y), $p = 0.006$	late ChRT 23.8% (2 y), $p = 0.12$	
Work, retrospective 1996	133 patients: 118 without BM at diagnosis			MS	Rates of BM	
	Group I – 23 CR with PCI			16.1 m	21.7%	
	Group II – 23 CR without PCI			13.8 m	26.1%	
	Group III – 72 not achieve CR, and no PCI			8.4 m (n.s.)	22.2% (n.s.)	
Work, Aurhus Lung Cancer Group 1997	199 LD patients			Initial ChRT 20%,	BM – Initial ChRT 19%,	
	99 initial ChRT, 100 late ChRT. Initial PCI always given to initial ChRT patients. After 1984, initial PCI was given also to late ChRT group			late ChRT 19% (2 y), $p = 0.4$	late ChRT 13% (2 y), $p = 0.24$	
	Used split course ChRT (20–22.5 Gy/11f separated by 21 days)					
Auperin, meta-analysis 1999, 2000	847 LD, 140 ED patients in 7 randomized trials				RR of	
	Time between start of induction	PCI+	PCI–		Death	BM
	therapy & randomization	$n =$	$n =$			
	<4 m	84	77		0.92	0.27
	4–6 m	127	152		0.79	0.50
	>6 m	102	91		1.01	0.69
					$p = 0.39, 0.01$	

Schild, phase 2 NCCTG 2007	76 LD patients: 6 cycles of EP. PCI 25 Gy/10f during cycle 3 to responding patients. Cycles 4 and 5 included concurrent chemo and chest (30 Gy/20f BID, a 2-week break, and another 30 Gy/20f BID)	24% (5 y)	Toxicity – 97% ≥Gr 3, 80% ≥Gr 4
Sas-Korczynska, phase 2 2010	41 LD patients: early PCI 30 Gy/15f, immediately after end of ChRT 54 Gy/27–30f, prior to last chemo (EP) cycles	25.5% (4 y)	3/41 (7.3%) vs 9/45 (20%) developed BM, $p = 0.009$
	45 late PCI 30 Gy/15f, after chemoRT		
Ramlov, retrospective 2012	118 patients received PCI: 74 LD, 44 ED. Medium follow up 16.6 m	MS:	5/21 of BM were within limbic system
	21 (17.8%) had brain relapse, at 4–27 m	all patients 16 m, LD 24 m,	
		ED 12 m	
Tai, retrospective population database 2013	289 LD patients treated with sequential or concurrent chemoradiation: 177 CR, 88 IR	MS: CR – PCI+ 21.6 (5.0–256.0) m	Incidence of BM and median time to symptoms: CR – PCI+ 19% BM, at 21 m; IR – PCI+ 28% at 19 m
		IR – PCI+ 14.3 (4.0–102.6) m	

BM: brain metastases; chemo: chemotherapy; ChRT: chest radiation therapy; CR: complete response; ED: extensive disease; EP: etoposide and cisplatin; f: fractions; Gr: grade; Gy: Gray (radiotherapy absorbed dose); IR: incomplete response; LD: limited disease; m: months; MS: median survival; n: number of patients; NCCTG: North Central Cancer Treatment Group; NCIC: National Cancer Institute of Canada; n.s.: non-significant; PCI+: received prophylactic cranial irradiation; PCI–: not received prophylactic cranial irradiation; RR: relative risk; SWOG: Southwest Oncology Group; y: year.

dealing with smaller micrometastases in the brain. A smaller number of patients developed BM if PCI starts at the third chemotherapy cycle than by the completion of chemoradiation. (2) Radiotherapy helps to increase the permeability of the blood–brain barrier (van Vulpen et al., 2002). The remaining chemotherapy then can treat the brain. (3) Patients develop BM when chemoradiation is all completed – 13/40 (32.5%) were found to have brain relapse immediately before PCI (Manapov et al., 2008). Murray et al. (1993) reported the National Cancer Institute of Canada (NCIC) study results with a higher rate of BM at 2 years despite PCI, compared to other studies using early chest RT and PCI (see Table 18.1). The authors proposed that a difference in the brain failure rate may explain different long-term outcomes.

However, early PCI concurrent with chemotherapy is usually not delivered because of the following reasons: (1) neurocognitive functions deteriorated in a large prospective CALGB study, in which PCI was given concurrently with chemotherapy (Ahles et al., 1998). (2) Partial responders may not benefit from PCI. When PCI is given too early, oncologists do not have time to assess any response and may waste resources. (3) If CR had not been achieved in the chest, reseeding to the brain after PCI may occur. (4) PCI would delay the delivery of chemotherapy and reduce the dose-intensity of subsequent chemotherapy. The toxicity of PCI given between chemotherapy cycles is more than when given after all chemotherapy is finished. There will be a decrease in quality of life during the intensive treatment period. The general condition may decline after PCI and thoracic RT, if given early in the chemotherapy schedule.

Rosen et al. (1983) found that patients who received PCI (Group I, early PCI and group II, late PCI, in Table 18.1) had significantly longer times to CNS relapse than the control patients of Group III with no PCI ($p < 0.001$ and 0.026, respectively), and patients in Group I tended to have prolonged time to CNS relapse compared with patients in Group II ($p = 0.07$). After adjustment was made for the most influential prognostic factors, stage of disease, and liver involvement, the overall significant differences remained among the three groups ($p = 0.049$). However, there was no longer a significant difference between the two groups of patients who received PCI at different times (Group I and Group II, $p = 0.23$). In all groups, CNS relapse continued to occur over time until 24 to 30 months, when there was a suggestion of a plateau in the survival curve.

The more recent studies use modern chemotherapy and RT techniques. An example is the Polish study by Sas-Korczynska et al. (2010). It had a median follow up of 19 (range: 4–135) months. None of their 86 patients with PCI developed neurotoxicity, despite 41 receiving PCI during the chemoradiotherapy period (see Table 18.1). In summary, the current Canadian standard of practice is to finish the induction chest radiotherapy and chemotherapy before starting PCI.

Does the Timing of Chest RT Affect the Rate of Brain Relapse after PCI?

El Sharouni et al. (2009) reported a relatively large series which used sequential chemoradiation before 2001: radical chest radiotherapy, 16 × 2.5 Gy, concurrently with PCI of 15 × 2 Gy after CR ($n = 111$). After 2001, 40 patients received four to five cycles of chemotherapy concurrently with RT of 25 × 1.8 Gy, and PCI was applied to patients with CR. Median survivals of the two groups were 14.0 and 21.8 months, and 5-year overall survivals 10.5 and 26.9%, respectively. Frequencies of BM after PCI were 16.4% and 8.7%, respectively.

Therefore, concurrent chemoradiation resulted in longer median survival and higher overall survival than sequential chemoradiation.

Is the Rate of Brain Relapse Affected by the Dose of PCI?

The randomized United Kingdom Coordinating Committee for Cancer Research (UKCCCR) and the European Organization for Research and Treatment of Cancer (EORTC) trial comparing no PCI, PCI with 24 Gy (in 2-Gy fractions) and PCI with 36 Gy (in 2-Gy fractions) suggested a possible dose-response effect (Gregor et al., 1997). The decrease in the incidence of BM with 24 Gy of PCI versus no PCI was not significant (hazard ratio [HR] 0.71). In contrast, there was a significant reduction in BM with 36 Gy of PCI compared to no PCI (HR 0.16).

A retrospective analysis of PCI doses demonstrated an approximately linear dose-response relationship for reduced BM with increasing dose ranging from 0 to 35 Gy (in 2-Gy fractions) (Suwinski et al., 1998). Then a randomized trial was launched between September 1999 and December 2005. It recruited 720 patients with limited-stage SCLC in CR after chemotherapy and thoracic radiotherapy from 157 centers in 22 countries (Le Péchoux et al., 2009). Patients were randomly assigned to a standard (n = 360, 25 Gy in 10 daily fractions of 2.5 Gy) or higher PCI total dose (n = 360, 36 Gy) delivered using either conventional (18 daily fractions of 2 Gy) or accelerated hyperfractionated (24 fractions in 16 days with two daily sessions of 1.5 Gy separated by a minimum interval of 6 hours) radiotherapy. There was no significant difference in the 2-year incidence of BM between the standard PCI dose group and the higher-dose group, at 29% and 23%. Therefore, the recommended radiation dose for PCI in most cancer centers is now 25 Gy in 10 daily fractions given over 2 weeks.

When do they Occur after PCI?

A German study reported that 30/125 limited stage SCLC patients (24%) developed BM after chemoradiation, of whom there are 10 CR, five partial response (PR), and 15 non-response (NR) of primary tumor after chemoradiotherapy (Manapov et al., 2012). Five of these 30 (17%) patients had PCI before. BM-free survival time for the entire cohort was 298 days (95% CI: 218–377): 567 days (95% CI: 322–811) in CR, 298 days (95% CI: 244–351) in PR and 252 days (95% CI: 217–286) in NR ($p < 0.0001$). PCI prolonged BM-free survival time in CR patients: 640 days (95% CI: 483–796) with PCI versus 482 days (95% CI: 111–926) without PCI ($p = 0.047$) versus 273 days (95% CI: 243–302) for PR and non-responders. The duration of BM-free survival was shown to correlate with long-term outcome ($p < 0.0001$).

The timeline for BM is interesting. Among the 332 patients with SCLC treated on National Cancer Institute protocols between 1970 and 1980, there were 33 cases of CNS failure in patients with CR, of whom two developed in the first 6 months after therapy, but all occurred within 30 months (Rosen et al., 1983). The most striking differences were seen after 30 months, when 70–75% of patients who received PCI, but only 50% of patients who did not receive PCI, were free from CNS metastases.

Hoskin et al. (1986) observed that brain relapse after PCI occurred earlier than expected from published clinical data of tumor doubling times. Between August 1981 and December 1983, 30 patients with SCLC treated by induction chemotherapy, followed by high-dose cyclophosphamide (7 mg/m^2), were selected for PCI on the basis of clinical, radiologic, and bronchoscopic CR. Pretreatment CT brain scans were normal in all patients, and 20 Gy mid-plane dose in five daily fractions were delivered by lateral fields to whole brain. Progressive focal neurologic signs of BM developed in 7/30 (23%) patients 3–11 months after PCI, confirmed on CT scanning in four patients. Relapse at other sites, predominantly the thorax, occurred in all seven patients at intervals of 1–6 months prior to CNS relapse. It is likely that the usual dose of PCI was inadequate to eradicate microscopic tumor deposits in the brain. Unfortunately, higher doses cannot be used due to concerns of toxicity, as dementia will affect the quality of life and patients can become institutionalized.

How to Detect them?

Currently, brain imaging is often not part of the routine in many countries for SCLC follow up post-therapy. BM are generally found when there are clinical symptoms and then scans are ordered to confirm clinical suspicion. It is impossible to estimate the cost-effective analysis of routine brain CT or MRI as most of these patients are elderly and even if BM are detected, treatment would not result in a very long quality-adjusted survival time.

TREATMENT OPTIONS

Patients should be given supportive treatments including steroids. Generally, surgery is not used for treatment of BM after PCI due to the elderly age of patients, poor salvage outcome, and chemo- and radiosensitivity of SCLC.

Stereotactic Radiotherapy

The term "stereotactic" means precise localization of tissue and hence the radiotherapy treatment is minimally invasive by focusing on the tumor with a small margin. Stereotactic radiosurgery (SRS) uses a single fraction of radiation treatment, achieving the effect of brain surgery without opening the skull. The term "stereotactic radiotherapy" means multiple fractions of treatment, though generally five fractions or less.

When there are a few BM, SRS can be employed. Typical doses of SRS after previous PCI, is 16 Gy at 50% (isodose prescription). If the lesion is smaller (<1 cm), 16 Gy at 70% is used. If the lesion is near the brainstem, 14 Gy at 50% is used. After prior PCI, oncologists may give 30 Gy in five fractions for patients with a reasonable performance status and minimum disease burden. A Japanese study reported on salvage gamma knife radiosurgery (GKS) for BM of SCLC after whole brain radiotherapy (Nakazaki et al., 2013). The median prescribed dose and number of lesions treated with the initial GKS were 20.0 Gy and 3.5, respectively, and the tumor control rate was 95.8% (median follow-up period, 4.0 months). The 6-month new lesion-free survival, functional preservation rates, and overall survival were 50.0%, 94.7%, and 5.8 months, respectively. Neurologic death occurred in 17.9% of cases. The poor prognostic factor for new lesion-free survival time was more than five BM and functional preservation was carcinomatous meningitis, respectively. Poor prognostic factors for survival time were Karnofsky performance status <70, >10 BM, diameter of the largest tumor >20 mm, and carcinomatous meningitis. Median OS from BM diagnosis was 16.9 months. The authors conclude that GKS may be an effective option for controlling SCLC-associated BM after whole brain radiotherapy and for preventing neurologic death in patients without carcinomatous meningitis. The best treatment result appears to be achieved by combined whole brain radiotherapy and SRS. The experience from the University of Pittsburgh showed that Karnofsky performance status and combined treatment involving whole brain radiotherapy and SRS within 4 weeks were the two factors identified as being significant predictors of increased overall survival ($p = 0.033$ and 0.040, respectively) (Wegner et al., 2011).

Most complications of radiosurgery occur after 6–12 months and some long-term complications up to after 5–10 years. Oncologists should watch for complications of acute edema or hydrocephalus. Although severe, immediate side effects are rare when large volumes are irradiated, especially in the posterior fossa, and such a case was reported (Wolff et al., 2003). After intubation and external ventricular cerebrospinal fluid drainage, a permanent shunt was inserted. The edema resolved, and the patient recovered to her pretreatment condition within 10 days. So prophylactic shunt insertion or hospitalization the night following the treatment should be considered.

Whole Brain Re-Irradiation

The standard radiation treatment to the whole brain in most radiation oncology centers entails patients to be simulated with a head mask for immobilization. Radiation beams were directed in opposed lateral portals for whole brain irradiation (Figure 18.1). The treatment volume included a 1.5–2 cm margin of the cranium that is the clinical target volume (CTV) in laterals, anterior, posterior, superior, and covers the temporal lobes, base of the skull and the first cervical vertebral body inferiorly. The eyes, nose, maxillary sinuses and oral cavity are often shielded. Radiation energy is often 4–6 MV photons.

Most Canadian cancer centers will recommend brain re-irradiation at least 6 months after PCI. The recommended dose often ranges from 20 Gy to 22.5 Gy in 10 fractions over 2 weeks if the initial PCI was 25 Gy in 10 fractions over 2 weeks. Common side effects of whole brain

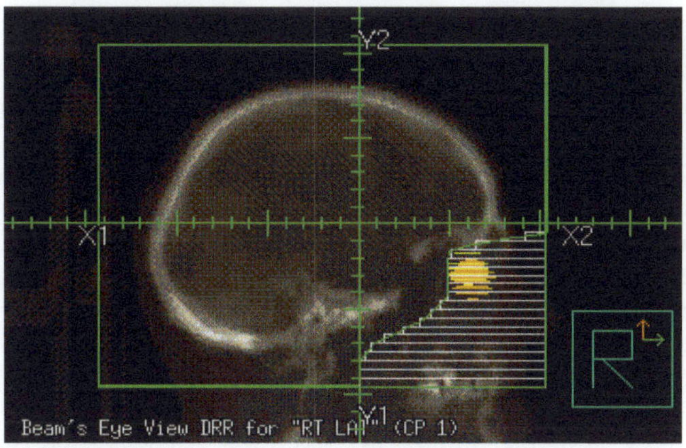

FIGURE 18.1 Re-irradiation to whole brain with 6 MV photons, 20 Gy/10 f.

TABLE 18.2 Acute and Chronic Side Effects of Whole Brain Radiotherapy

Acute
1. Nausea & vomiting, anorexia
2. Mild headache
3. Forehead skin & scalp irritation due to radiation dermatitis
4. Hair loss
5. Mucositis – pharyngitis, esophagitis, laryngitis as a result of steroid given to prevent 1 and 2 above
6. Fatigue
7. Bone marrow suppression with potential pancytopenia
Chronic
1. Brain – cognitive impairment, very mild change in recent memory
2. Potential cataract formation
3. Hair loss
4. Secondary malignancy – meningioma, sarcoma

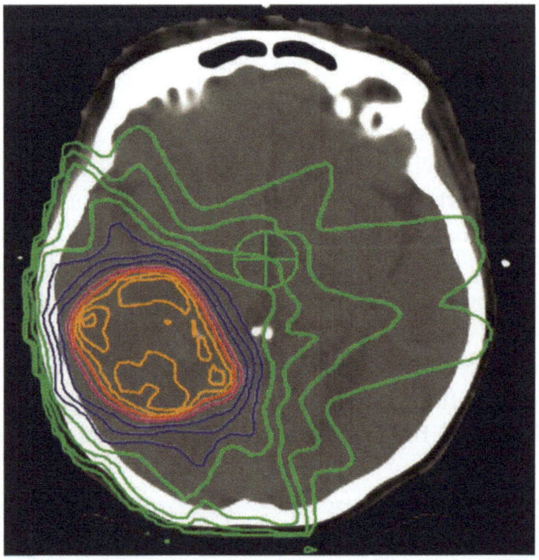

FIGURE 18.2 Re-irradiation to a brain metastasis using intensity-modulated radiotherapy technique with 6 MV photons, 20 Gy/10 f.

radiotherapy are listed in Table 18.2. The acceptable tolerance dose for the lens in most centers is 6 Gy. When stereotactic radiotherapy capability is not available, small local field(s) can be given by using an intensity-modulated radiotherapy technique (Figure 18.2). The latter is delivered by small beamlets given over different angles from a radiotherapy machine (linear accelerator).

Chemotherapy

The topoisomerase-I inhibitor, topotecan, produces cerebrospinal fluid concentrations exceeding 30% of the corresponding plasma concentrations (Korfel et al., 2002). A multicenter phase II study evaluated the efficacy and toxicity of topotecan in 30 pretreated SCLC patients who relapsed with symptomatic BM, of whom 22 patients received the initially planned dose of 1.5 mg/m^2 topotecan as a 30-min intravenous infusion for 5 consecutive days every 3 weeks. Due to thrombocytopenia, the dose was reduced to 1.25 mg/m^2 in the last eight patients. All 30 patients were pretreated with chemotherapy: 14 with one and 16 with at least two protocols. Eight patients had prior whole brain irradiation (WBI): seven in the prophylactic and one in the palliative setting. The median age was 62 years. Concomitant systemic metastases were recorded in 24 patients at the time of brain relapse. BM responded in 33% of patients (10/30: three CR and seven PR). Response was achieved in four of eight patients pretreated by WBI (three in prophylactic and one in palliative setting). The systemic response rate was 29% (7/24). Median time to progression was 3.1 months (range 0.25–14.2+ months), median survival from the beginning of the study was 3.6 months (range 0.25–14.2+). Therapy was generally well tolerated, with myelotoxicity being the most common adverse event. Grade 3 leukocytopenia according to the Common Toxicity Criteria (CTC) occurred in 28% (23/83) of the courses and grade 4 in 22% (18/83). Grade 3 thrombocytopenia was observed in 17% of the courses (14/83) and grade 4 in 11% (9/83). Five of 30 (17%) patients had a documented grade 3 infection. These results using topotecan are promising in heavily pretreated patients with BM and merit further evaluation. This is an important study as limited options are available for patients previously given PCI. Although topotecan may potentiate the effects of radiation, concurrent chemoradiation would not be used clinically as it increases the risk of brain necrosis.

OUTCOME AND CONCLUSION

The reported median survival time from diagnosis of BM ranges from 2.6 (95% CI, 0.97–4.3) months (Manapov et al., 2012) to 16.9 months (Nakazaki et al., 2013). As the general condition of patients deteriorates, physicians at some point may have to make a decision to stop all treatments. Although PCI is a relatively simple radiotherapy procedure among many sophisticated radiotherapy treatment technologies to be delivered to patients, there are still controversies regarding the optimal time, dose and patient selection for its administration. BM post-PCI often are associated with poor prognosis as the brain is frequently not the only site of relapse. A randomized trial on treatment of BM after PCI is unlikely to be started or complete enrolment soon, meanwhile oncologists have to exercise judgment on individual patients based on the best evidence discussed above. Prognosis is dismal.

References

Ahles, T.A., Silberfarb, P.M., Herndon, J., et al., 1998. Psychologic and neuropsychologic functioning of patients with limited small-cell lung cancer treated with chemotherapy and radiation therapy with or without warfarin: a study by the Cancer and Leukemia Group B. J. Clin. Oncol. 16, 1954–1960.

Arriagada, R., Le Chevalier, T., Borie, F., et al., 1995. Prophylactic cranial irradiation for patients with small-cell lung cancer in complete remission. J. Natl. Cancer Inst. 87, 183–190.

Arriagada, R., Le Chevalier, T., Rivière, A., et al., 2002. Patterns of failure after prophylactic cranial irradiation in small-cell lung cancer: analysis of 505 randomized patients. Ann. Oncol. 13, 748–754.

Aupérin, A., Arriagada, R., Pignon, J.P., et al., 1999. Prophylactic cranial irradiation for patients with small-cell lung cancer in complete remission. Prophylactic Cranial Irradiation Overview Collaborative Group. N. Engl. J. Med. 341, 476–484.

El Sharouni, S.Y., Kal, H.B., Barten-Van Rijbroek, A., Struikmans, H., Battermann, J.J., Schramel, F.M., 2009. Concurrent versus sequential chemotherapy and radiotherapy in limited disease small cell lung cancer: a retrospective comparative study. Anticancer Res. 29, 5219–5224.

Felletti, R., Souhami, R.L., Spiro, S.G., et al., 1985. Social consequences of brain or liver relapse in small cell carcinoma of the bronchus. Radiother. Oncol. 4, 335–339.

Gregor, A., Cull, A., Stephens, R.J., et al., 1997. Prophylactic cranial irradiation is indicated following complete response to induction therapy in small cell lung cancer: results of a multicentre randomised trial. United Kingdom Coordinating Committee for Cancer Research (UKCCCR) and the European Organization for Research and Treatment of Cancer (EORTC). Eur. J. Cancer 33, 1752–1758.

Hansen, H.H., 1973. Should initial treatment of small cell carcinoma include systemic chemotherapy and brain irradiation? Cancer Chemother. Rep. 4, 239–241.

Hoskin, P.J., Yarnold, J.R., Smith, I.E., Ford, H.T., 1986. CNS relapse despite prophylactic cranial irradiation (PCI) in small cell lung cancer (SCLC). Int. J. Radiat. Oncol. Biol. Phys. 12, 2025–2028.

Korfel, A., Oehm, C., von Pawel, J., et al., 2002. Response to topotecan of symptomatic BM of small-cell lung cancer also after whole-brain irradiation. a multicentre phase II study. Eur. J. Cancer 38, 1724–1729.

Le Péchoux, C., Dunant, A., Senan, S., Prophylactic Cranial Irradiation (PCI) Collaborative Group, 2009. Standard-dose versus higher-dose prophylactic cranial irradiation (PCI) in patients with limited-stage small-cell lung cancer in complete remission after chemotherapy and thoracic radiotherapy (PCI 99-01, EORTC 22003-08004, RTOG 0212, and IFCT 99-01): a randomised clinical trial. Lancet Oncol. 10, 467–474.

Lewiński, T., Zuławski, M., Meder, J., et al., 1990. Elective (prophylactic) brain irradiation in small cell lung cancer patients treated with chemotherapy combined with surgery. Nowotwory 40, 254–259.

Lucas, C.F., Robinson, B., Hoskin, P.J., Yarnold, J.R., Smith, I.E., Ford, H.T., 1986. Morbidity of cranial relapse in small cell lung cancer and the impact of radiation therapy. Cancer Treat. Rep. 70, 565–570.

Manapov, F., Klautke, G., Fietkau, R., 2008. Prevalence of BM immediately before prophylactic cranial irradiation in limited disease small cell lung cancer patients with complete remission to chemoradiotherapy: a single institution experience. J. Thorac. Oncol. 3, 652–655.

Manapov, F., Klöcking, S., Niyazi, M., et al., 2012. Primary tumor response to chemoradiotherapy in limited-disease small-cell lung cancer correlates with duration of brain-metastasis free survival. J. Neurooncol. 109, 309–314.

Marsh, J.C., Herskovic, A.M., Gielda, B.T., et al., 2010. Intracranial metastatic disease spares the limbic circuit: a review of 697 metastatic lesions in 107 patients. Int. J. Radiat. Oncol. Biol. Phys. 76, 504–512.

Murray, N., Coy, P., Pater, J.L., et al., 1993. Importance of timing for thoracic irradiation in the combined modality treatment of limited-stage small-cell lung cancer. The National Cancer Institute of Canada Clinical Trials Group. J. Clin. Oncol. 11, 336–344.

Nakazaki, K., Higuchi, Y., Nagano, O., Serizawa, T., 2013. Efficacy and limitations of salvage gamma knife radiosurgery for BM of small-cell lung cancer after whole-brain radiotherapy. Acta Neurochir. (Wien) 155, 107–114.

Newman, S.J., Hansen, H.H., 1974. Frequency, diagnosis, and treatment of BM in 249 consecutive patients with bronchogenic carcinoma. Cancer 33, 492–496.

Pedersen, A.G., Kristjansen, P.E., Hansen, H.H., 1988. Prophylactic cranial irradiation and small cell lung cancer. Cancer Treat. Rev. 15, 85–103.

Ramlov, A., Tietze, A., Khalil, A.A., Knap, M.M., 2012. Prophylactic cranial irradiation in patients with small cell lung cancer. A retrospective study of recurrence, survival and morbidity. Lung Cancer 77, 561–566.

Rosen, S.T., Makuch, R.W., Lichter, A.S., et al., 1983. Role of prophylactic cranial irradiation in prevention of central nervous system metastases in small cell lung cancer. Potential benefit restricted to patients with complete response. Am. J. Med. 74, 615–624.

Sas-Korczyńska, B., Korzeniowski, S., Wójcik, E., 2010. Comparison of the effectiveness of "late" and "early" prophylactic cranial irradiation in patients with limited-stage small cell lung cancer. Strahlenther. Onkol. 186, 315–319.

Schild, S.E., Bonner, J.A., Hillman, S., et al., 2007. Results of a phase II study of high-dose thoracic radiation therapy with concurrent cisplatin and etoposide in limited-stage small-cell lung cancer (NCCTG 95-20-53). J. Clin. Oncol. 25, 3124–3129.

Slotman, B., Faivre-Finn, C., Kramer, G., EORTC Radiation Oncology Group and Lung Cancer Group, 2007. Prophylactic cranial irradiation in extensive small-cell lung cancer. N. Engl. J. Med. 357, 664–672.

Stiess, J., Kiricuta, I.C., Mueller, G., Bohndorf, W., 1995. Usefulness of prophylactic whole brain irradiation in small-cell bronchial carcinoma. Strahlenther. Onkol. 171, 284–289.

Suwinski, R., Lee, S.P., Withers, H.R., 1998. Dose-response relationship for prophylactic cranial irradiation in small cell lung cancer. Int. J. Radiat. Oncol. Biol. Phys. 40, 797–806.

Tai, P., Assouline, A., Joseph, K., Stitt, L., Yu, E., 2013. Prophylactic cranial irradiation for patients of limited stage small cell lung cancer with response to chemoradiation. Clin. Lung Cancer 14, 40–44.

van Vulpen, M., Kal, H.B., Taphoorn, M.J., El-Sharouni, S.Y., 2002. Changes in blood-brain barrier permeability induced by radiotherapy: implications for timing of chemotherapy? Oncol. Rep. 9, 683–688.

Wegner, R.E., Olson, A.C., Kondziolka, D., Niranjan, A., Lundsford, L.D., Flickinger, J.C., 2011. Stereotactic radiosurgery for patients with brain metastases from small cell lung cancer. Int. J. Radiat. Oncol. Biol. Phys. 81, e21–e27.

Wolff, R., Karlsson, B., Dettmann, E., Böttcher, H.D., Seifert, V., 2003. Pertreatment radiation induced oedema causing acute hydrocephalus after radiosurgery for multiple cerebellar metastases. Acta Neurochir. (Wien) 145, 691–696.

Work, E., Bentzen, S.M., Nielsen, O.S., Fode, K., Michalski, W., Palshof, T., 1996. Prophylactic cranial irradiation in limited stage small cell lung cancer: survival benefit in patients with favourable characteristics. Eur. J. Cancer 32A, 772–778.

Work, E., Nielsen, O.S., Bentzen, S.M., Fode, K., Palshof, T., 1997. Randomized study of initial versus late chest irradiation combined with chemotherapy in limited-stage small-cell lung cancer. J. Clin. Oncol. 15, 3030–3037.

CHAPTER

19

Brain Metastasis from Small-Cell Lung Cancer with High Levels of Placental Growth Factor

Yu-Hua Chen and Bo Li

OUTLINE

Introduction 213

Placental Growth Factor 215

Placental Growth Factor in Normal and Tumor Cells 215

PLGF and Vascular Permeability 216

Roles of PLGF in SCLC Metastasis to the Brain 216

Levels of PLGF Expression in SCLC Patients 217

Effects of PLGF on SCLC Migration across the Brain Endothelium 219

PLGF-Induced Changes in Tight Junctions between Brain Endothelial Cells 220

Discussion 221

Acknowledgments 224

References 224

INTRODUCTION

Small cell lung cancer (SCLC) is the most aggressive histologic subtype of lung cancer, with a strong predilection for metastasizing early. About 10% of patients with SCLC develop brain metastasis at the time of diagnosis, and the majority of these patients will be symptomatic. The progressive growth of metastasis in the brain is often associated with the terminal stage of the disease, and the prognosis of most patients is consistently poor, with median survival duration of 4–6 months. Additionally, brain metastasis (BM) occurs during the course of the

M.A. Hayat (ed): *Brain Metastases from Primary Tumors, Volume 1*
DOI: http://dx.doi.org/10.1016/B978-0-12-800896-6.00019-X

© 2014 Elsevier Inc. All rights reserved.

disease in over 50% of SCLC patients surviving 2 years or more (Castrucci and Knisely, 2008; Dowell, 2010). Obviously, it is necessary to prevent BM in SCLC management. Although BM can be surgically removed without producing severe neurologic complications, the prognosis of the disease is still very poor. Therefore, a better understanding of the mechanisms of SCLC metastasis to the brain is important to improve current therapies and design new treatment modalities.

The brain is a common site of metastasis in SCLC. It is important for successful BM formation that SCLC cells migrate across the blood–brain barrier (BBB), which is constituted with the endothelium and the surrounding cells. The unique anatomical structure of BBB isolates central cells from peripheral tissue and maintains highly stable conditions (Abbott et al., 2010). Owing to the existence of the BBB, the mechanism of SCLC metastasis to the brain is believed to be different from that to other tissues. SCLC cells adhesion to and migration through this barrier require complex molecular interactions, and the detailed understanding of these events may lead the way to target inhibition of BM formation. However, in-depth knowledge about these mechanisms is largely lacking. In many patients, the BBB has failed to block the invasion of metastatic SCLC cells into brain parenchyma, suggesting the presence of some mechanisms that facilitate invasion of cancer cells into the brain parenchyma through the BBB. Moreover, the BBB is breached in metastases as evidenced by magnetic resonance imaging, which shows that more than 70% of SCLC brain metastases have leakage of contrast agent from blood vessels (Langley and Fidler, 2011). It is likely that the increased BBB permeability plays a crucial role in the process. However, the detailed mechanism remains a mystery.

A major anatomical feature regulating BBB permeability is the presence of closely associated areas called tight junctions (TJs) between opposing endothelial cells. The TJs are the main components that confer the low paracellular permeability and high electrical resistance. TJs function both as a "zipper" and a "fence" that limit paracellular permeability and are composed of transmembrane proteins, such as claudins and occludin, joining the cytoskeleton via cytoplasmic proteins, such as zonula occludin proteins (ZO-1 and ZO-2). Thus, the regulation of TJ protein expression and/or subcellular distribution plays a key role in the alteration of the BBB permeability.

Our previous studies had clearly indicated that SCLCs could trigger the disassembly of TJs between brain microvascular endothelial cells resulting in the enhancement of the BBB permeability (Li et al., 2006). So, the "opening" of TJs seemed to be a key event in SCLC cell transendothelial migration. Then, how do SCLC cells "open" the TJs between brain endothelium? Recent investigations were beginning to provide insight into how several cytokines and their signaling pathways participate in breast cancer and melanoma cell metastatic colonization in the brain. A variety of the factors were postulated to be involved in altering BBB permeability when these tumor cells metastasized to brain. Bos et al. (2009), performed comparative genome-wide expression analysis on breast cancer cell brain metastatic variants and identified the cyclooxygenase COX2, as a critical mediator of extravasation through the blood–brain barrier; Lee et al. (2004) determined that stromal cell-derived factor 1α (SDF-1α) induced blood vessel instability, through increased vascular permeability, resulting in the penetration of breast tumor cells through the human brain microvascular endothelial cells. Overexpression of transforming growth factor-β2 (TGF-β2) in murine B16 melanoma cells induced parenchymal micrometastases but had no effect on the leptomeningeal lesions (Zhang et al., 2009). It was reported that vascular endothelial growth factor (VEGF) is an important regulator for breast cancer cell migration across the brain endothelial cells (Lee et al., 2003). In a brain metastatic variant of MDA-MB-231 cells, there was a significant increase in VEGF production, and inhibition of VEGFR activity significantly reduced brain tumor burden after intracarotid injection in mice (Kim et al., 2004). However, some studies demonstrated that VEGF expression was not sufficient for BM production. When lung adenocarcinoma cells (PC14PE6) transfected with antisense VEGF165 were injected into the carotid artery of nude mice, the formation of brain metastases was substantially decreased compared with untransfected cells. However, in lung squamous carcinoma cells (H226) transfected with VEGF121 or VEGF165, no increase in metastasis was observed (Yano et al., 2000). Therefore, another vascular permeability factor beside VEGF might facilitate tumor cell migration across the BBB and metastasize to the brain. The alteration of BBB permeability between brain endothelium was an important biological event during SCLC cell transendothelial migration. However, the detailed molecular mechanism which contributes to the pathological process needs to be elucidated.

PLACENTAL GROWTH FACTOR

Placental Growth Factor in Normal and Tumor Cells

Placental growth factor (PLGF) is the second member of VEGF family. The name refers to the placenta since it was cloned from a human placental cDNA library (Maglione et al., 1993). The human *plgf* gene mapped to chromosome 14q24, and was formed by seven exons spanning 13.7kb, excluding the upstream and downstream regulatory sequences. PLGF is highly expressed in placenta throughout all stages of gestation. It has been proposed to control trophoblast growth and differentiation. In addition, PLGF is expressed at a low level in several other organs including the heart, lung, thyroid, skeletal muscle, and adipose tissue under normal physiologic conditions. The major function of PLGF is as a pro-angiogenic factor for pathologic angiogenesis in adults and is not produced by the majority of normal human tissues. Additionally, PLGF also stimulates leukocyte infiltration, stromal cell migration, and revascularization of ischemic tissues, indicating that PLGF has a biological activity *in vivo* (De Falco, 2012).

The role of PLGF in tumor progression has been explored extensively in a large body of clinical and experimental research. A prognostic implication of PLGF expression independent of conventional pathologic prognosticators has been demonstrated in a variety of cancers. PLGF expression in tumor tissues has been found to be correlated with tumor stage and patient survival in gastric cancer and colorectal cancer, with tumor stage in lung cancer, with recurrence and metastasis in breast cancer, and even with postoperative early recurrence in hepatocellular carcinoma (Kim et al., 2012). More importantly, PLGF levels in plasma and tumors are also correlated with tumor stage, vascularity, recurrence, metastasis, and survival in various tumors. Plasma PLGF levels were upregulated and correlate with tumor grade and survival in patients with renal-cell carcinoma (Matsumoto et al., 2003), and the recurrence and survival in patients with colorectal cancer (Wei et al., 2005). However, controversial studies addressing the role of PLGF in various models yielded conflicting results. PLGF overexpression enhanced tumor growth in some models but, in others, PLGF paradoxically had an inhibitory effect (Kim et al., 2012). Up to now, the significance of this molecule is still a matter of debate. It remains to be determined whether PLGF acts as a positive regulator of cancer growth and metastasis.

In tumor tissues, PLGF is not only produced by malignant cells, but also by endothelial cells, smooth-muscle cells, pericytes, tumor-associated macrophages, and inflammatory cells. Some experimental studies showed that PLGF mediated a number of cellular activities to promote metastasis, including attraction of endothelial cells for establishment of a blood supply and enhanced cellular movement (Casalou et al., 2007; Taylor and Goldenberg, 2007; Taylor et al., 2010). Notably, recent studies showed that PLGF blockade had no significant effect on primary tumor growth but significantly inhibited melanoma cell extravasation into the lung (Bais et al., 2010). Altogether, these observations suggested that PLGF had more versatile roles in cancer pathology besides tumor angiogenesis.

PLGF and Vascular Permeability

PLGF is a homodimeric glycoprotein, structurally and functionally related to VEGF. Exogenous PLGF has been reported to have either an indirect or direct effect on *in vitro* or *in vivo* vascular permeability but most studies agree that PLGF enhances VEGF-induced vascular permeability (Carmeliet et al., 2001). Some evidence has shown that the absence of PLGF reduced vascular permeability and inflammation in pathological models of neoangiogenesis (Luttun et al., 2002). Transgenic mice overexpressing PLGF in the skin displayed a marked increase in dermal vascular permeability (Odorisio et al., 2002), while PLGF deficiency resulted in a diminished and abbreviated inflammatory response, together with a reduction of plasma extravasation and edema formation (Oura et al., 2003). Recombinant PLGF induced an increase of filtration in isolated cerebral vein of Galen in mice (Schreurs et al., 2012). These findings revealed that PLGF might be a potent vascular permeability factor, but the detailed mechanism was unclear.

Intercellular junctions, including adherens junctions (AJs) and TJs, between endothelial cells control vascular permeability and integrity. There has been no evidence up to now about the effect of PLGF on TJs between endothelial cells, but some evidence has been reported that PLGF mimics VEGF effects to regulate the external blood–retinal barrier function by a direct effect on retinal pigment epithelial cell TJs. Injection of PLGF into the rat eye vitreous induced an opening of the TJs between retinal pigment epithelial cells with subsequent subretinal fluid accumulation, retinal edema and cytoplasmic translocation of junction proteins (Miyamoto et al., 2007, 2008). These findings indicated that PLGF might be involved in the organization of TJs between the endothelium. Although PLGF has been shown to increase vascular permeability in peripheral tissue, whether PLGF affects the cerebral endothelium to enhance BBB permeability is unknown.

ROLES OF PLGF IN SCLC METASTASIS TO THE BRAIN

Brain metastasis is one of the major causes of morbidity and mortality in patients with SCLC. Therefore, a full understanding of these mechanisms is essential to controlling SCLC brain metastasis. Our previous studies had clearly indicated that the increase of brain endothelial permeability induced by SCLC cells was a key event in tumor cell transendothelial migration. Then, how do SCLC cells induce increased brain endothelial permeability? We pay close attention to the issue.

Levels of PLGF Expression in SCLC Patients

A variety of factors are involved in altering BBB permeability during tumor cell metastasis to brain, such as VEGF, SDF-1α, TGF-β2 and COX-2. So, which molecules contribute to SCLC cells migration across the BBB? To ascertain this question, we first examined the serum levels of several soluble factors in SCLC patients with or without BM. The collection of serum samples from 18 SCLC patients with BM, 27 SCLC patients without BM and 16 normal persons were used for ELISA analysis. The serum levels of PLGF and VEGF were significantly increased in SCLC patients with BM compared to SCLC patients without BM and normal specimens (Figure 19.1A), and the serum levels of SDF-1α, TGF-β2 and COX-2 were not elevated in SCLC patients with BM. PLGF is a member of the "VEGF family" of structurally related growth factors, which shares 42% amino acid sequence identity with VEGF and has a very similar biologic function. It had been reported that VEGF expression was necessary but not sufficient for the production of breast cancer cell BM. In our studies, the serum levels of PLGF and VEGF in SCLC patients with BM were significantly higher than SCLC patients without BM, which gives us a clue that PLGF might be

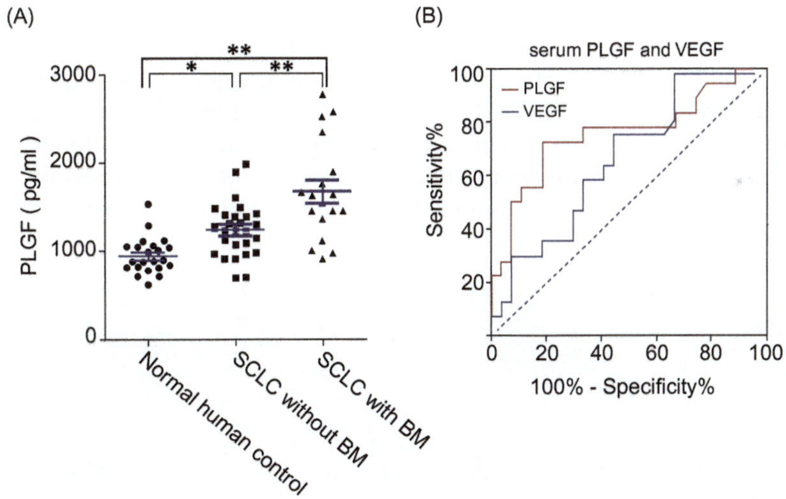

FIGURE 19.1 (A) The levels of PLGF in the serum of SCLC patients were associated with brain metastasis. The serum samples were collected from 18 SCLC patients with brain metastasis, 27 SCLC patients without brain metastasis and 16 normal persons. ELISA analysis for PLGF in the serum of SCLC patients with BM ($n = 18$) and SCLC patients without BM ($n = 27$) was performed. *, $p < 0.05$; **, $p < 0.01$. (B) The receiver operating curve (ROC) analysis of serum PLGF and VEGF in SCLC patients to predict brain metastasis ($n = 45$). The serum PLGF value (red line) of >136 ng/mL seemed to be the appropriate cutoff level for the prediction of brain metastasis with 77.78% of sensitivity, 66.67% of specificity, and 59.3% of accuracy. The area under the ROC of PLGF was 0.7562 ($p = 0.0039$, 95% confidence interval of 0.6013–0.9110) and the area under the ROC of VEGF (blue line) was 0.6862 ($p = 0.03607$, 95% confidence interval of 0.5309–0.8416), which indicates that PLGF was more valuable than VEGF to predict brain metastasis.

a potential factor associated with BM, especially for SCLC. To determine potential values of serum PLGF for prediction of BM, we further performed the receiver operating curve (ROC) analysis of serum PLGF. For the screening method, a serum PLGF value of >136 ng/mL seemed to be the appropriate cutoff level for the prediction of BM with 77.78% sensitivity, 66.67% specificity, and 59.3% accuracy. The area under the ROC was 0.7562 ($p = 0.0039$, 95% confidence interval of 0.6013–0.9110), which indicated the potential predictive value of BM. Even though the sensitivity or specificity of PLGF cutoff value was not relatively high, the area under the ROC and the p value indicated the potential promising predictive value. In addition, we compared the ROC of PLGF to VEGF. The area under the ROC of VEGF was 0.6862 ($p = 0.03607$, 95% confidence interval of 0.5309–0.8416), which indicates the PLGF was more valuable than VEGF to predict BM (see Figure 19.1B). Next, we sought to determine whether PLGF was increased in the specimens of SCLC BM. We also collected 21 SCLC BM specimens and 39 primary SCLC specimens, which were frequency matched by age and sex. None of the patients had received preoperative neo-adjuvant chemotherapy or radiation therapy. Immunohistochemical staining analysis showed that SCLC cells displayed strong positive staining for PLGF corresponding to the negative staining in no-tumor tissue of the lung. The immunostaining intensity of PLGF in tumor tissues was assessed as PLGF expression levels and was quantified by the integrated optical density (IOD) values. The results showed that the PLGF levels in SCLC BM specimens were significantly higher than primary SCLC specimens, which were consistent with the data of serum analysis (Figure 19.2). These clinical data suggested that PLGF was a correlative factor with SCLC BM.

Additionally, to demonstrate further the clinical relevance of PLGF levels and SCLC, a retrospective analysis for the expression of PLGF in SCLC primary tumor specimens was carried out. A total of 79 patients with SCLC were included. Clinicopathological characteristics were defined according to the TNM criteria of the Universal Integrated Circuit Card (UICC). The IOD values of PLGF for the tumor samples ranged from 1281.190 to 69 333.400, with a median value of 12 662.5. Patients were divided into low and high expression groups, based on whether PLGF levels were above or below the median value. Differences between groups

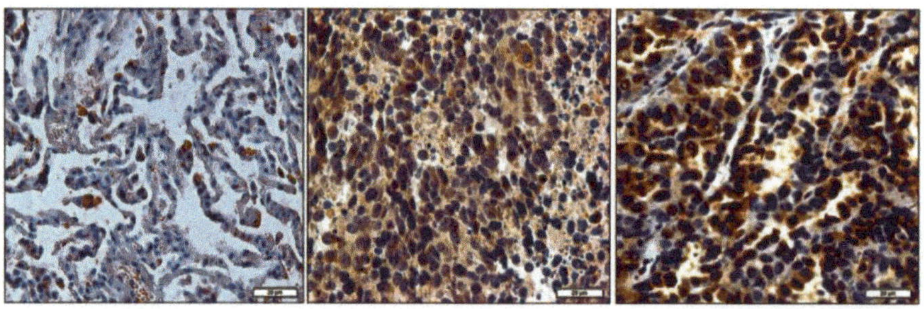

FIGURE 19.2 Immunohistochemical staining of normal lung tissue, SCLC tissue in the lung without BM and SCLC tissue in the brain with BM. Immunohistochemical staining analysis showed that SCLC cells displayed the positive cytoplasmic staining for PLGF in tumor tissue corresponding to the negative staining in the normal lung tissue. The PLGF immunostaining of SCLC tissue in brain was more strongly positive than that in lung. Scale bar, 20 μm.

were assessed using the Pearson chi-square test or Fisher exact test for the variables. There were significant correlation differences between the levels of PLGF expression and age ($p = 0.03$), nodal metastasis status ($p = 0.013$), UICC-TNM classification ($p = 0.022$) and the probabilities of cancer specific survival ($p = 0.0214$). For further comparison, patients were grouped according to tumor stages. Our results showed that the levels of PLGF in SCLC tumor tissues increased gradually from stages I to IV, with IOD mean values for each stage of 10303.77, 10858.03, 23110.74 and 29124.15, respectively. Patients with high PLGF expression were more likely to have advanced disease (stages III and IV) than those with low PLGF expression. Moreover, the PLGF levels of SCLC patients with nodal metastasis were significantly higher than those of SCLC patients with no nodal metastasis. Similarly, the difference between the PLGF levels in SCLC patients who had died and those who still survived was statistically significant. These data suggested that PLGF was associated with progression, and poor prognosis of SCLC, and might be an underlying prognostic factor for SCLC.

Effects of PLGF on SCLC Migration across the Brain Endothelium

To ascertain the effect of PLGF on SCLC metastasis to the brain, we selected six lung cancer cell lines, including SCLC cells and non-small cell lung cancer (NSCLC) cells. First, the expression of PLGF was elevated in the SCLC cells, but its expression was barely detectable in the NSCLC cells. Moreover, NCI-H250 cells, which were derived from an SCLC brain metastatic site, expressed the PLGF more abundantly than NCI-H209 and NCI-H446 cells, which were derived from an SCLC bone marrow metastatic site and a pleural effusion metastatic site, respectively. Transendothelial migration assay showed that SCLC cells which expressed the high level of PLGF, have strong transendothelial migration activity. Conversely, NSCLC cells, which expressed the low level of PLGF, showed poor transendothelial migration activity. Statistical analysis revealed that a significant correlation between the levels of PLGF mRNA and the cell numbers of cancer cell tranendothelial migration. SCLC cells, which expressed the high level of PLGF, preferred to migrate across the human brain microvascular endothelial cell (HBMEC). These results raised the possibility that PLGF might facilitate SCLC cells migration across the brain endothelial cells. Further experiments confirmed the speculation: treatment with recombinant human PLGF proteins significantly increased the transendothelial migration activity of NCI-H446 cells, which expressed the least level of PLGF; treatment with PLGF antibody, which has been shown specifically to neutralize the secreted form of PLGF, significantly decreased the migratory activity of NCI-H250 cells. As an alternative approach, the downregulation of PLGF expression in SCLC cells by RNAi could not only obviously reduce their transendothelial migration *in vitro* but also suppress the formation of SCLC cells metastatic colonization in an experimental BM *in vivo* mouse model. Thus, the results indicated that PLGF had a potential for promoting SCLC cell migration across brain endothelial cells.

Unlike VEGF, PLGF only binds to VEGFR-1, which is mainly expressed on the endothelial cells. PLGF signals can directly via VEGFR-1 act on the endothelial cells, which led to a significant increase in tyrosine phosphorylation of the VEGFR-1. To test the hypothesis that VEGFR-1 in HBMEC might be able to mediate the transendothelial migration of SCLC cells in the presence of PLGF, we first sought to determine whether SCLC cells can induce the activation of VEGFR-1 in HBMEC co-cultured with SCLC cells. SCLC cells, which have been shown to express an abundance of PLGF, could induce an evident increase in tyrosine phosphorylation of VEGFR-1 in HBMEC. However, the PLGF antibody, which specifically antagonizes the effects of PLGF in a co-culture system, effectively blocked the level of VEGFR-1 tyrosine phosphorylation in HBMEC induced by SCLC cells. These findings implied that VEGFR-1 in HBMEC was functionally active and fully responsive to PLGF during SCLC cell migration across the HBMEC monolayer. Treatment with anti-VEGFR-1 antibody caused a significant reduction in SCLC cell transendothelial migration. Meanwhile, the reduction in transendothelial migration following depletion of VEGFR-1 in HBMEC was also observed in SCLC cells. These findings suggested that PLGF promoted SCLC cell transendothelial migration through interaction with VEGFR-1 on HBMEC.

PLGF-Induced Changes in Tight Junctions between Brain Endothelial Cells

PLGF is an angiogenic cytokine that stimulates endothelial cell growth, migration, and survival and plays an important role in angiogenesis (De Falco, 2012). However, experimental brain metastasis *in vivo* studies using either breast cancer or melanoma showed that tumor cells were growing along the pre-existing vessels rather than inducing neoangiogenesis, which excluded the requirement for neoangiogenesis in brain metastatic tumor formation (Kienast et al., 2010). So, it seemed more important to influence cancer cell extravasation by breaching BBB integrity in brain metastases formation.

Our previous studies had clearly indicated that SCLC cells could increase the permeability of brain microvascular endothelial cells by inducing the TJs disassembly (Li et al., 2006). Therefore, we evaluated the effect of PLGF/VEGFR-1 axis on the integrity of TJs in HBMEC according to our previous work. PLGF significantly induced an increase of HRP flux across the brain endothelial monolayer and an obvious shift of occludin distribution from insoluble to soluble fractions prepared from HBMEC in a time- and dose-dependent manner. Meanwhile, the alterations of occludin and ZO-1 distribution, TJ structural proteins, were visualized by immunofluorescence. Treatment with PLGF could gradually make the continuous lines of occludin and ZO-1 staining become discontinuous, segmented and dotted. These results indicated that PLGF could specifically disrupt TJ complexes in HBMEC. Accumulating evidence suggested that the phosphorylation of occludin and claudin-5 might be an important molecular mechanism mediating TJs dysfunction in pathological disease, such as neuroinflammation (Stamatovic et al., 2006; Murakami et al., 2009). We found that PLGF could phosphorylate occludin and claudin-5 on Thr and Ser residues in a time-dependent manner to disrupt the integrity of brain endothelial TJs. Furthermore, knockdown of VEGFR-1 in HBMEC by specific shRNA abolished PLGF-induced alterations of TJs, that is, the changes of HRP flux, the redistribution of ZO-1 and occludin, the recruitment of detergent-soluble occludin, and the phosphorylation of occludin and claudin-5 on Thr and Ser residues. All these results demonstrated that the PLGF/VEGFR-1 axis mediated SCLC cell transendothelial migration through changing the integrity of TJs in HBMEC.

A significant body of evidence indicated that the assembly and the maintenance of TJs were regulated by several components of intracellular signaling pathways, such as Rho/ROCK, PI3K /Akt, protein kinase C, MAPK/ERK1/2and c-Src kinases (Guillemot et al., 2008). Our findings indicated that ROCK and ERK1/2 signaling pathways were involved in the disassembly of brain endothelial TJs induced by PLGF. Further insight into the role of Rho/ROCK signaling was derived from the results that PLGF-induced TJs disassembly was remarkably inhibited when HBMEC was transfected with a Rho binding-defective dominant negative mutant of ROCK. In addition, to provide enough evidence of the contribution of ERK1/2 signaling activation to PLGF-induced TJs disruption in HBMEC, the downregulation of ERK1/2 in HBMEC by specific different ERK1/2 siRNAs was carried out, and PLGF-induced changes of TJs in the brain endothelial barrier were also eliminated.

As further evidence for the involvement of ROCK/ERK1/2-dependent signaling in the process, a significant enhancement of Rho activation in HBMEC was observed at 5min after treatment with PLGF, followed by the increase of ERK1/2 activation at 15min after treatment with PLGF. Furthermore, when the activity of VEGFR-1 in brain endothelial cells was suppressed through downregulation of VEGFR-1 expression or inhibition of VEGFR receptor tyrosine kinase, the Rho and ERK1/2 activation were impaired. These suggested that Rho and ERK1/2 signaling acted as the downstream effectors of VEGFR-1 signaling and Rho might act as the upper signal of ERK1/2. Subsequently, we further confirmed the cross-talk between Rho/ROCK and ERK1/2 signaling in PLGF-induced TJs disruption in brain endothelial cells. When ERK1/2 activity in HBMEC was inhibited by PD98059, a specific inhibitor for ERK1/2, and siRNA, there were no changes in Rho activation. Conversely, ERK1/2 activation in HBMEC was significantly abolished when Rho kinase was inhibited by overexpression of dominant-negative ROCK and Y27632, a specific inhibitor for Rho kinase. Furthermore, the inhibition of ERK1/2 activation led to a pronounced reduction of SCLC transmendothelial migration. Thus, Rho activity is required for downstream constitutively active ERK1/2 in PLGF-induced TJs disruption in HBMEC.

DISCUSSION

Brain metastasis is one of the major causes of morbidity and mortality in patients with SCLC. Therefore, a full understanding of the mechanism is essential for controlling SCLC brain metastasis. Our previous study showed that the disassembly of TJs between brain endothelial cells was an important biological event during transendothelial migration of SCLC cells (Li et al., 2006). Our further studies displayed enough evidence that PLGF secreted by SCLC cells, promoted SCLC BM through TJs between brain endothelium. We provided clinical, experimental, and mechanistic evidence that PLGF played an important role in SCLC metastasis to the brain.

First, we screened some factors that were postulated to be involved in altering BBB permeability during SCLC cells metastasis to the brain. It was noticeable that the serum level of PLGF was significantly increased in SCLC patients with BM compared to SCLC patients without BM. Our further data revealed that PLGF expression was also increased in tumor tissue of SCLC patients, especially in the BM tissues. There was a significant correlation between the levels of PLGF expression in the primary tumor tissues and age, nodal metastasis status, UICC-TNM classification and the probabilities of cancer specific survival. These clinical characters strongly indicated that elevated PLGF levels in the serum, which were contributed by the primary tumor, might be a potential signature for SCLC BM.

Most of the studies focused on the function of PLGF in the angiogenesis of tumor progression. In our context, a novel role of PLGF in SCLC BM was identified. That is, PLGF directly promotes the penetration of SCLC cells through the BBB and metastaszes to the brain. Using an *in vitro* BBB model, we demonstrated that PLGF, derived from SCLC cells, acted on brain endothelial cells to promote SCLC cells transendothelial migration, which was effectively prevented by neutralization of PLGF in the medium and knockdown of PLGF in SCLC cells. Using an experimental BM mouse model *in vivo*, we found that down-regulation of PLGF in SCLC cells effectively blocked the formation of tumor nodules in the mouse brain. Experimental BM *in vivo* studies using either breast cancer or melanoma showed that tumor cells were growing along the pre-existing vessels rather than inducing neoangiogenesis, which excluded the requirement for neoangiogenesis in brain metastatic tumor formation (Kienast et al., 2010). These give us a clue to propose that the decreased BM in the mouse model caused by PLGF knockdown might be mainly due to the attenuated penetration of SCLC cells through the BBB, without the involvement of neoangiogenesis. These data suggested that PLGF is a novel target to block the penetration of SCLC cells through the BBB and metastasize to the brain.

So, how did PLGF promote the penetration of SCLC cells through the BBB and metastasize to the brain? The disassembly of TJs in brain endothelial cells was a key step for the transendothelial migration of SCLC cells (Li et al., 2006). Interestingly, our findings showed that PLGF secreted by SCLC cells directly triggered the disassembly of TJs in brain endothelial cells. These data highlighted that PLGF has a direct role in "opening" the BBB during SCLC cell extravasation to brain. It has been reported that the phosphorylation status of occludin at Ser/Thr residues is involved in maintaining TJs integrity in endothelial cells (Stamatovic et al., 2006; Murakami et al., 2009). We found that the Ser/Thr residues of occludin were phosphorylated in response to PLGF, which indicated that PLGF induced the Ser/Thr residue phosphorylation of occludin in brain endothelial cells, leading to TJ disassembly. It was noticed that there was a controversy over whether phosphorylation or dephosphorylation of occludin at Thr residues was linked to the integrity of TJs (Cipolla et al., 2004). Our data showed that the phosphorylation of occludin at Thr residues was associated with the disruption of TJs integrity, which might be due to the different types of cells and the different types of stimulus. We found that PLGF made a junction "porous" between the brain endothelium for SCLC cells infiltration into brain, which was dependent on the phosphorylation of TJ proteins.

Another interesting finding in our study was that PLGF-promoted SCLC cell transendothelial migration, which was driven by VEGFR-1 on brain endothelial cells. VEGFR-1 is one of the tyrosine kinase transmembrane receptors and the sole known high affinity receptor for PLGF. Initially, it was proposed that VEGFR-1 might not be primarily a receptor transmitting a mitogenic signal, but rather a "decoy" receptor, able to regulate in a negative fashion the activity of VEGF on the vascular endothelium, by preventing VEGF binding to VEGFR-2 (Carmeliet et al., 2001). Much evidence has focused on the role for VEGFR-1 in angiogenesis, whereas there was uncertainty concerning the role of individual VEGFR-1 for special biological functions, such as vascular permeability. To our knowledge, there was no report about the involvement of individual VEGFR-1 in TJs integrity. In our study, the role of individual VEGFR-1 in vascular permeability was identified. The activation of VEGFR-1 was observed in brain endothelial cells interacting with SCLC cells, and neutralization of PLGF secreted by SCLC cells almost completely blocked SCLC cell-induced VEGFR-1 activation in brain endothelial cells. Furthermore, we also demonstrated that VEGFR-1 was required for the PLGF-induced disruption of TJs integrity in brain endothelial cells. A recent study was consistent with our findings. Schreurs et al. (2012) found that recombinant PLGF induced an increase of filtration in isolated cerebral vein of Galen, which was abolished by neutralizing VEGFR-1. Thus, PLGF, via activation of VEGFR-1 on the brain endothelial cells, caused the alteration of TJs integrity to drive SCLC cells transendothelial migration.

The involvement of VEGFR-1 in TJs disassembly raised the question of which intracellular signal molecules participate in the process. It has been shown that intracellular signaling molecules, including phospholipase C (PLC), PI3K/Akt and Ras/Raf/MAPK were involved in VEGFR-1-mediated biological responses (Shibuya and Claesson-Welsh, 2006). Our data clearly indicated that the inhibition of Rho/ROCK or ERK1/2 completely prevented PLGF-induced functional, morphological and biochemical alterations of TJs in brain endothelial cells. Blockage of VEGFR-1 activity was obviously associated with inhibition of Rho and ERK1/2 activation induced by PLGF. The significance of these observations was that Rho and ERK1/2 signals could act as the intracellular signaling from VEGFR-1, which was not referred to in previous present studies.

It was well known that ERK activation was associated with loss of endothelial TJs integrity (Guillemot et al., 2008). We also observed the involvement of ERK1/2 activation in PLGF-induced TJs disassembly, which contributed to SCLC cells transendothelial migration. So, what is the mechanism of the cross-talk between Rho/ROCK and ERK1/2 signals in the process? The reciprocal relationship between Rho and ERK1/2 signaling pathway has already been reported, but studies obtained from various models yielded conflicting results. For example, Mavria et al. (2006) delineated a mechanism by which ERK-MAPK promotes endothelial cell survival and sprouting by downregulating Rho-kinase signaling. On the contrary, a study supported a model in which the Ras-ERK and Rho-Rho kinase pathways cooperate to promote cell migration (Jo et al., 2002). In our context, ERK1/2 activation was dependent on Rho activation, which was confirmed by the different inhibition experiments. Although the ERK pathway was reported to be activated by PLGF in leukemia cells and breast cancer cells and to be important for their migration (Casalou et al., 2007; Taylor et al., 2010), these pathways were not linked to downstream Rho GTPase or brain microvascular permeability. Our results demonstrated that PLGF/VEGFR-1-mediated Rho-ERK1/2 signal transduction contributed to the changes of vascular permeability under the pathological condition of SCLC BM.

Based on our findings, we propose a possible scenario for the PLGF-mediated SCLC cell migration across the brain endothelium: the early step is the interaction of PLGF secreted by SCLC cells with its receptor VEGFR-1, expressed on brain endothelial cells. This interaction in turn activates Rho/ROCK which further activates the ERK1/2 signaling pathway. Activation of ERK1/2 directly causes the Ser/Thr residue phosphorylation of TJ proteins, which results in TJ protein redistribution and an increase in paracellular permeability for SCLC cells transendothelial migration (Figure 19.3). Our studies provided clear evidence to delineate a function for PLGF in SCLC metastasis to brain, which would help us to develop better therapeutic strategies for SCLC BM, and to improve the survival and quality of life of SCLC patients. Further clinical large-sampled investigations should be done to confirm the value of PLGF as a biomarker of SCLC BM.

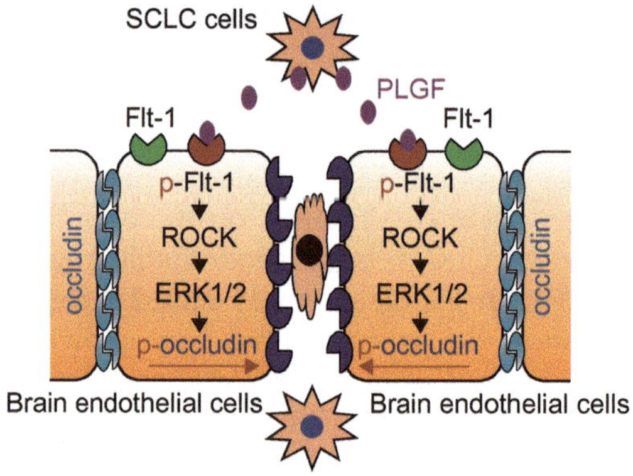

FIGURE 19.3 Proposed model for the role of PLGF in SCLC BM. PLGF derived from SCLC cells binds to its receptor VEGFR-1 (also named as Flt-1) on brain endothelial cells, then, the intracellular Rho kinase signaling is activated followed by ERK1/2 activation. Activated ERK1/2 causes Ser/Thr phosphorylation of TJ proteins (occludin), which results in TJ disassembly for the transendothelial migration of SCLC cells.

Acknowledgments

This work was supported by the Trans-Century Training Program Foundation for Talents, Ministry of Education of China (JJH2002-48), the Innovation Team Program Foundation of Liaoning Province (2006T131, LT2011011), the National Natural Science Foundation of China (30600270) and the Science and Technology Foundation of Liaoning Province (20102291).

References

Abbott, N.J., Patabendige, A.A., Dolman, D.E., Yusof, S.R., Begley, D.J., 2010. Structure and function of the blood-brain barrier. Neurobiol. Dis. 37, 13–25.

Bais, C., Wu, X., Yao, J., et al., 2010. PlGF blockade does not inhibit angiogenesis during primary tumor growth. Cell 141, 166–177.

Bos, P.D., Zhang, X.H., Nadal, C., et al., 2009. Genes that mediate breast cancer metastasis to the brain. Nature 459, 1005–1009.

Carmeliet, P., Moons, L., Luttun, A., et al., 2001. Synergism between vascular endothelial growth factor and placental growth factor contributes to angiogenesis and plasma extravasation in pathological conditions. Nat. Med. 7, 575–583.

Casalou, C., Fragoso, R., Nunes, J.F., Dias, S., 2007. VEGF/PLGF induces leukemia cell migration via P38/ERK1/2 kinase pathway, resulting in Rho GTPases activation and caveolae formation. Leukemia 21, 590–594.

Castrucci, W.A., Knisely, J.P., 2008. An update on the treatment of CNS metastases in small cell lung cancer. Cancer J. 14, 138–146.

Cipolla, M.J., Crete, R., Vitullo, L., Rix, R.D., 2004. Transcellular transport as a mechanism of blood-brain barrier disruption during stroke. Front Biosci. 9, 777–785.

De Falco, S., 2012. The discovery of placenta growth factor and its biological activity. Exp. Mol. Med. 44, 1–9.

Dowell, J.E., 2010. Small cell lung cancer: are we making progress? Am. J. Med. Sci. 339, 68–76.

Guillemot, L., Paschoud, S., Pulimeno, P., Foglia, A., Citi, S., 2008. The cytoplasmic plaque of tight junctions: a scaffolding and signalling center. Biochim. Biophys. Acta 1778, 601–613.

Jo, M., Thomas, K.S., Somlyo, A.V., Somlyo, A.P., Gonias, S.L., 2002. Cooperativity between the Ras-ERK and Rho-Rho kinase pathways in urokinase-type plasminogen activator-stimulated cell migration. J. Biol. Chem. 277, 12479–12485.

Kienast, Y., von Baumgarten, L., Fuhrmann, M., et al., 2010. Real-time imaging reveals the single steps of brain metastasis formation. Nat. Med. 16, 116–122.

Kim, K.J., Cho, C.S., Kim, W.U., 2012. Role of placenta growth factor in cancer and inflammation. Exp. Mol. Med. 44, 10–19.

Kim, L.S., Huang, S., Lu, W., Lev, D.C., Price, J.E., 2004. Vascular endothelial growth factor expression promotes the growth of breast cancer brain metastases in nude mice. Clin. Exp. Metastasis 21, 107–118.

Langley, R.R., Fidler, I.J., 2011. The seed and soil hypothesis revisited – The role of tumor stroma interactions in metastasis to different organs. Int. J. Cancer 128, 2527–2535.

Lee, B.C., Lee, T.H., Avraham, S., Avraham, H.K., 2004. Involvement of the chemokine receptor CXCR4 and its ligand stromal cell-derived factor 1alpha in breast cancer cell migration through human brain microvascular endothelial cells. Mol. Cancer Res. 2, 327–338.

Lee, T.H., Avraham, H.K., Jiang, S., Avraham, S., 2003. Vascular endothelial growth factor modulates the transendothelial migration of MDA-MB-231 breast cancer cells through regulation of brain microvascular endothelial cell permeability. J. Biol. Chem. 278, 5277–5284.

Li, B., Zhao, W.D., Tan, Z.M., Fang, W.G., Zhu, L., Chen, Y.H., 2006. Involvement of Rho/ROCK signalling in small cell lung cancer migration through human brain microvascular endothelial cells. FEBS Lett. 580, 4252–4260.

Luttun, A., Brusselmans, K., Fukao, H., et al., 2002. Loss of placental growth factor protects mice against vascular permeability in pathological conditions. Biochem. Biophys. Res. Commun. 295, 428–434.

Maglione, D., Guerriero, V., Rambaldi, M., Russo, G., Persico, M.G., 1993. Translation of the placenta growth factor mRNA is severely affected by a small open reading frame localized in the 5′ untranslated region. Growth Factors 8, 141–152.

Matsumoto, K., Suzuki, K., Koike, H., et al., 2003. Placental growth factor gene expression in human prostate cancer and benign prostate hyperplasia. Anticancer Res. 23, 3767–3773.

Mavria, G., Vercoulen, Y., Yeo, M., et al., 2006. ERK-MAPK signaling opposes Rho-kinase to promote endothelial cell survival and sprouting during angiogenesis. Cancer Cell 9, 33–44.

Miyamoto, N., de Kozak, Y., Jeanny, J.C., et al., 2007. Placental growth factor-1 and epithelial haemato-retinal barrier breakdown: potential implication in the pathogenesis of diabetic retinopathy. Diabetologia 50, 461–470.

Miyamoto, N., de Kozak, Y., Normand, N., et al., 2008. PlGF-1 and VEGFR-1 pathway regulation of the external epithelial hemato-ocular barrier. A model for retinal edema. Ophthal. Res. 40, 203–207.

Murakami, T., Felinski, E.A., Antonetti, D.A., 2009. Occludin phosphorylation and ubiquitination regulate tight junction trafficking and vascular endothelial growth factor-induced permeability. J. Biol. Chem. 284, 21036–21046.

Odorisio, T., Schietroma, C., Zaccaria, M.L., et al., 2002. Mice overexpressing placenta growth factor exhibit increased vascularization and vessel permeability. J. Cell Sci. 115, 2559–2567.

Oura, H., Bertoncini, J., Velasco, P., Brown, L.F., Carmeliet, P., Detmar, M., 2003. A critical role of placental growth factor in the induction of inflammation and edema formation. Blood 101, 560–567.

Schreurs, M.P., Houston, E.M., May, V., Cipolla, M.J., 2012. The adaptation of the blood-brain barrier to vascular endothelial growth factor and placental growth factor during pregnancy. FASEB J. 26, 355–362.

Shibuya, M., Claesson-Welsh, L., 2006. Signal transduction by VEGF receptors in regulation of angiogenesis and lymphangiogenesis. Exp. Cell Res. 312, 549–560.

Stamatovic, S.M., Dimitrijevic, O.B., Keep, R.F., Andjelkovic, A.V., 2006. Protein kinase C alpha-RhoA cross-talk in CCL2-induced alterations in brain endothelial permeability. J. Biol. Chem. 281, 8379–8388.

Taylor, A.P., Goldenberg, D.M., 2007. Role of placenta growth factor in malignancy and evidence that an antagonistic PlGF/Flt-1 peptide inhibits the growth and metastasis of human breast cancer xenografts. Mol. Cancer Ther. 6, 524–531.

Taylor, A.P., Leon, E., Goldenberg, D.M., 2010. Placental growth factor (PlGF) enhances breast cancer cell motility by mobilizing ERK1/2 phosphorylation and cytoskeletal rearrangement. Br. J. Cancer 103, 82–89.

Wei, S.C., Tsao, P.N., Yu, S.C., et al., 2005. Placenta growth factor expression is correlated with survival of patients with colorectal cancer. Gut 54, 666–672.

Yano, S., Shinohara, H., Herbst, R.S., et al., 2000. Expression of vascular endothelial growth factor is necessary but not sufficient for production and growth of brain metastasis. Cancer Res. 60, 4959–4967.

Zhang, C., Zhang, F., Tsan, R., Fidler, I.J., 2009. Transforming growth factor-beta2 is a molecular determinant for site-specific melanoma metastasis in the brain. Cancer Res. 69, 828–835.

CHAPTER

20

Brain Metastases from Lung Cancer

Amol J. Ghia and Ritsuko Komaki

OUTLINE

Introduction 227

Treatment Options 228

Surgical Resection 228

Stereotactic Radiosurgery 228

Whole-Brain Radiation Therapy 229

WBRT as Primary Therapy for Gross Disease 230

WBRT as an Adjuvant after Local Therapy 232

Prophylactic Cranial Irradiation 233

Toxicity of Radiation to the Brain 237

Conclusion 238

References 238

INTRODUCTION

Brain metastases from lung cancer represent a significant portion of all brain metastases. Between 10% and 25% of patients with lung cancer have brain metastases at diagnosis, and about 40–50% of all patients with lung cancer will develop brain metastasis during the course of the disease. Some evidence exists to suggest that improved control of locally advanced disease may be associated with increased incidence of brain metastases (Ceresoli et al., 2002). The prognosis for patients with brain metastasis is poor, with median survival times usually less than 1 year.

The manifestations of brain metastases vary and depend on the location and number of lesions and the amount of associated edema, hemorrhage, or both. Presenting symptoms can include headache, nausea and emesis, focal weakness, seizures, confusion, ataxia, visual disturbances or, occasionally, cranial nerve palsies. Magnetic resonance imaging (MRI) is currently the gold standard for identifying brain metastases and is more sensitive than computed tomography (CT) scanning for this purpose.

M.A. Hayat (ed): *Brain Metastases from Primary Tumors, Volume 1*
DOI: http://dx.doi.org/10.1016/B978-0-12-800896-6.00020-6

© 2014 Elsevier Inc. All rights reserved.

Initial management of brain metastases usually involves oral or intravenous corticosteroids (Coia et al., 1992). Patients with seizures should be treated with antiseizure medications. However, prophylactic use of antiseizure medication is controversial because of the high risk of adverse effects. Subsequent management of brain metastases depends on the size, number, and location of the lesions as well as the presence of extracranial disease and the general condition of the patient. Whole brain radiation therapy (WBRT) can be used as primary therapy for brain metastases, as adjuvant treatment after surgery or stereotactic radiosurgery (SRS), or as salvage therapy after local treatment. SRS can produce local control rates that are comparable to those after surgery with minimal toxicity, and SRS can be used as primary therapy or salvage therapy. Its versatility makes SRS useful for multiple or deep-seated lesions and for patients with medical conditions that render them poor candidates for surgery. Surgery provides rapid relief of mass effects and may be the best choice for large single metastases.

This chapter focuses on the roles of various forms of therapy for treatment of brain metastases from lung cancer, including surgical resection, SRS, WBRT, and prophylactic cranial irradiation (PCI).

TREATMENT OPTIONS

Surgical Resection

The surgical resection of brain metastases has traditionally been reserved for palliation of symptomatic lesions or for situations in which pathologic confirmation is necessary. However, some subsets of patients with favorable prognostic factors have undergone surgical resection with the intent of improving survival. A pivotal trial conducted in the 1980s by Patchell et al. (1990) evaluated the use of surgery for 48 patients with a single brain metastasis who were also receiving WBRT. Specifically, patients with a suspected brain metastasis were randomly assigned to undergo either biopsy followed by WBRT or surgical resection followed by WBRT. WBRT was to be delivered to a dose of 36 Gy in 12 fractions. Resection was found to improve local recurrence rates (52% vs 20%) and quality of life (9 months vs 2 months of functional independence). Surgery was also found to extend overall survival time (9 months vs 3 months) and time to death from neurologic causes (14 months vs 6 months). Rates of operative mortality (4%) and morbidity (8%) in that study were deemed acceptable.

Another phase III trial conducted in the Netherlands involved patients with a single brain metastasis who were given WBRT (40 Gy in 2-Gy fractions twice a day) either alone or with surgical resection (Noordijk et al., 1994). Surgical resection was again associated with extended median survival time (10 months vs 6 months), with particular benefit seen among those with stable extracranial disease. Indeed, local therapy is generally advocated for those with favorable performance status, a single brain metastasis, and stable extracranial disease. The need for adjuvant radiotherapy after surgical resection to maintain intracranial disease control is discussed further later in this chapter.

Stereotactic Radiosurgery

The neurosurgeon Lars Leksell formulated the principles of radiosurgery in 1951, about 17 years before the launch of the first Gamma knife prototype at the Karolinska Institute. SRS is commonly defined as a single high dose of radiation directed by stereotaxis conformally to the target, minimizing the dose to the normal surrounding tissue. The first Gamma knife unit in the USA was installed at the University of Pittsburgh Medical Center in 1987. Today, brain metastases represent the most common indication for SRS (Jayarao et al., 2009). The goals of SRS can be achieved with several types of technologies, including the Gamma knife, linear accelerators, or the Cyberknife.

The Radiation Therapy Oncology Group (RTOG) has conducted several trials investigating SRS for brain metastases. The prospective trial RTOG 90-05 sought to determine the optimal dose for radiosurgery of brain metastases by evaluating the maximum tolerated radiosurgical dose in 168 patients who had previously undergone irradiation for primary or metastatic brain lesions (Shaw et al., 2000). The maximum tolerated doses depended on the size of the lesion, being 24 Gy for tumors ≤20 mm in diameter, 18 Gy for those 21–30 mm, and 15 Gy for tumors 31–40 mm. However, the actual maximum tolerated dose for lesions ≤20 mm was not met because the investigators were reluctant to exceed 24 Gy. Notably, the rate of radionecrosis at 2 years was 11%. Subsequent research suggested that treating tumors ≤20 mm with 20 Gy rather than 24 Gy produced equivalent control with lower complication rates (Shehata et al., 2004; Elliott et al., 2011).

RTOG 95-08 was a randomized controlled trial comparing WBRT alone versus WBRT with SRS for 333 patients with one to three brain metastases (Andrews et al., 2004). The WBRT dose was 37.5 Gy delivered in 15 fractions, and the SRS dose was delivered according to the guidelines established by RTOG 90-05. Although no difference was found in overall survival between the two groups, subgroup analyses revealed that SRS improved overall survival for patients with a single brain metastasis. The addition of SRS to WBRT also led to higher response rates and better local control rates at 1 year (82% vs 71%); receipt of SRS was the only factor predictive of local control in a Cox proportional hazards analysis. The risk of developing a local recurrence was 43% greater in the WBRT-alone group relative to the WBRT with SRS group. Moreover, patients receiving SRS were more likely to have had stable or improved Karnofsky performance status scores at 6 months after treatment.

To date, no randomized controlled trials have been undertaken to compare surgery with SRS for single brain metastases. Findings from retrospective analyses are mixed and fraught with selection bias. The indications for SRS remain controversial, with factors contributing to the choice of treatment including the number of metastases, performance status, status of extracranial disease, and tumor histology. Further clinical trials are necessary to define an SRS treatment algorithm for patients with brain metastases.

Whole-Brain Radiation Therapy

WBRT has been used to treat brain metastases since the early 20th century. The first report of its efficacy in a large series came from Memorial Hospital, where 38 patients with brain metastases were treated from 1949 to 1953 with fractionated WBRT. Palliation was successful for 63% of patients so treated, and the recommended dose was 30–40 Gy given over 3–5 weeks. A subsequent report, published in the early 1960s, of an additional 218 patients at Memorial Hospital given WBRT to a goal dose of 30 Gy in 3 weeks revealed a survival benefit among those who responded to this therapy, further establishing the role of WBRT in the treatment of intracranial metastatic disease. WBRT is still used for palliation of gross brain metastases and as prophylaxis against the development of new brain metastases. These topics are described further in the following sections.

WBRT as Primary Therapy for Gross Disease

Prospective trials led by the RTOG have been used to help ascertain the optimal dose and fractionation for WBRT. In general, WBRT to a dose of 20–40 Gy given over 1–4 weeks has resulted in median survival times of 4–6 months for patients with brain metastases (Table 20.1) (Sneed et al., 1996). Although the treatment schedules varied somewhat among studies, they were comparable with regard to the incidence and the duration of improvement, time to

TABLE 20.1 Studies of Postoperative Whole-Brain Radiation Therapy for Brain Metastases by the Radiation Therapy Oncology Group

Protocol	Period of Study	No. of Patients	Treatment Scheme	Median Survival Time
RTOG 6901	1971–1973	233	30 Gy in 10 Fx over 2 wks	21 wks
		217	30 Gy in 15 Fx over 3 wks	18 wks
		233	40 Gy in 15 Fx over 3 wks	18 wks
		227	40 Gy in 20 Fx over 4 wks	16 wks
RTOG 7361	1973–1976	447	20 Gy in 5 Fx over 1 wk	15 wks
		228	30 Gy in 10 Fx over 2 wks	15 wks
		227	40 Gy in 15 Fx over 3 wks	18 wks
RTOG 6901 ultra-rapid	1971–1973	26	10 Gy in 1 Fx over 1 day	15 wks
RTOG 7361 ultra-rapid	1973–1976	33	12 Gy in 2 Fx over 2 days	13 wks
RTOG 7606 favorable pts	1976–1979	130	30 Gy in 10 Fx over 2 wks	18 wks
		125	50 Gy in 20 Fx over 4 wks	17 wks
RTOG 8528	1986–1989	30	48 Gy in 1.6-Gy bid	4.8 months
Accelerated		53	54.5 Gy in 1.6-Gy bid	5.4 months
HFX		44	64 Gy in 1.6-Gy bid	7.2 months
		36	70.4 Gy in 1.6-Gy bid	8.2 months
RTOG 9104	1991–1995	213	30 Gy in 10 Fx	4.5 months
		216	54.4 Gy in 1.6-Gy fx bid	4.5 months
RTOG 7916	1979–1983	193	30 Gy in 10 Fx over 2 wks	4.5 months
Misonidazole		200	5 Gy in 6 Fx over 3 wks	4.1 months
		196	30 Gy in 10 Fx + Miso	3.1 months
		190	5 Gy in 6 Fx + Miso	3.9 months
RTOG 8905	1989–1993	36	37.5 Gy in 15 Fx over 3 wks	6.1 months
BrdU		34	37.5 Gy in 15 Fx + BrdU	4.3 months

Modified from Sneed P.K., Larson D.A., Wara W.M. (1996). Neurosurg. Clin. N. Am. 7:505–515. Fx: fraction; pts: patients; wks: weeks; HFX: hyperfractionated; BrdU: bromodeoxyuridine.

progression, survival, and palliative index. In RTOG 7361, approximately 900 patients were randomly assigned to receive 20 Gy in five fractions over 1 week, 30 Gy in 10 fractions over 2 weeks, or 40 Gy in 15 fractions over 3 weeks. The median survival times were similar among the three treatment groups, at 15 weeks for the 20-Gy and 30-Gy groups and 18 weeks for the 40-Gy group. WBRT was shown to improve neurologic function for about half of the patients in this study, without much improvement in survival, depending on dose or fractionation. Another randomized comparison of an ultra-rapid high-dose radiation schedule (10 Gy in one fraction or 12 Gy in two fractions) revealed median survival times that were not much different than those in RTOG 7361; however, patients who received the ultra-rapid high-dose WBRT had more treatment-related neurologic toxicity. The rapidity of the response to therapy was also similar between the two treatment groups in this study, but the duration of improvement, time to worsening of neurologic status, and rate of complete disappearance of neurologic symptoms were generally less for patients receiving 10–12 Gy in one or two fractions than for those receiving more prolonged treatment such as 30 Gy in 10 fractions.

The RTOG 8528 trial investigated accelerated hyperfractionated WBRT, with patients receiving 1.6-Gy twice-daily fractionation to a total dose of 48 Gy, 54.4 Gy, 64 Gy, or 70.4 Gy. Although median survival times seemed to increase with increasing dose (4.8 months, 5.4 months, 7.2 months and 8.2 months), this apparent difference was not statistically significant. A follow-up randomized phase III RTOG study included 445 patients with Karnofsky performance status scores of ≥60 who were given either hyperfractionated RT at 1.2-Gy twice-daily fractionation to a total tumor dose of 54.4 Gy or 30 Gy in 10 fractions (Murray et al., 1997). The median survival time was 4.5 months in both treatment groups. Given the lack of superiority of the hyperfractionated regimens and the toxicity of ultra-rapid high-dose fractionations, modern clinical trials involving WBRT for gross disease typically use either 30 Gy in 10 fractions or 37.5 Gy in 15 fractions.

Various radiosensitizers have also been investigated in prospective randomized clinical trials. The RTOG 7916 trial evaluated one such radiosensitizer, misonidazole, in patients with brain metastases. This study involved 779 patients who received 30 Gy in 10 fractions over 2 weeks with or without $1\,g/m^2$ of misonidazole or 30 Gy in six fractions over 3 weeks with or without $2\,g/m^2$ misonidazole. The median survival times ranged from 3.1 months to 4.5 months and were not affected by the use of misonidazole. Other sensitizers tested have included the halogenated pyrimidine bromodeoxyuridine (BrdU) and gadolinium texaphyrins. To investigate the role of BrdU as a radiosensitizer for brain metastases, RTOG 89-05 enrolled 72 patients and treated them with WBRT to 37.5 Gy in 15 fractions over 3 weeks, with BrdU at $0.8\,g/m^2$ per day for 4 days given each week for 3 weeks. Five patients who received BrdU manifested significant grade 4 and 5 hematologic or skin toxicity, and no significant survival benefit was found from BrdU.

Another randomized controlled trial, RTOG 9801, evaluated the role of motaxefin gadolinium (MGd) as a radiosensitizer for patients with brain metastases treated with WBRT (Mehta et al., 2003). In that study, 401 patients received either WBRT alone (30 Gy in 10 fractions) or WBRT with MGd, injected intravenously at a dose of 5 mg/kg/d at 2–5 hours before each fraction. Receipt of MGd did not affect median survival times, at 5.2 months for MGd and WBRT and 4.9 months for WBRT alone. Regression after WBRT correlated with survival and preservation of neurocognitive function (Li et al., 2007); in that analysis, time to neurologic progression was longer among patients with metastatic lung cancer receiving MGd. In a subsequent phase III study, 554 patients with brain metastases from non-small cell lung cancer (NSCLC) were randomly assigned to receive the same treatments as those given in RTOG 9801 (Mehta et al., 2009). The median interval to neurologic progression seemed to be better in the MGd group (15.4 months vs 10.0 months), although this apparent difference was not statistically significant at $p = 0.11$.

Thalidomide was investigated as a radiosensitizer in patients with brain metastases in RTOG 0118 (Knisely et al., 2008), in which patients were randomly assigned to receive WBRT alone (37.5 Gy in 15 fractions) or WBRT with thalidomide. Nearly half of the patients had to discontinue thalidomide because of side effects, and no survival benefit was noted. In the latest published study of radiosensitizers with WBRT, temozolomide or erlotinib was given concurrently with WBRT and SRS for patients with NSCLC and one to three brain metastases in RTOG 0320 (Sperduto et al., 2013). In that phase III trial, the addition of radiosensitizer increased the rates of grade 3–5 toxicity (11% control vs 41% temozolomide vs 49% erlotinib, $p < 0.001$) and seemed to reduce the median survival time (13.4 months control vs 6.3 months temozolomide vs 6.1 months erlotinib). Other radiosensitizers continue to be investigated for their potential efficacy in combination with WBRT.

WBRT as an Adjuvant after Local Therapy

WBRT AFTER SURGERY

WBRT has an established role in preventing local recurrence after surgical resection of brain metastases. In one prospective, randomized trial reported by Patchell et al. (1998), 95 patients with a single brain metastasis underwent complete resection followed by either observation or postoperative WBRT to a dose of 50.4 Gy. Receipt of WBRT led to a significant reduction in recurrence anywhere in the brain compared with the observation group (18% vs 70%; $p < 0.001$). Rates of local recurrence in the tumor bed were reduced from 46% to 10%, and rates of regional recurrence within the brain and outside the tumor bed were reduced from 37% to 14%. WBRT also reduced the rate of deaths from neurologic causes from 44% to 14% but did not affect median survival.

Most of the retrospective studies evaluating the role of WBRT after surgical resection (Komaki and Chang, 2004) found no significant reduction in brain recurrence after postoperative WBRT except for a study by DeAngelis et al. ($p = 0.03$) (DeAngelis et al., 1989). Only two retrospective studies have shown an improvement in median survival time after postoperative WBRT ($p = 0.02$) (Smalley et al., 1987; Skibber et al., 1996).

In general, more patients who receive WBRT at recurrence die from neurologic causes than do those given WBRT immediately after surgery, findings that support the immediate postoperative delivery of WBRT. Although the routine use of postoperative WBRT seems to prevent deaths from neurologic causes, this practice has become controversial because of growing concerns about the long-term toxicity of WBRT, including neurocognitive decline and dementia. Withholding postoperative WBRT carries the risk of increased neurologic morbidity from tumor recurrence within the brain; thus, if postoperative WBRT is to be given, it should be given promptly, usually within a few weeks of resection, depending on the aggressiveness of the surgical procedure and the patient's rate of postoperative recovery.

WBRT AFTER STEREOTACTIC RADIOSURGERY

WBRT after SRS has also been evaluated in prospective clinical trials. In a study reported by Aoyama et al. (2006), 132 patients with one to four brain metastases smaller than 3 cm in diameter were randomly assigned to undergo SRS or SRS followed by WBRT to a total dose of 30 Gy in 10 fractions. The SRS dose was reduced by 30% for the patients who were to be given WBRT. The addition of WBRT to SRS improved the 1-year local control rate (89% vs 73%) and decreased the incidence of new brain metastases at 1 year (42% vs 63.7% for SRS alone). Because no differences were found in median survival times, percentages with neurologic death, or neurocognitive outcomes, the authors concluded that SRS alone could be considered a reasonable strategy, with WBRT reserved for salvage therapy as needed.

In a similar study, Chang et al. (2009) enrolled 58 patients with one to three brain metastases and RTOG recursive partitioning analysis class 1 or 2 status to receive either SRS alone or SRS followed by WBRT to a dose of 30 Gy in 12 fractions. Notably, the primary endpoint in this study was neurocognitive function as defined by the Hopkins Verbal Learning Test-Revised (HVLT-R) of total recall at 4 months. The study was stopped early when it became clear that SRS followed by WBRT led to declines in learning and memory function. Indeed, the addition of WBRT led to a significant decline in HVLT-R 4-month recall (52% vs 24%); however, use of WBRT led to improved rates of local control at 1 year (100% vs 67%) and distant brain control at 1 year (73% vs 45%). Conversely, median overall survival time was longer in the SRS-only group (15 months vs 6 months SRS + WBRT).

The European Organisation for Research and Treatment of Cancer (EORTC) also undertook a randomized trial with 359 patients undergoing either SRS ($n = 199$) or surgery ($n = 160$) for one to three brain metastases who were then randomly assigned to receive WBRT (30 Gy in 10 fractions) or observation (Kocher et al., 2011). Those who went on to receive WBRT had reduced rates of relapse at initial sites at 2 years (surgery: 27% vs 59%; SRS: 19% vs 31%) and relapse at new sites (surgery: 23% vs 42%; SRS: 33% vs 48%). The rates of neurologic death were also lower among those who received WBRT (28% vs 44%). No differences were found in time to worsening performance status or overall survival.

The need for WBRT after SRS for the initial treatment of brain metastases continues to be debated. Although distant intracranial control is undoubtedly improved by the addition of WBRT, the lack of survival benefit and toxicity argue against the routine use of WBRT after SRS. Clinical trials are ongoing to evaluate survival, quality of life, and functional independence for such patients.

Prophylactic Cranial Irradiation

PCI has been noted to improve survival among children with acute lymphocytic leukemia by preventing the disease from involving the central nervous system (CNS). With the increasing use of more effective types of systemic chemotherapy, isolation of the malignancy in the CNS has become more common among patients with acute lymphocytic leukemia, a phenomenon that has also been noted in patients with small cell lung cancer (SCLC).

PCI has been proposed for patients with SCLC since the 1970s because of the high incidence of brain metastases from SCLC. Approximately half of patients with SCLC who do not receive PCI will develop clinically significant brain metastases. However, the incidence of microscopic brain metastases and extracranial CNS metastases had been underestimated given the relatively short survival duration for such patients, and PCI became more important when improvements in systemic treatment and earlier use of thoracic RT were shown to improve survival rates for patients with limited-stage SCLC (Kumar, 1997). Because PCI can be neurotoxic and because it had not improved overall survival times, it generally had not been considered for routine use despite its ability to reduce the number of brain metastases until neuropsychological testing of patients before and after PCI revealed no significant mental deterioration (Komaki et al., 1995).

Trials of PCI for SCLC date back to the late 1970s, when the Veterans Affairs Lung Study Group found that giving PCI to a dose of 20 Gy in five fractions did not reduce brain metastasis. At the time, this was thought to have resulted from the low total dose of RT (20 Gy), although the fraction size was considerably larger than the 2- to 3-Gy fractions in subsequent trials of PCI. Indeed, subsequent studies involving 24 to 30 Gy, delivered in 3-Gy fractions, have shown that PCI can reduce the incidence of brain metastases, although this effect is generally not associated with prolonged overall survival. Other groups have also found that PCI produced statistically significant reductions in brain metastasis but did not affect overall survival. Use of radiation doses in excess of 30 Gy seemed to reduce brain tumor recurrence in studies conducted in the late 1980s, although this may also have been related to the advent of more sensitive means of detecting brain metastases, improvements in systemic chemotherapy, and the use of thoracic RT (Gregor et al., 1999). Hirsch et al. (1979) reported a series of 111 patients randomly assigned to receive or not receive PCI to 40 Gy, which did not significantly reduce the incidence of brain metastasis (9% with PCI vs 13% without PCI). This finding was thought to be related to the late use of the PCI, which was begun 12 weeks after completion of the prolonged systemic treatment.

Twenty years after publication of the previous report, a meta-analysis by Auperin et al. (1999) showed a survival benefit from PCI for patients with SCLC in complete remission. That analysis involved individualized data from 987 patients who had participated in seven clinical trials comparing PCI with no PCI from 1977 to 1994 (Table 20.2) (Arriagada et al., 1995; Gregor et al., 1997). A minority of patients (12–17%) had extensive-stage disease. An absolute increase of 5.4% in survival rate at 3 years was noted for patients undergoing PCI (20.7% vs 15.3% no PCI), and the relative risk of death for the treatment group compared with the control group was 0.84 (95% confidence interval 0.73–0.97, $p = 0.01$). PCI also led to a significant increase in the rate of brain metastasis-free survival at 3 years (22.3% vs 13.5% in control patients, $p < 0.001$), and PCI reduced the cumulative incidence of brain metastasis at 3 years from 58.6% to 33.3% ($p < 0.001$). Analysis of four total radiation doses (8 Gy, 24–25 Gy, 30 Gy, and 36–40 Gy) revealed that the larger doses led to greater decreases in the risk of brain metastasis ($p = 0.02$), but the effect on survival was not proportional to the dose administered. This meta-analysis also confirmed the finding reported by Hirsch et al. (1979) that earlier use of PCI after induction chemotherapy reduces the risk of brain metastasis ($p = 0.01$ for <4 months vs 4–6 months vs >6 months after chemotherapy). No significant neuropsychological deterioration after PCI was noted, but most of these studies did not include systematic evaluations with neuropsychological testing before and after PCI.

TABLE 20.2 Characteristics of Seven Trials Included in a Meta-Analysis of the Effects of Prophylactic Cranial Irradiation for Small-Cell Lung Cancer

Trial Name and Site	Enrollment Period	Median Follow-Up Time (Years)	Induction Therapy	Total Dose/ No. of Fractions (Dose/ Fraction)	Median Time from Start of Induction Therapy to Enrollment (Months)	Total No. of Patients	No. of Surviving Patients
U Maryland Cancer Ctr	1977–1980	18.5	CT	30 Gy/10 (3 Gy)	3.6	29	2
Okayama University	1981–1986	11.7	CT or CT + RT	40 Gy/20 (2 Gy)	2.5	46	4
PCI-85	1985–1993	8.4	CT or CT + RT	24 Gy/8 (3 Gy)	5.3	300	32
Danish-National Cancer Institute (unpublished)	1985–1991	8.8	CT	24 Gy/8 (3 Gy)	4.4	55	7
UKCCR–EORTC	1987–1995	3.5	CT or CT + RT	8–36 Gy/1–18*	NA	314	54
PCI-88	1988–1994	5.1	CT or CT + RT	24 Gy/8 (3 Gy)	5.1	211	37
ECOG–RTOG	1991–1994	3.9	CT or CT + RT	25 Gy/10 (2.5 Gy)	NA	32	5

**The first part of the trial included three treatment groups: no PCI, PCI to 24 Gy in 12 fractions, and PCI to 36 Gy in 18 fractions; the second part of the trial involved only two treatment groups: no PCI and PCI at various doses.*

PCI: prophylactic cranial irradiation; UKCCR-EORTC: United Kingdom Clinical Cancer Research – European Organization for Research and Treatment of Cancer; ECOG-RTOG: Eastern Cooperative Oncology Group-Radiation Therapy Oncology Group; CT: chemotherapy; RT: thoracic radiation therapy.

Modified from Auperin et al., 1999.

In addition to limited-stage SCLC, PCI seems to have a role in extensive-stage SCLC as well. The EORTC conducted a prospective randomized trial in which 286 patients with extensive-stage SCLC who had shown any response to four to six cycles of chemotherapy were assigned to receive PCI (20Gy in five fractions or 30Gy in 12 fractions) or no PCI (Slotman et al., 2007). Those who received PCI had lower rates of symptomatic brain metastases (15% vs 40%) and improved overall survival (27% vs 13%) at 1 year. Notably, no brain imaging had been required before randomization in this study, and a follow-up report suggested that those who received PCI had worse health-related quality of life (Slotman et al., 2009).

Ongoing debate regarding the optimal dose for PCI led to an Intergroup trial that enrolled 720 patients with limited-stage SCLC in complete response after chemotherapy and thoracic RT to receive PCI at either a standard dose (25Gy in 10 fractions) or one of two higher doses (36Gy in 18 fractions daily or 36Gy in 24 fractions twice daily) (Le Pechoux et al., 2009). Brain imaging was used in all cases. No difference was found in the 2-year incidence of brain metastases, but the standard dose produced a better overall survival rate (42% vs 37%; $p = 0.05$). A subsequent analysis revealed no significant difference between the low-dose versus high-dose groups in quality of life, neurologic function or cognitive function over the 3-year study period (Le Pechoux et al., 2011). Thus, at this time, the standard fractionation regimen for PCI remains a dose of 25Gy given in 10 fractions.

Randomized studies have also been done to evaluate PCI for patients with NSCLC. One such study was RTOG 84-03, in which patients whose primary tumors were of adenocarcinomatous or large-cell histology and had been controlled were randomly assigned to receive or not receive PCI to a dose of 30Gy in 10 fractions. The results, reported in 1991, indicated that patients given PCI had fewer brain metastases but no significant improvement in overall survival, an outcome that could reflect either the ineffectiveness of the systemic chemotherapy or the timing of the PCI. A subsequent multicenter study from Germany on neoadjuvant and adjuvant therapies for operable stage IIIA NSCLC offered additional information regarding the role of PCI in NSCLC (Pottgen et al., 2007). In that study, 112 patients were randomly assigned to undergo either primary thoracic resection followed by adjuvant thoracic RT or preoperative chemotherapy followed by concurrent chemoradiotherapy to the primary site and definitive surgery at the primary site. The latter group also received postoperative PCI (30Gy in 15 fractions). Receipt of PCI reduced the probability of brain metastases as the first site of failure at 5 years (8% vs 35%) without a discernible difference in neurocognitive toxicity. The RTOG then attempted a phase III trial (RTOG 0214) comparing PCI versus observation for patients with locally advanced NSCLC (Gore et al., 2011). In that study, 340 eligible patients who had been treated for stage III NSCLC and had no disease progression after primary therapy were randomly assigned to PCI (30Gy in 15 fractions) or observation. Overall survival and disease-free survival rates were the same in the two groups, but the 1-year rate of brain metastases was lower in the PCI group (8% vs 18%). In subsequent analyses of neurocognition and quality of life, no differences were found at 1 year in global cognitive function or quality of life, although memory (measured by the HVLT) had declined significantly (Sun et al., 2011). Based on these prospective findings, the routine use of PCI for NSCLC is not warranted at this time.

In summary, PCI can effectively reduce the incidence of brain metastases without evidence of serious PCI-related complications if it is given appropriately. The use of PCI extends survival times among patients with limited-stage SCLC who achieve a complete response to primary therapy as well as those with extensive-stage SCLC who achieve any response to primary therapy (Auperin et al., 1999; Slotman et al., 2007). Dose escalation beyond 25 Gy in 10 fractions offers no additional benefit (Le Pechoux et al., 2009). The use of PCI does not seem to confer a survival advantage for patients with NSCLC.

TOXICITY OF RADIATION TO THE BRAIN

Complications of RT are generally divided into acute effects (those occurring during the course of radiation), early-delayed effects (at 2–4 months after radiation), and late effects (at months or years after radiation). Common acute effects include reversible alopecia, mild radiation dermatitis, and mild fatigue. Acute encephalopathy is exceedingly rare with the use of modern-day fractionation schedules, although fatal encephalopathy was reported after receiving 10 Gy in a single fraction. Somnolence syndrome, described as persistent fatigue, anorexia, and irritability (especially in children), can occur 3–10 weeks after WBRT but usually resolves within 6 months.

Among long-term survivors after WBRT, some of whom received multiple chemotherapeutic drugs, a syndrome consisting of progressive dementia, ataxia, and urinary incontinence was reported to cause severe disability and the deaths of seven of 12 patients in one report (DeAngelis et al., 1989). CT scans of the brains of those patients showed cortical atrophy and hypodense white matter. All 12 patients had received daily fractions of at least 3 Gy, and nine patients received some daily fractionation of 5 Gy or more during treatment. On the basis of these findings, the authors of this report advocated the use of smaller fractions, 1.8–2 Gy per day, for a total dose of 40–45 Gy to reduce long-term sequelae among patients with more favorable prognostic factors. More recently, recursive partitioning analyses have identified subgroups of patients who are likely to experience extended survival. In the Graded Prognostic Assessment, clinical characteristics including age, performance status, number of CNS metastases, and the presence of extracranial metastases are scored to characterize the prognosis of patients with brain metastases (Sperduto et al., 2008). The subgroup with the most favorable prognosis was noted to have a median survival time of 11 months compared with 2.6 months for the subgroup with the least favorable prognosis. For patients with favorable clinical factors, we advocate a dose per fraction of 3 Gy or less.

The relationship between WBRT, intracranial disease control, and neurocognitive function is complicated. Briefly, intracranial disease progression and WBRT may be competing risk factors in the development of neurocognitive dysfunction (Meyers et al., 2004; Corn et al., 2008; Li et al., 2008; Chang et al., 2009). Further studies are necessary to characterize adequately the relative risks of these competing factors to help guide therapeutic recommendations for patients with a favorable prognosis.

Within the PCI literature, concerns have also been expressed regarding neuropsychological toxicity not only from WBRT but also from systemic treatment. Johnson et al. (1990) described the frequency of neuropsychological deficits in orientation, memory, and language function as occurring in 86% of patients with SCLC who survived for 6–13 years after treatment. Factors or conditions contributing to these impairments include immunologic dysfunction, opportunistic infection, microscopic brain metastasis, toxicity from large irradiated field volumes, use of a neurotrophic chemotherapeutic agent in combination with PCI, and the total dose of RT. Particular concern has been expressed for children with acute lymphocytic leukemia who undergo PCI while receiving methotrexate, and also for patients with SCLC who undergo PCI combined with lomustine. However, at least one group has found a lack of clinical findings corresponding to CT abnormalities among patients who received prophylactic CNS radiation and experienced unexplained late neurologic sequelae (Catane et al., 1981). However, in a subsequent prospective evaluation of 30 patients with limited SCLC and no evidence of brain metastasis that involved neuropsychological testing before any treatment and after PCI, 29 patients were found to have had had minor cognitive dysfunction before the PCI. The most common impairment was in verbal memory, followed by frontal lobe dysfunction and fine-motor incoordination. No significant deterioration attributable to the PCI was found after the PCI (Komaki et al., 1995). Similar results were found in two subsequent randomized trials of PCI for SCLC with prospectively evaluated neurocognitive endpoints (Arriagada et al., 1995; Gregor et al., 1997); that is, neurocognitive impairments were noted before the PCI, but PCI had no detected effects on neurocognitive function.

As systemic therapies continue to improve and patients survive for longer periods, the late effects of WBRT will become increasingly relevant. A recently closed phase III trial by the RTOG randomly assigned patients to receive or not receive memantine, an N-methyl-D-aspartate receptor agonist approved for use in patients with Alzheimer's disease, with WBRT. Results of this study are pending. Conformal RT techniques are also being investigated as a way of sparing critical structures involved in neurocognition, as dose to the hippocampus has been implicated in neurocognitive dysfunction (Cheung and Chan, 2003; Gondi et al., 2010, 2012). The RTOG is currently conducting a phase II trial to assess whether hippocampal-sparing WBRT can help to preserve neurocognitive function.

CONCLUSION

In summary, WBRT is a valuable tool for treating gross brain metastases, for preventing the recurrence of brain metastases after local therapy, and for preventing the development of brain metastases in patients with SCLC. Many prospective clinical trials have been conducted to identify the ideal dose and fractionation schedules, to clarify the potential role of concurrent systemic agents, and to assess the risk of toxicity. Further advances in neuroimaging, neuropsychological testing, and SRS delivery will direct the optimal implementation of WBRT in the future.

References

Andrews, D.W., Scott, C.B., Sperduto, P.W., et al., 2004. Whole brain radiation therapy with or without stereotactic radiosurgery boost for patients with one to three brain metastases: phase III results of the RTOG 9508 randomised trial. Lancet 363, 1665–1672.

Aoyama, H., Shirato, H., Tago, M., et al., 2006. Stereotactic radiosurgery plus whole-brain radiation therapy vs stereotactic radiosurgery alone for treatment of brain metastases: a randomized controlled trial. J. Am. Med. Assoc. 295, 2483–2491.

Arriagada, R., Le Chevalier, T., Borie, F., et al., 1995. Prophylactic cranial irradiation for patients with small-cell lung cancer in complete remission. J. Natl. Cancer Inst. 87, 183–190.

Auperin, A., Arriagada, R., Pignon, J.P., et al., 1999. Prophylactic cranial irradiation for patients with small-cell lung cancer in complete remission. Prophylactic Cranial Irradiation Overview Collaborative Group. N. Engl. J. Med. 341, 476–484.

Catane, R., Schwade, J.G., Yarr, I., et al., 1981. Follow-up neurological evaluation in patients with small cell lung carcinoma treated with prophylactic cranial irradiation and chemotherapy. Int. J. Radiat. Oncol. Biol. Phys. 7, 105–109.

Ceresoli, G.L., Reni, M., Chiesa, G., et al., 2002. Brain metastases in locally advanced nonsmall cell lung carcinoma after multimodality treatment: risk factors analysis. Cancer 95, 605–612.

Chang, E.L., Wefel, J.S., Hess, K.R., et al., 2009. Neurocognition in patients with brain metastases treated with radiosurgery or radiosurgery plus whole-brain irradiation: a randomised controlled trial. Lancet Oncol. 10, 1037–1044.

Cheung, M.C., Chan, A.S., 2003. Memory impairment in humans after bilateral damage to lateral temporal neocortex. Neuroreport 14, 371–374.

Coia, L.R., Aaronson, N., Linggood, R., Loeffler, J., Priestman, T.J., 1992. A report of the consensus workshop panel on the treatment of brain metastases. Int. J. Radiat. Oncol. Biol. Phys. 23, 223–237.

Corn, B.W., Moughan, J., Knisely, J.P., et al., 2008. Prospective evaluation of quality of life and neurocognitive effects in patients with multiple brain metastases receiving whole-brain radiotherapy with or without thalidomide on Radiation Therapy Oncology Group (RTOG) trial 0118. Int. J. Radiat. Oncol. Biol. Phys. 71, 71–78.

DeAngelis, L.M., Delattre, J.Y., Posner, J.B., 1989. Radiation-induced dementia in patients cured of brain metastases. Neurology 39, 789–796.

Elliott, R.E., Rush, S.C., Morsi, A., et al., 2011. Local control of newly diagnosed and distally recurrent, low-volume brain metastases using fixed dose (20 Gy) gamma knife radiosurgery. Neurosurgery 68, 921–931.

Gondi, V., Tome, W.A., Mehta, M.P., 2010. Why avoid the hippocampus? A comprehensive review. Radiother. Oncol. 97, 370–376.

Gondi, V., Hermann, B.P., Mehta, M.P., Tome, W.A., 2012. Hippocampal dosimetry predicts neurocognitive function impairment after fractionated stereotactic radiotherapy for benign or low-grade adult brain tumors. Int. J. Radiat. Oncol. Biol. Phys. 83, e487–e493.

Gore, E.M., Bae, K., Wong, S.J., et al., 2011. Phase III comparison of prophylactic cranial irradiation versus observation in patients with locally advanced non-small-cell lung cancer: primary analysis of radiation therapy oncology group study RTOG 0214. J. Clin. Oncol. 29, 272–278.

Gregor, A., Cull, A., Stephens, R.J., et al., 1997. Prophylactic cranial irradiation is indicated following complete response to induction therapy in small cell lung cancer: results of a multicentre randomised trial. United Kingdom Coordinating Committee for Cancer Research (UKCCCR) and the European Organization for Research and Treatment of Cancer (EORTC). Eur. J. Cancer 33, 1752–1758.

Gregor, A., Cull, A., Lung, P., Klastersk, J., Van, C., Rocmans, P., 1999. Role of prophylactic cranial irradiation: benefits and late effects. In: Van Houtte, P., Klastersk, J., Rocmans, P. (Eds.), Progress and Perspectives in the Treatment of Lung Cancer Springer Verlag, Berlin, pp. 139–149.

Hirsch, F.R., Hansen, H.H., Paulson, O.B., 1979. Development of brain metastasis in small cell anaplastic carcinoma of the lung. In: Whitehouse, J.M.A., Kay, H.E.M. (Eds.), CNS Complications of Malignant Disease Springer-Verlag, Berlin, pp. 175–184.

Jayarao, M., Chin, L.S., Regine, W.F., 2009. Stereotactic radiosurgery for brain metastases. In: Lundsford, L.D., Sheehan, J. (Eds.), Intracranial Stereotactic Radiosurgery Thieme Medical Publishers, New York, pp. 151–162.

Johnson, B.E., Patronas, N., Hayes, W., et al., 1990. Neurologic, computed cranial tomographic, and magnetic resonance imaging abnormalities in patients with small-cell lung cancer: further follow-up of 6- to 13-year survivors. J. Clin. Oncol. 8, 48–56.

Knisely, J.P., Berkey, B., Chakravarti, A., et al., 2008. A phase III study of conventional radiation therapy plus thalidomide versus conventional radiation therapy for multiple brain metastases (RTOG 0118). Int. J. Radiat. Oncol. Biol. Phys. 71, 79–86.

Kocher, M., Soffietti, R., Abacioglu, U., et al., 2011. Adjuvant whole-brain radiotherapy versus observation after radiosurgery or surgical resection of one to three cerebral metastases: results of the EORTC 22952-26001 study. J. Clin. Oncol. 29, 134–141.

Komaki, R., Chang, E., 2004. Whole-brain radiation therapy. In: Sawaya, R. (Ed.), Intracranial Metastases: Current Management Strategies Blackwell Publishing, Malden, MA, pp. 126–138.

Komaki, R., Meyers, C.A., Shin, D.M., et al., 1995. Evaluation of cognitive function in patients with limited small cell lung cancer prior to and shortly following prophylactic cranial irradiation. Int. J. Radiat. Oncol. Biol. Phys. 33, 179–182.

Kumar, P., 1997. The role of thoracic radiotherapy in the management of limited-stage small cell lung cancer: past, present, and future. Chest 112 (Suppl.), 259S–265S.

Le Pechoux, C., Dunant, A., Senan, S., Prophylactic Cranial Irradiation (PCI) Collaborative Group, 2009. Standard-dose versus higher-dose prophylactic cranial irradiation in patients with limited-stage small-cell lung cancer in complete remission after chemotherapy and thoracic radiotherapy (PCI 99-01, EORTC 22003-08004, RTOG 0212, and IFCT 99-01): a randomised clinical trial. Lancet Oncol. 10, 467–474.

Le Pechoux, C., Laplanche, A., Faivre-Finn, C., Prophylactic Cranial Irradiation (PCI) Collaborative Group, 2011. Clinical neurological outcome and quality of life among patients with limited small-cell cancer treated with two different doses of prophylactic cranial irradiation in the intergroup phase III trial (PCI99-01, EORTC 22003-08004, RTOG 0212 and IFCT 99-01). Ann. Oncol. 22, 1154–1163.

Li, J., Bentzen, S.M., Renschler, M., Mehta, M.P., 2007. Regression after whole-brain radiation therapy for brain metastases correlates with survival and improved neurocognitive function. J. Clin. Oncol. 25, 1260–1266.

Li, J., Bentzen, S.M., Renschler, M., Mehta, M.P., 2008. Relationship between neurocognitive function and quality of life after whole-brain radiotherapy in patients with brain metastasis. Int. J. Radiat. Oncol. Biol. Phys. 71, 64–70.

Mehta, M.P., Rodrigus, P., Terhaard, C.H., et al., 2003. Survival and neurologic outcomes in a randomized trial of motexafin gadolinium and whole-brain radiation therapy in brain metastases. J. Clin. Oncol. 21, 2529–2536.

Mehta, M.P., Shapiro, W.R., Phan, S.C., et al., 2009. Motexafin gadolinium combined with prompt whole brain radiotherapy prolongs time to neurologic progression in non-small-cell lung cancer patients with brain metastases: results of a phase III trial. Int. J. Radiat. Oncol. Biol. Phys. 73, 1069–1076.

Meyers, C.A., Smith, J.A., Bezjak, A., et al., 2004. Neurocognitive function and progression in patients with brain metastases treated with whole-brain radiation and motexafin gadolinium: results of a randomized phase III trial. J. Clin. Oncol. 22, 157–165.

Murray, K.J., Scott, C., Greenberg, H.M., et al., 1997. A randomized phase III study of accelerated hyperfractionation versus standard in patients with unresected brain metastases: a report of the Radiation Therapy Oncology Group (RTOG) 9104. Int. J. Radiat. Oncol. Biol. Phys. 39, 571–574.

Noordijk, E.M., Vecht, C.J., Haaxma-Reiche, H., et al., 1994. The choice of treatment of single brain metastasis should be based on extracranial tumor activity and age. Int. J. Radiat. Oncol. Biol. Phys. 29, 711–717.

Patchell, R.A., Tibbs, P.A., Walsh, J.W., et al., 1990. A randomized trial of surgery in the treatment of single metastases to the brain. N. Engl. J. Med. 322, 494–500.

Patchell, R.A., Tibbs, P.A., Regine, W.F., et al., 1998. Postoperative radiotherapy in the treatment of single metastases to the brain: a randomized trial. J. Am. Med. Assoc. 280, 1485–1489.

Pottgen, C., Eberhardt, W., Grannass, A., et al., 2007. Prophylactic cranial irradiation in operable stage IIIA non small-cell lung cancer treated with neoadjuvant chemoradiotherapy: results from a German multicenter randomized trial. J. Clin. Oncol. 25, 4987–4992.

Shaw, E., Scott, C., Souhami, L., et al., 2000. Single dose radiosurgical treatment of recurrent previously irradiated primary brain tumors and brain metastases: final report of RTOG protocol 90-05. Int. J. Radiat. Oncol. Biol. Phys. 47, 291–298.

Shehata, M.K., Young, B., Reid, B., et al., 2004. Stereotatic radiosurgery of 468 brain metastases < or =2 cm: implications for SRS dose and whole brain radiation therapy. Int. J. Radiat. Oncol. Biol. Phys. 59, 87–93.

Skibber, J.M., Soong, S.J., Austin, L., Balch, C.M., Sawaya, R.E., 1996. Cranial irradiation after surgical excision of brain metastases in melanoma patients. Ann. Surg. Oncol. 3, 118–123.

Slotman, B., Faivre-Finn, C., Kramer, G., EORTC Radiation Oncology Group and Lung Cancer Group, 2007. Prophylactic cranial irradiation in extensive small-cell lung cancer. N. Engl. Med. 357, 664–672.

Slotman, B.J., Mauer, M.E., Bottomley, A., et al., 2009. Prophylactic cranial irradiation in extensive disease small-cell lung cancer: short-term health-related quality of life and patient reported symptoms: results of an international Phase III randomized controlled trial by the EORTC Radiation Oncology and Lung Cancer Groups. J. Clin. Oncol. 27, 78–84.

Smalley, S.R., Schray, M.F., Laws, E.R., O'Fallon, J.R., 1987. Adjuvant radiation therapy after surgical resection of solitary brain metastasis: association with pattern of failure and survival. Int. J. Radiat. Oncol. Biol. Phys. 13, 1611–1616.

Sneed, P.K., Larson, D.A., Wara, W.M., 1996. Radiotherapy for cerebral metastasis. Neurosurg. Clin. N. Am. 7, 505–515.

Sperduto, P.W., Berkey, B., Gaspar, L.E., Mehta, M., Curran, W., 2008. A new prognostic index and comparison to three other indices for patients with brain metastases: an analysis of 1,960 patients in the RTOG database. Int. J. Radiat. Oncol. Biol. Phys. 70, 510–514.

Sperduto, P.W., Wang, M., Robins, H.I., et al., 2013. A phase 3 trial of whole brain radiation therapy and stereotactic radiosurgery alone versus WBRT and SRS with temozolomide or erlotinib for non-small cell lung cancer and 1 to 3 brain metastases: Radiation Therapy Oncology Group 0320. Int. J. Radiat. Oncol. Biol. Phys. 85, 1312–1318.

Sun, A., Bae, K., Gore, E.M., et al., 2011. Phase III trial of prophylactic cranial irradiation compared with observation in patients with locally advanced non-small-cell lung cancer: neurocognitive and quality-of-life analysis. J. Clin. Oncol. 29, 279–286.

CHAPTER

21

Lambert–Eaton Myesthenic Syndrome and Brain Metastasis from Occult Small Cell Lung Carcinoma: A Clinician's Perspective

Arunansu Talukdar, Nikhil Sonthalia, Sayantan Ray and Supratip Kundu

OUTLINE

Introduction 244

Lambert–Eaton Myesthenic Syndrome 244

Paraneoplastic and Non-Paraneoplastic LEMS 244

Pathophysiology 245

Clinical Features 245

Investigations 246

Treatment 246

Management of PLEMS 246

Management of NPLEMS 247

LEMS and Small Cell Lung Carcinoma 247

DELTA-P Score 249

Brain Metastasis 249

Brain Metastasis with Unknown Primary 250

Brain Metastasis in Occult Small Cell Lung Carcinoma 251

Our Experience 252

References 253

M.A. Hayat (ed): *Brain Metastases from Primary Tumors, Volume 1*
DOI: http://dx.doi.org/10.1016/B978-0-12-800896-6.00021-8

© 2014 Elsevier Inc. All rights reserved.

INTRODUCTION

Small cell lung carcinoma (SCLC) is a highly aggressive tumor, with a high proliferative capability, rapid tumor doubling time, and early onset of metastases carrying a poor prognosis. These features make SCLC a systemic disease in most cases, with 70% of SCLC patients presenting with extensive disease (ED) on diagnosis. The median overall survival of treated patients in the ED stage varies between 6 and 11 months, whereas 2- and 5-year survival rates hardly reach 5% and 1%, respectively, as reported by Stupp et al. (2004). In spite of these discouraging statistical data, cases of long survivors have been reported, although no predictors of such a course have been identified. There are case reports to show that the prognosis in a patient with a solitary brain metastasis and occult small cell lung carcinoma is not always as dismal compared with the patients with brain metastasis occurring after the evidence of SCLC and synchronous metastasis to other sites (Harrison and Goldstein, 2002).

Lambert–Eaton myasthenic syndrome (LEMS), on the other hand, is an autoimmune disease occurring in association with a carcinoma in ≈60% of patients, the majority of which constitutes SCLC (O'Neill et al., 1988). SCLC is a tumor of neuroendocrine origin which shows many features of a neuron including expression of voltage-gated calcium channel (VGCC) on the tumor cells. Antibody response to these channels triggers paraneoplastic LEMS (PLEMS). Long-term survival of patients with PLEMS associated with SCLC has been reported (Roberts et al., 1985). Rarely, both a paraneoplastic syndrome in the form of LEMS and solitary brain metastasis can occur in a patient before the primary SCLC causing its detection. Long-term follow up with palliative care is the cornerstone in managing these patients. Our experience with such a case suggests that these patients carry a better prognosis than patients with full-blown metastasis detected after the evidence of SCLC.

LAMBERT–EATON MYESTHENIC SYNDROME

LEMS is an antibody-mediated autoimmune disorder of neuromuscular transmission characterized by muscle weakness, hyporeflexia or areflexia and autonomic dysfunction. Anderson et al. (1953) reported the case of a 47-year-old man with a bronchial neoplasm, progressive proximal muscle weakness and hyporeflexia. They concluded that there was "strong clinical evidence for believing that the severe muscle weakness was of the myasthenic type". This patient showed the features of what we today call LEMS. In 1957, Eaton and Lambert summarized the clinical and electrophysiological characteristics of this myasthenic syndrome and concluded that the features are distinct from what is expected in cases of myasthenia gravis (Eaton and Lambert, 1957).

Paraneoplastic and Non-Paraneoplastic LEMS

LEMS is rare with a prevalence of ≈1 per 100000, equally common in men and women. There are two types of LEMS – LEMS associated with malignancy (PLEMS) and LEMS without malignancy (NPLEMS). Patients with either type have an autoimmune basis and similar electrophysiological characters. Approximately 60% of LEMS patients have associated SCLC. Other less commonly associated malignancy includes lymphoproliferative disorder, papillary carcinoma of thyroid, thymoma, colonic carcinoma, renal-cell carcinoma, intrathoracic carcinoid, and adenocarcinoma of lungs, pancreas, and prostate (O'Neill et al., 1988).

NPLEMS is characterized by the presence of various other autoimmune diseases such as thyroiditis, Addison's disease, vitiligo, pernicious anemia, systemic lupus erythematosus/discoid lupus erythematosus (SLE/DLE), rheumatoid arthritis and other immunological disorders which provides further evidence for autoimmunity involved in the pathogenisis of LEMS. Overall, approximately 25% of patients with LEMS have other associated autoimmune disease and approximately 35–45% have circulating organ-specific antibodies. Prevalence of autoantibodies is higher in the NPLEMS group (Lennon et al., 1982). Generally, NPLEMS occurs at a younger age as compared to PLEMS (mean ages 48 and 57.9 years, respectively). However, 80% of patients with LEMS are older than 40 years (Seneviratne and de Silva, 1999). O'Neill et al. (1988) in their series of 50 cases, found a statistically significant male predominance in the group without associated carcinoma and when both groups were considered together. There is a significant association noted with HLA-B8 in both groups, which appears to be stronger in the NPLEMS group. The levels of immunoglobulin G (IgG) heavy chain marker G1m(2) are also found to be increased in both groups (Willcox et al.,1985).

Pathophysiology

The common pathogenic mechanism involved in both groups of LEMS includes antibody-mediated blockage of voltage-gated calcium channels (VGCC) at the presynaptic neurons. This results in failure of calcium influx at the channels in response to the stimulus, thereby decreasing the neurotransmitter release at the presynaptic motor nerve terminals of the neuromuscular junction and autonomic neurons producing symptoms of weakness and autonomic dysfunction (Kim and Neher, 1988).

The VGCC based on their electrophysiological and pharmacological characteristics are classified as L, N, P/Q, R and T. In LEMS, IgG autoantibodies against P/Q type VGCC result in decreased release of acetylcholine both at the motor nerve terminals and at the postganglionic sympathetic and parasympathetic neurons.

The SCLC tumor cells have been shown to express VGCCs of L, N and P/Q subtypes. In patients with SCLC, LEMS is initiated by an immune reaction to these VGCC expressed on the surface of the tumor cells. The resulting antibodies react with VGCC at the presynaptic nerve terminal of the neuromuscular junction resulting in PLEMS (Roberts et al., 1985). Similarly, VGCCs are expressed in the cerebellum and patients with SCLC, with or without LEMS, may also have cerebellar dysfunction.

Clinical Features

The cardinal clinical features described by Lambert and Eaton were weakness and fatiguability of muscles, temporary increase in strength after voluntary exercise, diminished or absent tendon reflexes, marked sensitivity to curare (as in myasthenia gravis) and relatively poor response to neostigmine. Tendon reflexes show marked potentiation after sustained contraction of the appropriate muscle for ≈10–15 s (O'Neill et al., 1988). It is usually gradual and insidious in onset. The weakness usually starts with the lower limbs and involves proximal more than distal muscle groups. Cranial nerve involvement is seen in ≈70% of patients which produces symptoms such as diplopia, ptosis, dysphagia, nasal regurgitation, and weakness of neck flexion. Autonomic symptoms such as dry mouth, dry eyes, and orthostatic hypotension are seen in ≈80% of patients. Autonomic dysfunction can be elicited by testing even when the symptoms are mildly present (O'Neill et al., 1988).

Investigations

SERUM ANTIBODIES TO VGCC

Antibodies against P/Q type VGCCs are detected in ≈90% of patients with LEMS belonging to both groups. This finding appears to be particularly strong in carcinoma-associated LEMS where almost all patients are found positive for antibodies against the P/Q type of VGCCs. Antibodies to N-type VGCCs are detected in <50 % of cases, but more commonly in patients with underlying lung carcinoma. Therefore, detection of this type of antibody increases the possibility of an underlying primary lung carcinoma (Lennon et al., 1995).

ELECTRODIAGNOSTIC TESTS

Electrophysiological tests are used both for the diagnosis and monitoring the course of the illness. Compound muscle action potential (CMAP) after a supramaximal stimulus, postactivation potentiation (increase in the CMAP amplitude immediately after maximal voluntary contraction), repetitive nerve stimulation, and single fiber electromyography are the modalities that help to differentiate LEMS from myasthenia gravis. Postactivation exhaustion (decrease in the CMAP amplitude 2–4 min after maximal voluntary muscle contraction) can be seen in both LEMS and myasthenia gravis. The results should be interpreted taking the entire picture, including the clinical presentation, into consideration. Electrophysiological tests reveal characteristic features such as a low CMAP amplitude at rest, a decremental response at low stimulation frequency, and an incremental response at high-rate stimulation and post-tetanic potentiation (Figure 21.1).

Treatment

The treatment strategy in patients with LEMS depends on the severity of symptoms, the degree of response to symptomatic treatment, and the presence or absence of an associated malignancy. 3,4 Diaminopyridine (DAP), guanidine, pyridostigmine, steroids, immunosuppresives, plasma exchange, and intravenous immunoglobulins are some of the therapeutic options available for patients with LEMS which needs to be used according to the clinical settings and availability. Except for 3,4 DAP, all others are associated with significant side effects and poor responses (Seneviratne and de Silva, 1999).

Management of PLEMS

3,4-diaminopyridine is the drug of choice in these patients for symptomatic relief of weakness and autonomic dysfunction. The specific treatment of the underlying tumor usually results in improvement or remission of symptoms. In such patients, the only further treatment required may be continuation of 3, 4 DAP. When the specific tumor therapy fails to resolve symptoms, further treatment with prednisolone should be considered. Those who present with severe weakness will benefit from plasma exchange or intravenous immunoglobulin (IVIG). Bain et al. (1996) reported an onset of effect of IVIG in their patients at

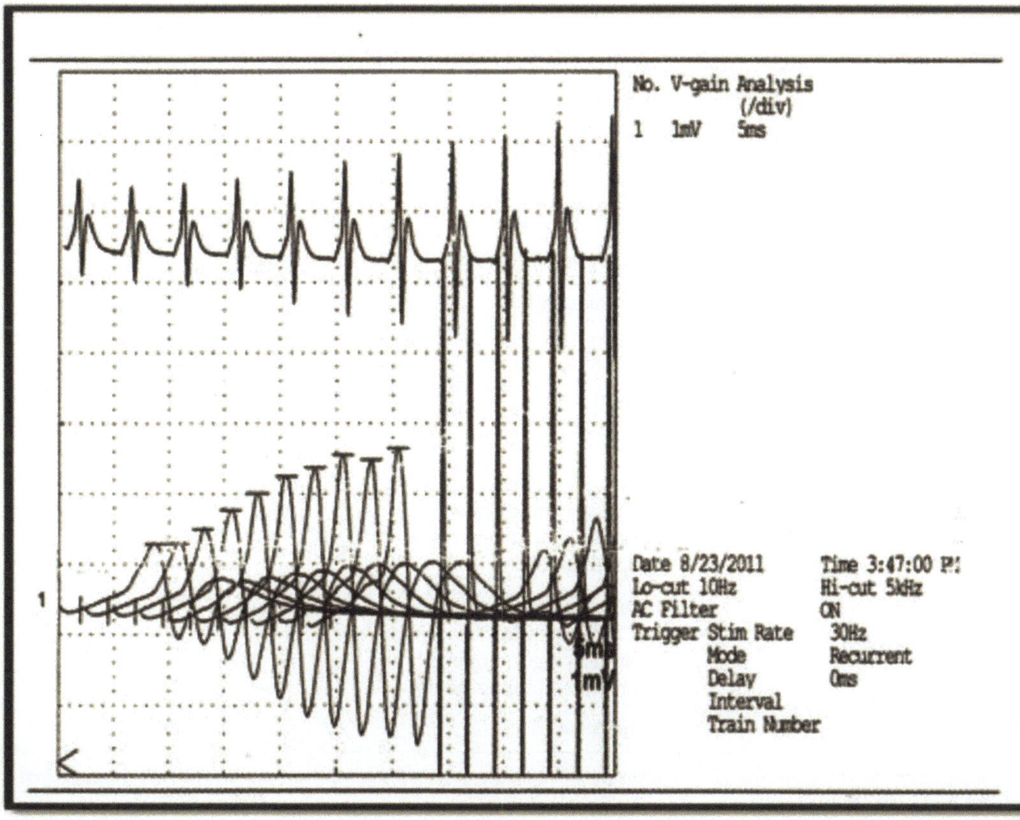

FIGURE 21.1 An incremental response as manifested by increase in area under curve for amplitude of about 300% at high-rate stimulation (30 Hz). Gain is 1 mV per division and a sweep speed of 5 milliseconds.

2–4 weeks. Severity of symptoms should be the guide for the choice of therapies in these patients.

Management of NPLEMS

3,4 DAP therapy is useful in this group for symptomatic relief and, if successful, no additional treatment is required. Those who have not responded should be treated with prednisolone and/or azathioprine as long-term therapy. Once remission is achieved, prednisolone could be tapered to the minimum maintenance dose. If the weakness is severe, plasma exchange or IVIG should also be considered in this group.

Table 21.1 summarizes the distinguishing features between PLEMS and NPLEMS.

LEMS and Small Cell Lung Carcinoma

Only 1–3% of patients with SCLC have LEMS. Between 40% and 60% of LEMS patients have SCLC, which results in an *a priori* chance of 50% of having an SCLC at the moment of

TABLE 21.1 The Distinguishing Features between PLEMS and NPLEMS

Features	Paraneoplastic LEMS	Non-Paraneoplastic LEMS
Age at diagnosis (median)	57.9	48
Sex	Male predominance	Female predominance (less compared to PLEMS)
Smoking history	Present	Usually absent
Associated other autoimmune diseases	Usually less frequent	Strong association
Immunoglobulin G (IgG) heavy chain marker G1m and HLA-B8/DR3 association	Less frequently	More frequently
Significant weight loss	Present	Absent
Disease onset and progression	Subacute and progressive	Chronic and progressive
Laboratory investigations	Raised ESR, LDH Reduced hemoglobin, variation in total leukocyte count (high or low)	Usually absent
Treatment	Less satisfactory response to 3, 4 DAP. Requires treatment of underlying tumor and aggressive immunotherapy	Good response to 3, 4 DAP.
DELTA-P score	Usually >4	<2

LEMS: Lambert–Eaton myasthenic syndrome; ESR: erythrocyte sedimentation rate; LDH: lactate dehydrogenase; DELTA-P: Dutch–English LEMS Tumor Association Prediction score.

diagnosis of LEMS (Maddison et al., 1999). This is a major clinical concern for the patient as well as for the doctors. Smoking and the absence of HLA-B8 are risk factors associated with a higher risk of having an underlying malignancy (Wirtz et al., 2005a). Most SCLCs are found within 2 years of diagnosis of LEMS. Discovery of a tumor has been described at >5 years after diagnosis of LEMS, and one anecdotal case with an interval of 12 years exists (Ramos-Yeo and Reyes, 1987).

The diagnosis of LEMS should prompt clinicians for a careful search for an SCLC. Screening for SCLC should be done by: computed tomography (CT) of thorax, ^{18}F labeled 2-deoxy-D glucose (FDG) positron emission tomography (PET), and bronchoscopy. As the SCLC may be too small to detect initially, these investigations need to be repeated every 6 months for at least 2 years from the initial diagnosis of LEMS. With this approach ≈96% of SCLC is found within a year of diagnosing LEMS, while a delay of >2 years is extremely rare; nevertheless, some patients undergo many procedures with associated anxiety and costs (Titulaer et al., 2008). Care would be improved if those who require intensive investigations as well as those no longer at risk could be identified. Some of the factors to be kept in mind in evaluating for a cancer in a patient with LEMS include old age, smoking, development of multiple clinical symptoms within 6 months after onset, raised erythrocyte sedimentation rate (ESR), and Sry-like high-mobility group box protein 1 antibodies (SOX1)

(Wirtz et al., 2005b). Absence of an underlying SCLC is suggested at young age, no smoking history, slow evolution of clinical symptoms, and the 8.1 HLA haplotype. A recent Dutch–English LEMS Tumor Association Prediction score was published by Titulaer et al. (2011) which predicts the association of SCLC in a patient diagnosed with LEMS.

An SCLC has a profound impact on therapy and prognosis. Therapy in patients with LEMS with an underlying SCLC is focused on the tumor. Survival of SCLC-associated LEMS is poor, compared to patients with NPLEMS who are thought to have a normal life expectancy. However, long-term survival in patients with SCLC who have an associated LEMS has been advocated compared to other patients with SCLC. The long-term survival in these patients, despite the presence of a highly malignant tumor, implies that the anti-VGCC antibodies may be playing a role in controlling tumor growth or, alternatively, that the small cell cancers that provoke LEMS may be of slow growth (Newsom-Davis, 1998).

DELTA-P Score

A Dutch–English LEMS Tumor Association Prediction score (DELTA-P score) was developed, allocating one point for the presence of each of the following items at or within 3 months from onset (Titulaer et al., 2011):

1. Age of onset ≥50 years
2. Smoking at diagnosis
3. Weight loss ≥5%
4. Bulbar involvement
5. Erectile dysfunction and
6. Karnofsky performance status <70.

The area under the curve of the receiver operating curve was 94.4% in the derivation cohort and 94.6% in the validation set. A DELTA-P score of 0 or 1 corresponded to a 0–2.6% chance of SCLC, whereas scores of 4, 5, and 6 corresponded to chances of SCLC of 93.5%, 96.6%, and 100%, respectively. In conclusion, the simple clinical DELTA-P score discriminated LEMS patients with or without SCLC with high accuracy early in the course of LEMS.

The DELTA-P score can be easily applied in the clinic to predict with higher than 94% reliability the likelihood of SCLC in patients with LEMS early in the course of their neurologic disease. The DELTA-P score can be used in routine clinical practice to prioritize high-risk patients for intensive tumor screening, while it also identifies those with very low tumor risk, who can be reassured in an early phase of the screening process.

BRAIN METASTASIS

The metastatic dissemination of a solid tumor to the brain is generally associated with a poor prognosis. Approximately, 10% of SCLC patients present with brain metastases at the time of diagnosis, and >50% will develop symptomatic brain metastases during their remaining lifetime (Hirsch et al., 1983). Here we discuss the clinical approach and therapeutic modalities in patients with brain metastasis presenting with an occult primary with special reference to SCLC.

Brain Metastasis with Unknown Primary

In up to 15% of the patients presenting with brain metastases, the site of the primary tumor is not detected despite thorough investigations (Nussbaum et al., 1996). Some authors find a better prognosis for patients presenting with brain metastases as the only manifestation of an unknown primary tumor than for patients with brain metastases and known primary (Nguyen et al., 1998). These results represent only a subset of patients with brain metastases and cancer of unknown primary (CUP). In the majority of the patients, extracerebral metastases are present on diagnosis of brain metastases which carries a dismal prognosis. Aggressive treatment or even an extensive search for the primary cancer in these patients may be of no benefit considering the often strongly limited prognosis of an advanced tumor. The period of time after which a patient is considered to have an "unknown primary" has no generally accepted definition. It varies from no exact definition to a period of 2 months (Nguyen et al., 1998). The reports in the literature on patients with brain metastases from an unknown primary tumor are all retrospective. They include patients in whom the brain metastases were the first symptom of a tumor discovered at diagnosis (most often a lung tumor) as well as patients whose primary tumor remained undetected after a thorough investigation (Takeshima et al., 2002).

Serial follow up and screening for underlying lung cancer in patients with a solitary brain metastasis (SBM) is mandatory as bronchogenic carcinoma is the commonest malignancy detected in patients of SBM with an occult primary (Salvati et al., 1995). In a prospective series, Ruda et al. (2001) found lung tumors to be the commonest culprit primary tumor followed by that of colon, thyroid, and pancreas detected in the course of time in cases of CUP with brain metastasis. The histological patterns of brain metastasis observed by them included most commonly adenocarcinoma, followed by squamous cell carcinoma. Median survival in their series was 10 months with 76% alive at 6 months, 42% at 1 year and 15% at 2 years in patients with brain metastasis whose primary tumor was still undiagnosed at first investigation. Melanoma and breast carcinoma have been rarely found as the primary tumor undetected at the time of brain metastasis (Salvati et al., 1995). Breast carcinoma is the second most common primary site in patients with known malignancy: its rarity in patients with an unknown primary tumor may be attributed to its tendency to metastasize to the brain later on in its natural history.

The treatment options in these patients include gross total resection when possible, followed by radiotherapy or radiotherapy alone. The superiority of the combination of surgery and whole brain radiotherapy (WBRT) over WBRT alone in patients with a single brain metastasis from both a known and an unknown origin has been confirmed by recent randomized trials in terms of duration of survival and quality of life, with the exception of patients with active systemic disease (Mintz et al., 1996). Among brain metastases as a whole, multiple lesions have a shorter survival compared to a single lesion. Van de Pol et al. (1996) in their series have found that survival rates among patients with brain metastases from an unknown primary tumor were similar between those with diagnosed and those with undetected tumor. So it is a matter of debate as to whether to do costly extensive evaluation for an undetected primary tumor during the follow up until more effective cancer therapy is available.

Brain Metastasis in Occult Small Cell Lung Carcinoma

In cases of SCLC with brain metastasis, the vast majority of the patients have synchronous metastases at other sites (Takeshima et al., 2002). Only a few case reports of a solitary brain metastasis with an occult primary lung tumor at the time of diagnosis of SCLC have been reported in the medical literature. There are no data pertaining to the incidence of SBM in occult primary lung cancer available in the literature. Harrison and Goldstein (2002) reported a case of a 30-year-old male whose SBM preceded a diagnosis of the primary SCLC. The treatment involved brain tumor resection, WBRT, chest irradiation, and carboplatin-based chemotherapy. The patient survived for 5 years and died because of the local recurrence and progression of the disease. Imai et al. (2001) described the case of a 59-year-old male with an SBM as the only clinical presentation of SCLC. The treatment consisted of subtotal excision of the metastatic brain tumor followed by adjuvant brain irradiation and irradiation of the primary lung tumor, discovered soon after metastasectomy. The patient refused to complete systemic chemotherapy and was followed-up for 5 years. These cases show that the prognosis for patients with brain metastases and occult small cell lung carcinoma may not always be dismal.

Now the dilemma arises in these cases with regards to their treatment modalities. Whether to treat them as a latent disease (LD) or extensive disease (ED) is a matter of debate. Aggressive treatment in ED SCLC does not improve survival as mentioned above and standard treatment of newly diagnosed SCLC with symptomatic brain metastases is palliative and consists of WBRT and chemotherapy. Although recently published practice guidelines based on randomized trials recommend the use of surgical resection plus postoperative WBRT, rather than WBRT alone, to improve local control and overall outcome in patients with newly diagnosed, single, resectable brain metastases, good performance status, and no or limited extracranial disease, the data clearly indicate that the recommendation does not apply to comparatively radiosensitive tumor histology such as SCLC (Kalkanis et al., 2010). The alternative treatment option in such cases could be stereotactic radiosurgery (SRS), either as sole treatment or in addition to WBRT. Unfortunately, there is still no evidence either from prospective studies or retrospective cohorts that SRS is more efficient in local tumor control than surgery + WBRT.

As far as the treatment of the primary site is concerned chemotherapy with thoracic radiotherapy remains the gold standard of treatment. However, there has recently been a growing number of articles underlining the need for a re-evaluation of the role of surgery in SCLC (Schreiber et al., 2010). The application of surgery involves the use of the TNM staging system in clinical practice and especially patients with T1–T2N0 lung primary, should be referred for surgery. Patients with a solitary brain metastasis from small cell lung cancer should, in our opinion, be treated radically, especially those at younger age with small lung primary tumors, good performance status, and a lack of systemic dissemination. There are articles reporting unexpectedly prolonged survival achieved by combined radical treatment of resectable lung primary and solitary brain metastasis which supports this approach (Abratt et al., 1995).

Usually, diagnosis of SCLC indicates a relatively large primary tumor mass. However, there are reports of slow-growing SCLC tumors in the presence of a solitary brain metastasis. This is unusual considering the high proliferative potential of the cancer cells in SCLC.

Some authors suggest that a subtype of slow-growing neuroendocrine small cell cancer should be distinguished from the common type of SCLC (Imai et al., 2001). The long-term survival in these patients, despite the presence of highly malignant tumor, implies that the anti-VGCC antibodies may be playing a role in controlling tumor growth or, alternatively, that the small cell cancers that provoke LEMS may be of slower growth.

OUR EXPERIENCE

We describe a case of a 60-year-old male patient who presented with a 6-month history of progressive weakness of all four limbs, ataxia, droopy eyelids, and bulbar features. Further laboratory and electrodiagnostic studies confirmed the diagnosis of LEMS. MRI of the brain showed a cerebellar tumor (Figure 21.2A) which, following surgery was revealed to be a metastatic small cell lung carcinoma. Paraneoplastic LEMS together with a solitary cerebellar metastasis was diagnosed but no evidence of primary malignancy was detected. An extensive search for related malignancies failed to get any clue. The patient underwent a total surgical excision of tumor and the histopathology revealed a metastatic small cell carcinoma (Figure 21.2B). 3, 4 DAP was not commercially available to us, so we put the patient on oral pyridostigmine (60 mg four times daily) and oral prednisolone (1 mg/kg) on alternate days. As the weakness was worsening with evidence of respiratory compromise, IVIG at a dose of 1 g/kg for 2 consecutive days was administered. Two weeks after IVIG, the patient showed satisfactory improvement in strength. The patient received whole brain irradiation at a total dose of

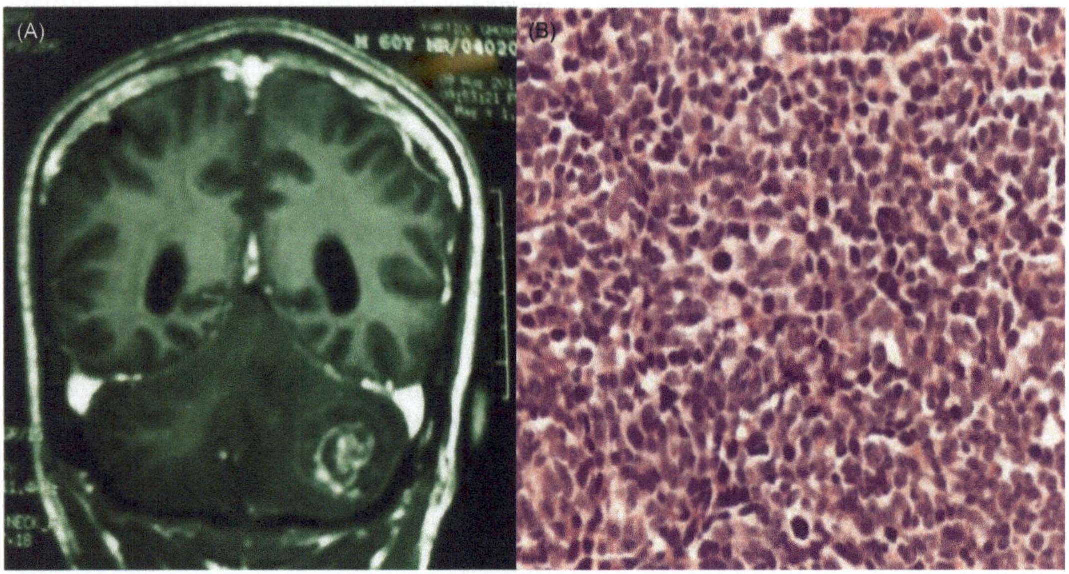

FIGURE 21.2 (A) Coronal T1W MR showing a focal rounded heterogeneous mass (2.7 cm × 2.9 cm × 2.6 cm) in the left cerebellar hemisphere with patchy and perifocal enhancement after contrast; (B) H&E, small cell carcinoma, brain metastasis ×400.

30Gy in 10 fractions with good tolerance following the complete excision of the tumor. The patient was followed up for 6 months without evidence of underlying primary lung tumor. Thereafter, the patient was lost to follow up. This case highlights that rarely both paraneoplastic LEMS and a cerebellar mass can together precede the primary malignancy causing them. Kuwata et al. (2011) reported a case of cerebellar metastasis of unknown origin, in which a primary lung adenocarcinoma was diagnosed by pathological examination of a cerebellar metastatic tumor, using immunohistochemical markers and epidermal growth factor receptor (EGFR) mutation of primary lung cancer. The pathological examination of the cerebellar metastatic tumor of our patient revealed features of metastatic small cell carcinoma which on immunohistochemistry showed positivity for dot-like staining pattern with pan-cytokeratin antibody AE1/AE3. Tumor cells showed positivity for cytokeratin 7 but were immunonegative for cytokeratin 20. Neuroendocrine differentiation was demonstrated using immunopositivity for synaptophysin. Our experience was the first case of a solitary brain metastasis together with a paraneoplastic syndrome (LEMS) occurring before the primary tumor could be diagnosed on first investigations.

References

Abratt, R.P., de Groot, M., Willcox, P.A., 1995. Resection of a solitary brain metastasis in a patient with small cell lung cancer – long-term survival. Eur. J. Cancer 31A, 419.

Anderson, H.J., Churchill-Davidson, H.C., Richardson, A.T., 1953. Bronchial neoplasm with myasthenia: prolonged apnoea after administration of succinylcholine. Lancet 2, 1291–1293.

Bain, P.G., Motomura, M., Newsom-Davis, J., et al., 1996. Effects of intravenous immunoglobulin on muscle weakness and calcium-channel autoantibodies in the Lambert-Eaton myasthenic syndrome. Neurology 47, 678–683.

Eaton, L.M., Lambert, E.H., 1957. Electromyography and electrical stimulation of nerves in diseases of the motor unit: observations on a myasthenic syndrome associated with malignant tumours. J. Am. Med. Assoc. 163, 1117–1124.

Harrison, M.L., Goldstein, D., 2002. Prolonged survival in a patient with an occult primary small-cell lung cancer and a solitary brain metastasis at diagnosis. Intern. Med. J. 32, 621–622.

Hirsch, F.R., Paulson, O.B., Hansen, H.H., Larsen, S.O., 1983. Intracranial metastases in small cell carcinoma of the lung: prognostic aspects. Cancer 51, 529–533.

Imai, R., Hayakawa, K., Sakurai, H., Nakayama, Y., Mitsuhashi, N., Niibe, H., 2001. Small cell lung cancer with a brain metastasis controlled for 5 years: a case report. Jap. J. Clin. Oncol. 31, 116–118.

Kalkanis, S.N., Kondziolka, D., Gaspar, L.E., et al., 2010. The role of surgical resection in the management of newly diagnosed brain metastases: a systematic review and evidence-based clinical practice guideline. J. Neurooncol 96, 33–43.

Kim, Y.I., Neher, E., 1988. IgG from patients with Lambert-Eaton syndrome blocks voltage-dependent calcium channels. Science 239, 405–408.

Kuwata, T., Iwata, T., Iwanami, T., 2011. Napsin A and thyroid transcription factor-1-positive cerebellar tumor with epidermal growth factor receptor mutation. Case Rep. Oncol. 4, 564–568.

Lennon, V.A., Lambert, E.H., Wittingham, S., Fairbanks, V., 1982. Autoimmunity in the Eaton Lambert myasthenic syndrome. Muscle Nerve. 5, S21–S25.

Lennon, V.A., Kryzer, T.J., Griesmann, G.E., et al., 1995. Calcium-channel antibodies in the Lambert- Eaton syndrome and other paraneoplastic syndromes. N. Engl. J. Med. 332, 1467–1474.

Maddison, P., Newsom-Davis, J., Mills, K.R., Souhami, R.L., 1999. Favourable prognosis in Lambert-Eaton myasthenic syndrome and small-cell lung carcinoma. Lancet 353, 117–118.

Mintz, A.H., Kestle, J., Rathbone, M.P., et al., 1996. A randomized trial to assess the efficacy of surgery in addition to radiotherapy in patients with a single cerebral metastasis. Cancer 78, 1470–1476.

Newsom-Davis, J., 1998. A treatment algorithm for Lambert-Eaton myasthenic syndrome. Ann. NY Acad. Sci. 841, 817–822.

Nguyen, L., Maor, M., Oswald, M.J., 1998. Brain metastases as the only manifestation of an undetected primary tumor. Cancer 83, 2181–2184.

Nussbaum, E., Djalilian, H., Cho, K., Hall, W., 1996. Brain metastases. Histology, multiplicity, surgery, and survival. Cancer 78, 1781–1788.

O'Neill, J.H., Murray, N.M., Newsom-Davis, J., 1988. The Lambert-Eaton myasthenic syndrome. A review of 50 cases. Brain 111, 577–596.

Ramos-Yeo, Y.L., Reyes, C.V., 1987. Myasthenic syndrome (Eaton-Lambert syndrome) associated with pulmonary adenocarcinoma. J. Surg. Oncol. 34, 239–242.

Roberts, A., Perera, S., Lang, B., Vincent, A., Newsom-Davis, J., 1985. Paraneoplastic myasthenic syndrome IgG inhibits 45Ca2+ flux in a human small cell carcinoma line. Nature 317, 737–739.

Ruda, R., Borgognone, M., Benech, F., Vasario, E., Soffietti, R., 2001. Brain metastases from unknown primary tumour: a prospective study. J. Neurol. 248, 394–398.

Salvati, M., Cervoni, L., Raco, A., 1995. Single brain metastases from unknown primary malignancies in CT-era. J. Neuro-Oncol. 23, 75–80.

Schreiber, D., Rineer, J., Weedon, J., et al., 2010. Survival outcomes with the use of surgery in limited-stage smallcell lung cancer: should its role be re-evaluated? Cancer 116, 1350–1357.

Seneviratne, U., de Silva, R., 1999. Lambert-Eaton myasthenic syndrome. Postgrad. Med. J. 75, 516–520.

Stupp, R., Monnerat, C., Turrisi 3rd, A.T., Perry, M.C., Leyvraz, S., 2004. Small cell lung cancer: state of the art and future perspectives. Lung Cancer 45, 105–117.

Takeshima, H., Kuratsu, J., Nishi, T., Ushio, Y., 2002. Prognostic factors in patients who survived more than 10 years after undergoing surgery for metastatic brain tumors. Report of 5 cases and review of the literature. Surg. Neurol. 58, 118–123.

Titulaer, M.J., Wirtz, P.W., Willems, L.N., van Kralingen, K.W., Smitt, P.A., Verschuuren, J.J., 2008. Screening for small-cell lung cancer: a follow-up study of patients with Lambert-Eaton myasthenic syndrome. J. Clin. Oncol. 26, 4276–4281.

Titulaer, M.J., Maddison, P., Sont, J.K., et al., 2011. Clinical Dutch-English Lambert-Eaton myasthenic syndrome (LEMS) tumor association prediction score accurately predicts small-cell lung cancer in the LEMS. J. Clin. Oncol. 29, 902–908.

Van de Pol, M., van Aalst, V.C., Wilmink, J.T., Twijnstra, A., 1996. Brain metastases from an unknown primary tumour: which diagnostic procedures are indicated? J. Neurol. Neurosurg. Psychiatr. 61, 321–323.

Willcox, N., Demaine, A.G., Newsom-Davis, J., Welsh, K.I., Robb, S.A., Spiro, S.G., 1985. Increased frequency of IgG heavy chain marker G1m(2) and of HLA B8 in Lambert Eaton myasthenic syndrome with and without associated lung carcinoma. Hum. Immunol. 14, 29–36.

Wirtz, P.W., Willcox, N., van der Slik, A.R., et al., 2005a. HLA and smoking in prediction and prognosis of small cell lung cancer in autoimmune Lambert-Eaton myasthenic syndrome. J. Neuroimmunol. 159, 230–237.

Wirtz, P.W., Lang, B., Graus, F., et al., 2005b. P/Q-type calcium channel antibodies, Lambert-Eaton myasthenic syndrome and survival in small cell lung cancer. J. Neuroimmunol. 164, 161–165.

Index

Note: Page numbers followed by *"f"* and *"t"* refer to figures and tables respectively.

A

Acute lymphoblastic leukemia (ALL), 4–5, 67
Adherens junctions (AJs), 216
Adults, incidence of brain metastasis in, 15–20
  breast cancer, 17
  choriocarcinoma, 19
  colorectal cancer (CRC), 18
  esophageal cancer, 19
  lung cancer, 16–17
  melanoma, 17–18
  ovarian cancer, 19
  prostate cancer, 18–19
  renal cancer, 18
  testicular cancer, 19–20
Afatinib, 152, 170
Age, incidence by, 14
AMD3100, 27
Anaplastic lymphoma kinase (ALK) rearrangements, 123–124
ANG1005, 57
Angiogenesis, 54
Angiogenesis/vascular remodeling, 38
Anti-angiogenic drugs, 54–55
Ataxia telangiectasia mutated (ATM) activity, 116
Autologous bone marrow transplantation (ABMT), 68

B

B1 integrin, 54
Bcl-2 antisense oligonucleotide therapy, 97
Bevacizumab, 54–55
Bioluminescence, 163*f*
Bioluminescent imaging (BLI), 162
Biopsy of brain metastases, 5
Blood–brain barrier (BBB), 8–9, 39, 50, 56–58, 76–77, 87, 116, 148–149, 158, 165, 214, 217–218, 222
Blood–tumor barrier, 39
Brain endothelial cells, tight junctions between, 220–223
Brain local vulnerability/resistance to metastases, 46
Brain metastases (BM), 106, 118
  in occult small cell lung carcinoma, 251–252
  with unknown primary, 250
Brain re-irradiation, 207–208
Brain synovial sarcomas, 93–94
  classification, 99
Breast cancer, 4, 12, 17, 45, 78
Breast cancer resistance protein (BCRP), 173

C

Cancer cell metastatization, 124
Cancer of unknown primary (CUP), 250
Carcinoembryonic antigen (CEA), 96
CC chemokines, 25–26
Cediranib, 55
Central nervous system (CNS), 4, 233
  CXCR4 in, 28
  epidemiology of, 11–12
  incidence, 12–13
    by demographic features, 13–15
    by specific cancer types, 15–21
  metastatic lesions, 145
  obstacles to drug activity within, 148–149
Cerebral metastases, 124
Cerebrospinal fluid (CSF), 145, 173
Chemokine receptors, 26, 125
Chemokine signaling pathways, 124–126
Chemokines, 25, 31, 125
Chemotherapy, for brain metastases, 75–76, 208–209
  breast cancer, 78
  melanoma, 78
  non-small cell lung cancer, 78
  options, 77
  rare tumors, 78
  second malignant neoplasia, 68
Children, incidence of brain metastasis in, 20–21
Choriocarcinoma, 19
Colon cancer, 45–46
Colorectal cancer (CRC), 18
Combined modality therapy, 69
Compound muscle action potential (CMAP), 246
Computed tomography (CT), 5, 116
  contrast-enhanced, 39
Convection enhanced delivery (CED), 158, 165
Corynebacterium diphtheriae, 159–160
Cranial radiotherapy (RT), 145
Crizotinib (Xalkori), 146
Crizotinib, 153
CX3C chemokines, 25–26
CX3CR1, 126–128

CXC chemokines, 25–26
CXCL12, 26–27
 axis in brain, 28
 receptors, 27
CXCL12/CXCR4/CXCR7
 brain metastasis and, 31–33
 and metastasis, 28–31
CXCR3 ligand, 27
CXCR4, 27–28
CXCR4/CXCL12 axis, 29
CXCR7, 27, 30
CXCR7 overexpression, 30–31
Cyber knife System, 132–133
Cyclooxygenase (COX2), 214–215
Cytokeratins, 96, 252–253

D

de novo angiogenesis, 6
Dementia, 88, 114
Diagnosis of brain metastases, 5–6
3, 4 Diaminopyridine (DAP), 246–247
Diphtheria toxin (DT), 158–160, 159*f*
 recombinant, 160
DNA-PK, 115
 catalytic subunit (DNA-PKc), 115
Docetaxel, 174–176
Double-strand break (DSB), 115
Drugs, prophylactic role of, 151
DTATEGF, 158
 bioluminescent imaging (BLI), 162
 body weights, histology, and statistical analysis, 162–163
 construction, 160
 in vitro and *in vivo* results, 163–164
 in vitro DTATEGF efficacy, 161
 intracranial NSCLC tumor model, 161–162
 NSCLC cell preparation, 161
 pump Implantation and DTATEGF delivery, 162
DTEGF13, 164–165
Dural metastases, 41
Dutch–English LEMS Tumor Association Prediction score (DELTA-P score), 249

E

Efaproxiral, 56
EGFR and radiation-induced DNA damage
 preclinical study and mechanism, 115
EGFR-mutated NSCLC, 172, 175
Electrodiagnostic tests, 246
Elongation factor-2 (EF2), 159
Enzyme-inducing antiepileptic drugs (EIAEDs), 173
Epidemiology and clinical presentation of brain metastases, 37–38
Epidermal growth factor receptor (EGFR), 78, 97, 114–115, 146
Epidermal growth factor receptor (EGFR) mutations, 17, 106
 brain metastasis and, 114–115
 clinical implications of, 150–151
 miliary brain metastases and, 108
 multiple brain metastases and, 107
 neurologically asymptomatic NSCLC patients with, 109
 neurologically symptomatic NSCLC patients with, 109
 and radiotherapy
  clinical study, 116–118
  preclinical study and mechanism, 115–116
Epidermal growth factor receptor tyrosine kinase inhibitors (EGFR TKIs), 106, 110, 145, 148–149, 157–158, 174–175
 clinical study, 118–119
 preclinical study and mechanism, 116
Epipodophyllotoxins, 70
Epithelial growth factor receptor (EGFR) activating mutations, 123–124
Epithelial-to-mesenchymal transition (EMT), 125
ErbB2 overexpression, 114–115
ERK pathway, 223
Erlotinib, 106, 110, 118, 144*f*, 149–151, 157–158, 172–174, 176–177
 adverse reactions of, 151–152
 combining radiotherapy with, 175–176
 future directions, 152–153
 rechallenge and pulsed dose escalation of, 176
 trials of, 148
Esophageal cancer, 19
Exon 19 deletion on radiographical features, 107
Extra-axial metastases, 41–43
 leptomeningeal metastases, 41–43
 pachymeningeal metastases, 41

F

"Fertile soil", 124
Flattening Filter Free (FFF) modality, 133–134
Fluid attenuation inversion recovery (FLAIR) image, 39–40, 43
Fotemustine, 77
Fractalkine, 126–127

G

G protein-coupled receptors (GPCRs), 26–27
Gadolinium-enhanced MRI, 41, 43
Gamma knife plans, 132–133
Gamma knife radiosurgery, 100
Gefitinib, 106, 110, 118, 146, 157–158, 173, 176
 adverse reactions of, 151–152
 trials of, 147

Gemcitabine, 170–171
Gender, incidence by, 14
Genomic aberrations and second malignancies, 67
Glioblastoma multiforme (GBM), 55
Glucocorticoid therapy, 7
Glycosaminoglycans (GAGs), 26
Gross disease, WBRT as primary therapy for, 230–232

H

Head and neck synovial sarcomas, 98
Hematogenous metastases to brain, 99
Hematopoietic stem cell transplantation (HSCT), 63
HER-2/neu, 97
Hexokinase 2 (HK2), 39
High-dose chemotherapy, 68–69
Homologous recombination, 115
Hopkins Verbal Learning Test (HVLT), 86
Hopkins Verbal Learning Test-Revised (HVLT-R), 87, 233
Hypoxia-induced HIF-1α activation and VEGF release, 29

I

I-metaiodobenzylguanidine (MIBG), 63–66, 70
Icotinib, 152–153
Image Guidance systems, 133
Immune-privileged site, 39
Immunotoxins, 158
Incidence of brain metastases, 12–13
  by age, 14
  by demographic features, 13–15
  by gender, 14
  onset of brain metastases from initial diagnosis, 14–15
  by race, 13
  SEER stage, 14
  by specific cancer types, 15–21
    breast cancer, 17
    choriocarcinoma, 19
    colorectal cancer (CRC), 18
    esophageal cancer, 19
    lung cancer, 16–17
    melanoma, 17–18
    ovarian cancer, 19
    prostate cancer, 18–19
    renal cancer, 18
    testicular cancer, 19–20
Intensity Modulated Radiation delivery (IMRT), 133
Interferon-γ (IFN-γ), 29
Interleukin-5 (IL5), 29
Interstitial lung disease (ILD), 151–152
Intra-axial metastases, 38–40, 40*f*
Intracranial diffusion, 124
Intracranial metastasis, in NSCLC patients, 170–171
Intracranial NSCLC tumor model, 161–162
Intracranial synovial sarcomas, treatment of, 99–100
Intrathecal therapy, 8
Italian Neuroblastoma Registry, 63

L

Lambert–Eaton Myesthenic Syndrome (LEMS), 244–249
  associated with malignancy (PLEMS), 244–245
  Dutch–English LEMS Tumor Association Prediction score (DELTA-P score), 249
  without malignancy, 244–245
  paraneoplastic and non-paraneoplastic, 244–247
  and small cell lung carcinoma, 247–249
Lapatinib, 8–9
Leksell, Lars, 132
Leptomeningeal metastases, 41–43
Leukemias and lymphomas, 63–66
LINAC-based stereotactic radiosurgery, 132–134
Lipoprotein receptor-related protein (LRP-1), 57
Lung adenocarcinoma, brain metastasis of patients with, 113
  brain metastasis and EGFR mutation, 114–115
  clinical study, 116–119
    EGFR mutation and radiotherapy, 116–118
    EGFR-TKIs combined with radiotherapy, 118–119
    EGFR-TKIs treatment for brain metastasis, 118
  preclinical study and mechanism, 115–116
    EGFR and radiation-induced DNA damage, 115
    EGFR mutation and radiotherapy, 115–116
    EGFR-TKIs combined with radiotherapy, 116
Lung cancer, 12, 16–17, 45, 106, 170
Lung cancer, brain metastases from, 227–228
  toxicity of radiation to the brain, 237–238
  treatment options, 228–237
    prophylactic cranial irradiation, 233–237
    stereotactic radiosurgery, 228–229
    surgical resection, 228
    whole-brain radiation therapy, 229–233
Lung carcinoma, organotropic spread of, 124–126
Lung metastases, 4

M

Magnetic resonance imaging (MRI), 5, 39, 54, 95, 116, 143*f*, 170, 227
  gadolinium-enhanced, 41, 43
Management of brain metastases in NSCLC patients, 182–187
  general considerations, 182–183
  multiple brain metastases, 184–185
    surgery for multiple brain metastases, 185
  prognostic factors specific to NSCLC patients, 187
  radiation management, 185
  single brain metastases, 183–184
    surgery vs SRS for single brain metastases, 184
  whole brain radiotherapy (WBRT), 185–186

Melanoma, 4, 17–18, 78, 87
Metabolic MIBG radiation therapy, 70
Metachronous BM, 108
Metastases, brain spatial distribution of, 43–48
  brain local vulnerability/resistance to metastases, 46
  primary tumor, role of, 45–46
  recurrent metastases, 46–48
Metastases in continuity through the skull base, 98–99
Metastases to the brain, 3
Metastatic diffusion, 124
Metastatic intracranial tumors, non-uniform distribution of, 37–38
Metastatic spread, 124–125
Microglia, 39
Micrometastatic tumors, 109
Miliary brain metastases and EGFR mutations, 108
Mini-mental status exam (MMSE), 88–89
Montexafin gadolinium (MGd), 55–56
Motaxefin gadolinium (MGd), 231–232
Multiple brain metastases and EGFR mutations, 107
Multiple brain metastases, management of, 184–185
  surgery for, 185

N

Nco I/ *Xho* I fragment gene, 160
Neoplastic cell meningitis, 4–5
Neuroblastoma
  second malignant neoplasia (SMN) and, 62–63
  targeted radiotherapy to, 70
Neurocognition, 88–89
Neuroimaging
  extra-axial metastases, 41–43
  intra-axial metastases, 38–40
Neurologic deficits, 5, 8
Non-homologous end-joining (NHEJ), 115
Non-paraneoplastic Lambert–Eaton Myesthenic Syndrome (NLEMS), 244–247, 248*t*
  management of, 247
Non-small cell lung cancer (NSCLC), 16–17, 55, 78, 106, 114, 117*t*, 123, 142, 146, 157–158, 164, 170, 182
  combining erlotinib with radiotherapy for, 175–176
  development and management of, 171–172
  EGFR mutated NSCLC patients, 172
  EGFR TKIs and, 174–175
  erlotinib, rechallenge and pulsed dose escalation of, 176
  first-line treatment for, 170–171
  management of brain metastases in, 182–187, 192*f*
    multiple brain metastases, 184–185
    prognostic factors specific to NSCLC patients, 187
    radiation management, 185
    single brain metastases, 183–184
    surgery for multiple brain metastases, 185
    whole brain radiotherapy (WBRT), 185–186
  oligometastatic NSCLC, 188–189
  optimal management of, 108
  role of prophylactic cranial irradiation (PCI) in, 236
  solitary brain metastasis from, 131
    patient selection, 136–137
    radiobiological issues and clinical data, 134–135
    radiosurgery alone/with whole-brain radiation therapy, 136
    surgery and whole-brain radiation therapy, 135–136
    technical and technological aspects, 132–134
    whole-brain radiation therapy, 135
Non-small cell lung cancer (NSCLC) cells, 219
Non-small cell lung cancer (NSCLC) with EGFR mutations
  brain metastases management from, 108–109
    asymptomatic, 109
    symptomatic, 109
  treatment of multiple brain metastases from, 109–110
NSCLC patients with synchronous brain metastases, management of, 187–194
  factors of undetermined or no prognostic significance, 189–191
  management algorithm for, 194
  oligometastatic NSCLC, 188–189
    future directions, 194
  prognostic factors, 191
  prognostic factors affecting survival, 189
  radiation management of thoracic disease, 191–192
  rationale for aggressive treatment of oligometastatic disease, 188
  staging workup of NSCLC patients with synchronous brain metastases, 193–194
  surgical management of thoracic disease, 193

O

Occult small cell lung carcinoma, brain metastasis in, 251–252
Oligometastatic NSCLC, management of, 188–189
Onset of brain metastases from initial diagnosis, 14–15
Origin of primary tumors, 3–4
OSI-774, 172–174
Ovarian cancer, 19

P

P-glycoprotein (P-gp), 57, 173
Pachymeningeal metastases, 41
Paraneoplastic Lambert–Eaton Myesthenic Syndrome (PLEMS), 244–247, 248*t*
Pathogenesis, 6
  extra-axial metastases, 41–43
  intra-axial metastases, 38–40
PC9-BrM3 cells, 161–162
Pemetrexed, 146, 170–171, 174–175
Percentage of brain metastases from different primary cancers, 15*t*

PgP transporters, 148–149
Placental growth factor (PLGF), 215–216
  in normal and tumor cells, 215–216
  in SCLC brain metastases, 216–221, 224*f*
  and vascular permeability, 216
Platinum-based regimens, 190–191
Post-surgery recurrent extra-axial metastases, 47*f*
Prednisolone, 246–247, 252–253
Prevention of BM, 9
Primary brain synovial sarcoma, 98
Prophylactic cranial irradiation (PCI), 200
  brain relapse after, 201
Prophylactic cranial irradiation, 233–237
Prophylactic cranial radiation (PCI), 88
Prophylactic radiation therapy, 9
Prostate cancer, 18–19
Pyridostigmine, 252–253

R

Race, incidence by, 13
Radiation, 7–8
  -related second malignant neoplasias, 69
  toxicity of, 237–238
Radiation management
  of brain metastases, 185
  of thoracic disease, 191–192
Radiosensitizing, 55–56
  whole brain radiation therapy and, 86–87
Radiosurgery
  Gamma knife radiosurgery, 100, 206
  stereotactic. *See* Stereotactic radiosurgery
  whole brain radiation therapy and, 85–86
Radiosurgery alone/with whole-brain radiation therapy, 136
Ras/Raf/MEK/ERK and STAT pathways, 115
Relapse rate, 200–201
Renal cell carcinoma (RCC), 4, 18
RTOG 95-08, 229

S

Second malignancies, 67
Second malignant neoplasia (SMN), 61–62
  clinical implications, 71–72
  factors increasing the risk of, 66–71
    chemotherapy, 68
    genomic aberrations and second malignancies, 67
    high-dose chemotherapy, 68–69
    metabolic MIBG radiation therapy, 70
    radiotherapy, 69
  incidence of, 63–66
    leukemias and lymphomas, 63–66
    solid tumors, 66
  risk in children treated for neuroblastoma, 62–63
  survival after, 71
"Seed and soil" hypothesis, 31, 38–39
SEER stage of cancer, 14
Sensitizing brain metastases to radiation, 55–56
Single brain metastases, management of, 183–184
  surgery vs SRS for, 184
Skull base surgery and neurosurgery, 98–99
Small and non-small cell lung cancer, 4
Small cell lung cancer (SCLC), 29, 200, 213–214, 244
  Lambert–Eaton Myesthenic Syndrome and, 247–249
  with placental growth factor, 216–221
  role of prophylactic cranial irradiation in, 233–234, 236–238
Small vessel ischemic disease (SVID), 49–50
Solid tumors, 66
Solitary brain metastasis (SBM), 250
Sorafenib, 55, 57
Sources of brain metastases, 12
SS18 gene, 96
Standard of care, for brain metastases, 76–77
Stereotactic ablative radiotherapy (SABR), 188, 191–192, 194
Stereotactic body radiotherapy (SBRT), 188
Stereotactic radiosurgery (SRS), 55, 131–134, 136, 145, 183, 206–207, 228–229
  for single brain metastases, 184
  WBRT after, 233
Stereotactic radiotherapy, 9, 206–209
Stromal cell-derived factor (SDF-1, CXCL12), 26
Stromal cell-derived factor 1α (SDF-1α), 214–215
Surgery, 7, 145, 228
  for multiple brain metastases, 185
  radiosurgery alone/with whole-brain radiation therapy, 136
  for single brain metastases, 184
  and whole-brain radiation therapy, 135–136
Surgical management of thoracic disease, 193
Synchronous brain metastases, 108
  management of, 187–194
  NSCLC patients with
    management algorithm for, 194
    radiation management of thoracic disease in, 191–192
    staging workup of, 193–194
    surgical management of thoracic disease in, 193
Synovial sarcoma, 93
  clinical features, 94–95
  epidemiology, 94
  future treatment issues, 97
  genetics, 96
  head and neck, 98
  pathology, 95–96
  prognosis, 97–98
  radiology, 95
  treatment, 96–97
Systemic therapy, 8, 145–146

T

Targeted therapy, 9, 146–148
Targeted toxins, 158
  limitations, 166
Targeting angiogenesis, 54–55
Temozolomide, 76–77, 87, 232
Testicular cancer, 19–20
Thalidomide, 55, 232
Therapy, 7–9
  intrathecal, 8
  radiation, 7–8
  surgery, 7
  systemic, 8
Thioredoxin reductase, 55–56
Tight junctions (TJs) between brain endothelial cells, 214, 216
  PLGF-induced changes in, 220–221
Topotecan, 146, 208–209
Total body irradiation (TBI), 63
Transforming growth factor-β2 (TGF-β2), 214–215
Treatment options for brain metastases, 145–146
  stereotactic radiosurgery (SRS), 145
  surgery, 145
  systemic therapy, 145–146
  whole brain radiotherapy (WBRT), 145
Tumor Node Metastasis (TNM) staging, 124
Tyrosine kinase inhibitors (TKIs), 151

U

University of Florida, 132
"Unknown primary", 250
Urokinase plasminogen activator receptor, 157–158

V

Vascular endothelial growth factor (VEGF), 54, 127, 214–215
Vascular permeability, PLGF and, 216
VEGFR-1, 219–221
Vinorelbine, 170–171
Voltage-gated calcium channel (VGCC), 244
  serum antibodies to, 246
Volumetric IMRT techniques, 133–134
Volumetric Modulation Arc Therapy, 133–134
Vorinostat, 56

W

Whole brain adjuvant radiotherapy, 131–132
Whole brain radiation therapy (WBRT), 46–48, 55–56, 81–84, 106, 109, 114, 117*t*, 118, 135, 145, 171–172, 174–175, 183–186, 228–233, 250
  as an adjuvant after local therapy, 232–233
  biologically effective dose (BED), 83–84
  expected survival after, 84
  future of, 89
  hypofractionated, 82
  as primary therapy for gross disease, 230–232
  and radiosensitizers, 86–87
  and radiosurgery, 85–86, 136
  re-irradiation, 88
  side effects, 88–89
    neurocognition, 88–89
  and surgery, 84–85, 135–136
Whole brain re-irradiation (WBI), 207–208

FSC
www.fsc.org
MIX
Papier | Fördert gute Waldnutzung
FSC® C083411

Kolibri 360 GmbH
Ferdinand-Jühlke-Straße 7
99095 Erfurt, Deutschland
produktsicherheit@kolibri360.de